The Biology of Chronic Pain:
Applications in Clinical Practice

The Biology of Chronic Pain: Applications in Clinical Practice

Editors

Andrea Polli
Jo Nijs

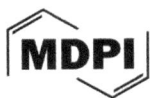

Basel • Beijing • Wuhan • Barcelona • Belgrade • Novi Sad • Cluj • Manchester

Editors

Andrea Polli
Vrije Universiteit Brussel
Brussels
Belgium

Jo Nijs
Vrije Universiteit Brussel
Brussels
Belgium

Editorial Office
MDPI
St. Alban-Anlage 66
4052 Basel, Switzerland

This is a reprint of articles from the Special Issue published online in the open access journal *Journal of Clinical Medicine* (ISSN 2077-0383) (available at: https://www.mdpi.com/journal/jcm/special_issues/9X62328772).

For citation purposes, cite each article independently as indicated on the article page online and as indicated below:

Lastname, A.A.; Lastname, B.B. Article Title. *Journal Name* **Year**, *Volume Number*, Page Range.

ISBN 978-3-7258-1351-3 (Hbk)
ISBN 978-3-7258-1352-0 (PDF)
doi.org/10.3390/books978-3-7258-1352-0

Contents

About the Editors vii

Preface ix

Alberto Herrero Babiloni, Andrée-Ann Baril, Camille Charlebois-Plante, Marianne Jodoin, Erlan Sanchez, Liesbet De Baets, et al.
The Putative Role of Neuroinflammation in the Interaction between Traumatic Brain Injuries, Sleep, Pain and Other Neuropsychiatric Outcomes: A State-of-the-Art Review
Reprinted from: *J. Clin. Med.* **2023**, *12*, 1793, doi:10.3390/jcm12051793 1

Arne Wyns, Jolien Hendrix, Astrid Lahousse, Elke De Bruyne, Jo Nijs, Lode Godderis and Andrea Polli
The Biology of Stress Intolerance in Patients with Chronic Pain—State of the Art and Future Directions
Reprinted from: *J. Clin. Med.* **2023**, *12*, 2245, doi:10.3390/jcm12062245 19

Giacomo Rossettini, Francesco Campaci, Joel Bialosky, Eva Huysmans, Lene Vase and Elisa Carlino
The Biology of Placebo and Nocebo Effects on Experimental and Chronic Pain: State of the Art
Reprinted from: *J. Clin. Med.* **2023**, *12*, 4113, doi:10.3390/jcm12124113 34

Kory Zimney, Wouter Van Bogaert and Adriaan Louw
The Biology of Chronic Pain and Its Implications for Pain Neuroscience Education: State of the Art
Reprinted from: *J. Clin. Med.* **2023**, *12*, 4199, doi:10.3390/jcm12134199 58

Maite M. van der Miesen, Catherine J. Vossen and Elbert A. Joosten
Habituation to Pain in Patients with Chronic Pain: Clinical Implications and Future Directions
Reprinted from: *J. Clin. Med.* **2023**, *12*, 4305, doi:10.3390/jcm12134305 72

Tomohiko Nishigami, Masahiro Manfuku and Astrid Lahousse
Central Sensitization in Cancer Survivors and Its Clinical Implications: State of the Art
Reprinted from: *J. Clin. Med.* **2023**, *12*, 4606, doi:10.3390/jcm12144606 97

Elin Johansson, Huan-Yu Xiong, Andrea Polli, Iris Coppieters and Jo Nijs
Towards a Real-Life Understanding of the Altered Functional Behaviour of the Default Mode and Salience Network in Chronic Pain: Are People with Chronic Pain Overthinking the Meaning of Their Pain?
Reprinted from: *J. Clin. Med.* **2024**, *13*, 1645, doi:10.3390/jcm13061645 110

Laura Agulló, Javier Muriel, César Margarit, Mónica Escorial, Diana Garcia, María José Herrero, et al.
Sex Differences in Opioid Response Linked to *OPRM1* and *COMT* genes DNA Methylation/Genotypes Changes in Patients with Chronic Pain
Reprinted from: *J. Clin. Med.* **2023**, *12*, 3449, doi:10.3390/jcm12103449 124

Irina T. Duff, Kristen N. Krolick, Hana Mohamed Mahmoud and Vidya Chidambaran
Current Evidence for Biological Biomarkers and Mechanisms Underlying Acute to Chronic Pain Transition across the Pediatric Age Spectrum
Reprinted from: *J. Clin. Med.* **2023**, *12*, 5176, doi:10.3390/jcm12165176 140

Thomas Matheve, Paul Hodges and Lieven Danneels
The Role of Back Muscle Dysfunctions in Chronic Low Back Pain: State-of-the-Art and Clinical
Implications
Reprinted from: *J. Clin. Med.* **2023**, *12*, 5510, doi:10.3390/jcm12175510 . . . . **168**

About the Editors

Andrea Polli

Dr. Andrea Polli is an FWO postdoctoral research fellow at the Vrije Universiteit Brussel and Katholieke Universiteit Leuven, Leuven, Belgium. He completed his PhD at the Vrije Universiteit Brussel, Brussels, Belgium, and has been awarded Awards and Honors. He worked at IRCCS San Camillo Hospital from 2012 to 2015. His research mainly focuses on exploring epigenetic and biological mechanisms in chronic pain, ME/CFS and Long-COVID.

Jo Nijs

Jo Nijs is full professor at the Vrije Universiteit Brussel (Brussels, Belgium), physiotherapist/ manual therapist at the University Hospital Brussels, holder of a Chair on oncological physiotherapy funded by the Berekuyl Academy, the Netherlands, and Visiting Professor at the University of Gothenburg (Sweden). Jo runs the Pain in Motion international and interdisciplinary research group. The primary aim of his research is improving care for patients with chronic pain. He has (co-)authored >300 peer reviewed publications, including first author papers in *The Lancet* and *The Lancet Rheumatology* (2x), and a senior author paper in *JAMA Neurology*. He supervised 29 PhD's to completion and served 400 times as an invited speaker at meetings in 31 countries (including 44 keynotes). He trained 4k clinicians in >100 courses held in 14 countries spread over 4 continents. Jo is ranked 2nd in the world among chronic pain researchers (1st in Europe), and 3rd in the world among musculoskeletal pain researchers (expertscape.com), and received the 2020 honorary Francqui Collen Chair awarded by the University of Hasselt, Belgium.

Preface

Chronic pain is one of the most prevalent diseases worldwide that lead to suffering, disability, and enormous social costs. Science has tremendously advanced our understanding of the pathophysiology of chronic pain. Breakthrough findings include functional and structural brain changes, neuro-inflammation, sensory changes, immune alterations, psychological problems, neurocognitive disorders, stress intolerance, sleep impairments, and (epi)genetic changes found in patients with chronic pain.

This *Journal of Clinical Medicine* Boutique Special Issue focuses on the exciting, broad field of the biology of chronic pain in humans. It includes invited state-of-the-art papers addressing key biological processes in patients with chronic pain and original research reports. The state-of-the-art papers were written by leading experts and key opinion leaders in the field. Topics addressed include biomarkers and mechanisms underlying acute to chronic pain transition across the pediatric age spectrum, a real-life understanding of the altered functional behavior of the default mode and salience network in chronic pain, central sensitization in cancer survivors and its clinical implications, habituation to pain in patients with chronic pain, the biology of chronic pain and its implications for pain neuroscience education, the biology of placebo and nocebo effects on experimental and chronic pain, the biology of stress intolerance in patients with chronic pain, the putative role of neuroinflammation in the interaction between traumatic brain injuries, sleep, pain, and other neuropsychiatric outcomes, sex differences in opioid response linked to OPRM1 and COMT genes, DNA methylation/genotypes changes in patients with chronic pain, and the role of back muscle dysfunctions in chronic low back pain. This Special Issue contributes to an exciting area of tremendous advancements and breakthrough research.

Andrea Polli and Jo Nijs
Editors

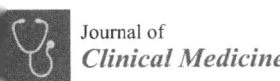

Journal of
Clinical Medicine

Review

The Putative Role of Neuroinflammation in the Interaction between Traumatic Brain Injuries, Sleep, Pain and Other Neuropsychiatric Outcomes: A State-of-the-Art Review

Alberto Herrero Babiloni [1,2,*], Andrée-Ann Baril [3,4], Camille Charlebois-Plante [2], Marianne Jodoin [2,5], Erlan Sanchez [6], Liesbet De Baets [7,8], Caroline Arbour [2,9], Gilles J. Lavigne [1,2,10], Nadia Gosselin [2] and Louis De Beaumont [2,11]

1   Division of Experimental Medicine, McGill University, Montreal, QC H3A 0C7, Canada
2   CIUSSS-NIM, Hôpital du Sacré-Coeur de Montréal, Montreal, QC H4J 1C5, Canada
3   Douglas Mental Health University Institute, Montreal, QC H4H 1R3, Canada
4   Faculty of Medicine and Health Sciences, McGill University, Montreal, QC H3G 2M1, Canada
5   Department of Psychology, University of Montreal, Montreal, QC H3T 1J4, Canada
6   Hurvitz Brain Sciences Program, Sunnybrook Research Institute, Toronto, ON M4N 3M5, Canada
7   Pain in Motion Research Group (PAIN), Department of Physiotherapy, Human Faculty of Medicine, University of Montreal, Montreal, QC H3T 1C5, Canada
8   Physiology and Anatomy, Faculty of Physical Education & Physiotherapy, Vrije Universiteit Brussel, 1050 Brussel, Belgium
9   Faculty of Nursing, Université de Montréal, Montreal, QC H3T 1J4, Canada
10 Faculty of Dental Medicine, University of Montreal, Montreal, QC H3T 1C5, Canada
11 Department of Surgery, University of Montreal, Montreal, QC H3T 1J4, Canada
*   Correspondence: alberto.herrerobabiloni@mail.mcgill.ca

Citation: Herrero Babiloni. A.; Baril, A.-A.; Charlebois-Plante, C.; Jodoin, M.; Sanchez, E.; De Baets, L.; Arbour, C.; Lavigne, G.J.; Gosselin, N.; De Beaumont, L. The Putative Role of Neuroinflammation in the Interaction between Traumatic Brain Injuries, Sleep, Pain and Other Neuropsychiatric Outcomes: A State-of-the-Art Review. *J. Clin. Med.* 2023, 12, 1793. https://doi.org/10.3390/jcm12051793

Academic Editor: Juan Sahuquillo

Received: 31 January 2023
Revised: 15 February 2023
Accepted: 21 February 2023
Published: 23 February 2023

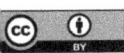
Abstract: Sleep disturbances are widely prevalent following a traumatic brain injury (TBI) and have the potential to contribute to numerous post-traumatic physiological, psychological, and cognitive difficulties developing chronically, including chronic pain. An important pathophysiological mechanism involved in the recovery of TBI is neuroinflammation, which leads to many downstream consequences. While neuroinflammation is a process that can be both beneficial and detrimental to individuals' recovery after sustaining a TBI, recent evidence suggests that neuroinflammation may worsen outcomes in traumatically injured patients, as well as exacerbate the deleterious consequences of sleep disturbances. Additionally, a bidirectional relationship between neuroinflammation and sleep has been described, where neuroinflammation plays a role in sleep regulation and, in turn, poor sleep promotes neuroinflammation. Given the complexity of this interplay, this review aims to clarify the role of neuroinflammation in the relationship between sleep and TBI, with an emphasis on long-term outcomes such as pain, mood disorders, cognitive dysfunctions, and elevated risk of Alzheimer's disease and dementia. In addition, some management strategies and novel treatment targeting sleep and neuroinflammation will be discussed in order to establish an effective approach to mitigate long-term outcomes after TBI.

Keywords: traumatic brain injury; headache; concussion; neuroinflammation; microglia; sleep; pain; Alzheimer's; dementia

1. Introduction

It has been reported that 69 million (95% CI 64–74 million) individuals are estimated to suffer traumatic brain injuries (TBI) from all causes each year, and that such injuries are associated with the development of consequences that may persist for years after the injury, such as pain, psychiatric, neurological, motor, and neurobehavioral issues, as well as with an increased risk of neurodegeneration [1–4]. Among the possible underlying pathological mechanisms of these consequences is neuroinflammation, which is an inflammatory response within the central nervous system (CNS) thought to be mediated by the production of cytokines, chemokines, reactive oxygen species (ROS) and other secondary messengers [5]. Although neuroinflammation is considered an adaptive and essential response following acquired traumatic injuries, edema, demyelination, and cellular and axonal damage were found to be associated with excessive neuroinflammation in chronic TBI [6]. Furthermore, evidence suggests that neuroinflammation secondary to acquired traumatic injuries, such as TBI, could play a central role in the development of chronic pain and also several tauopathies [7,8], such as Alzheimer's disease, Parkinson's disease, and chronic traumatic encephalopathy [6,9]. In this context, whether neuroinflammation could potentially precipitate or even cause neurodegenerative processes requires special attention.

In parallel, an important factor associated with TBI is disrupted sleep [10–17]. A recent meta-analysis showed that 50% of individuals with TBI report sleep disturbances, whereas approximately one-third of these patients report a sleep disorder [14]. Some of the sleep disturbances reported by those individuals include increased need for sleep even up to 6 months following the injury, obstructive sleep apnea, insomnia, narcolepsy-like symptoms, excessive daytime sleepiness, fatigue, and circadian-rhythm disturbances [16]. The causes of sleep disturbances following a TBI vary considerably: some might occur because of changes in patients' lifestyle, comorbidities caused by the trauma such as pain and mood changes, or CNS structural damage and pathophysiological mechanisms incurred following a TBI [11]. In addition, one cannot exclude the possibility that premorbid sleep disturbances were exacerbated by TBI. Given the known deleterious consequences of sleep disturbances on alertness, concentration, and vigilance, individuals experiencing sleep disturbances following traumatic injuries are also more prone to subsequent traumatic injuries [18]. Sleep disturbances are also associated with poor prognosis following TBI [14,16,19] as well as declining overall health [20]. Understanding the complex interaction between sleep and TBI is not only essential if we aim to design and implement new management strategies, but it may also be instrumental in understanding their potential mediating role on the development of TBI-prone chronic pain diseases and neuropsychiatric conditions. In that context, and based on emerging research, there is reason to believe that neuroinflammation could entail a promising mechanistic linkage underlying poor prognosis in TBI patients experiencing sleep disturbances [21,22].

In this state-of-the-art review, the objective is to explore the putative role of neuroinflammation from fundamental and clinical perspectives into the relationship between sleep and TBI, in particular to their complex interplay with TBI-prone chronic pain and other neuropsychiatric outcomes. For that purpose, the information is organized and grouped into three main sections: "State-of-the-art overview of mechanisms between TBI, neuroinflammation, and sleep", where a global perspective on mechanisms and outcomes (including chronic pain) of the multifaceted relationship between these conditions is described; "Neuroinflammation and other neuropsychiatric outcomes in the context of sleep disturbances and TBI", namely mood disorders, cognitive dysfunctions and neurodegeneration; and "Future directions for clinical practice: targeting neuroinflammation", which include sleep and neuroinflammation specific possible management options.

2. State-of-the-Art Overview of Mechanisms between TBI, Neuroinflammation, and Sleep

2.1. Mechanisms of Neuroinflammation Following TBI

Following tissue or nerve injury caused by a fracture or a TBI, a series of reactions generated by the body are triggered to allow the rapid return to homeostasis [23,24]. This inflammatory process can, in some cases, lead to an excessive and prolonged immune response, thus triggering a complex cascade of events such as chronic inflammation of the CNS (i.e., neuroinflammation) [25–27].

In acute and subacute neuroinflammation, microglia, which are the resident macrophages of the CNS, actively monitor the brain microenvironment and react when they encounter various elements of the CNS such as injured cells and pathogens, following TBI [5,28]. In response, microglia become activated and release cytokines (IL-1β, IL-6, TNF-a), nitric oxide (NO), and ROS, which are considered proinflammatory mediators [29]. This release leads to an acute neuroinflammatory response that is postulated to be beneficial to the CNS, in order to clear cellular debris via phagocytosis [28]. The resolution of the neuroinflammatory process is mediated by anti-inflammatory cytokines and the release of anti-inflammatory lipid mediators such as lipoxins, resolvins and neuroprotectins [28]. However, a neuroinflammatory response that persists over time may be detrimental and ultimately lead to neuronal death [30].

A growing body of evidence suggests that microglial activation is associated with synaptic dysfunction/dysregulation, mostly by altering long-term potentiation (LTP) [27]. These LTP, in turn, affect cognitive function, in particular long-term memory [9]. Synaptic dysfunction was also found to precede neuronal pathology such as tauopathies [31], and thus, such that neuroinflammation could be involved in both the onset and the progression of neurodegenerative diseases [6]. For instance, recent animal studies showed that rather than simply activating microglia, neuroinflammation can induce an exaggerated microglial response within the CNS thus "priming", the inflammatory system for an increased vulnerability to a "second hit", consequently favoring subsequent neuropsychiatric and neurodegenerative complications [32,33]. This inappropriate neuroinflammatory response activates several self-propagating cycles, causing apoptosis, synaptic dysfunction, impaired regeneration and the production of amyloid-beta (Aβ) and phosphorylated tau, thereby exacerbating behavioral and cognitive impairments [32].

2.2. TBI and Neuroinflammation

Brain damage related to the mechanical force applied to the brain in TBI is referred to as the primary insult (i.e., skull fractures, intracranial hematoma, lacerations, and contusions, diffuse axonal injury) [34]. The secondary insult refers to ischemia caused by various mechanisms, including intracranial hypertension, that compromise the balance between oxygen delivery to neurons and cerebral oxygen consumption [34]. It generates complex and interrelated neurochemical changes, including an extracellular increase in excitatory amino acids, ROS production, increased intracellular sodium and calcium concentration, mitochondrial dysfunction, and a long-lasting inflammatory response that may ultimately lead to cell death [34–36]. The significant activation of microglia, as part of the secondary insult, leads to the release of cytokines responsible for neuroprotection (anti-inflammatory process) and neurodestruction (toxic and pro-inflammatory process) [33,37,38]. The balance between the neuroprotective and neurodestructive components is precarious. When a misalignment between these two components occurs to the advantage of the latter, there is an increased risk of progressive brain damage that may persist and progress into chronic neurodegeneration [39]. Indeed, recent studies have found an increased levels of proteins involved in pathological processes of neurodegeneration, such as α-synuclein, Aβ, and tau in TBI patients, which play a major role in the development of neurodegenerative diseases such as Parkinson's and Alzheimer's diseases [40–43]. Given the high prevalence of TBI across the lifespan, understanding the complex interaction between neuroinflammation and its associated neurodegenerative processes is essential to improve patients' clinical outcomes.

Regarding polytrauma (i.e., the simultaneous traumatic injury of several regions of the body), numerous studies have shown a high incidence of TBI in individuals who have suffered orthopedic trauma, which is not surprising considering that they both share similar causative events (accidental falls, motor vehicle accidents, and accidents in a recreational setting) [44,45]. Therefore, the anatomical proximity of the upper extremities to the head is such that these two types of acquired traumatic injuries inevitably share somewhat comparable biomechanical characteristics [46]. Consequently, the occurrence of a polytrauma brings its share of challenges due to the overlapping pathophysiological mechanisms common to both injuries and their possible interactions. Indeed, the permeability of the blood–brain barrier (BBB) following a TBI facilitates peripheral factors to invade the CNS [47]. Thus, pro-inflammatory cytokines, such as IL-6, IL-1β, and TNF-α, released following a peripheral lesion lead to a significant increase in systemic inflammation [24,35]. Therefore, patients with a TBI and a concomitant peripheral injury are potentially at greater risk for an exacerbation of the ongoing neuroinflammatory response than patients with an isolated TBI or peripheral injury [48]. The latter becomes specially relevant in the context of chronic pain development, as the risk of neural sensitization is increased by the possibility of both peripheral and central neuroinflammation, which may be driving the onset of post-traumatic conditions such as post-traumatic headache and complex regional pain syndrome [49–51].

Importantly, attention needs to be directed toward pediatric populations as well, as childhood and adolescence is a time of elevated risk for TBI [52], and prognosis and treatment responses may differ from adults due to the neuronal and brain network developmental status [53,54]. For instance, TBI can influence hippocampal neuro-genesis, which can increase the risk of developing adult neurological and neurodegenerative diseases [55,56]. A recent large-scale study using diffusion-weighted imaging showed that children with persistent post-concussive symptoms (more than 6 months following mild TBI) had more white matter microstructural changes than those with less persistent symptoms or mild orthopedic injury, suggesting more neuroinflammation and axonal swelling [57]. Hence, future research on this population is encouraged, as one might suspect augmented risk for neurocognitive alterations, especially in cases where neuroinflammation persists.

2.3. TBI and Sleep

Sleep–wake disturbances, including excessive daytime sleepiness, fatigue, and insomnia, are frequently reported by patients with TBI [58], and actually patients with TBI are at higher risk of developing chronic sleep–wake disturbances [11,59]. These disturbances can occur immediately after the TBI and tend to persist over time, as longitudinal studies have reported these symptoms are presents 6 months, 12 months, and even 3 years after the TBI [11,60–63]. For instance, a meta-analysis in patients with chronic TBI (>6 months post-injury) showed that moderate-severe TBI was associated with elevated slow wave sleep (SWS), reduced stage 2, and reduced sleep efficiency [15], and a recent retrospective cohort study in war veterans, with a median follow-up rate of 8.4 years, showed that TBI was associated with insomnia at follow-up when compared with patients without TBI (hazard ratio = 2.07; 95%) [64]. Indeed, insomnia following mild TBI seems to be common and perhaps among the main causes of disability in these patients [65,66], and relevant factors such as female sex, black race, history of psychiatric illness, and intracranial injuries seem to lead towards different insomnia trajectories [67]. Another sleep-related consequence of TBI is increased sleepiness, especially in early stages, and research has highlighted the damage of orexin/hypocretin neurons, whose activation involve wakefulness, as a possible contributor of the association between this association [68]. For example, a study revealed that TBI patients in the acute stage of severe TBI showed increased sleep duration and earlier sleep onset, perhaps suggesting that in the short-term the injured brain enhances sleep need and/or decreases the ability to maintain wakefulness [69]. Importantly, mood disorders (e.g., anxiety and depression), which are also associated with neuroinflammation, have been suggested as potential mediators of this association, and as with many other chronic conditions, it is very difficult to disentangle their role and their respective contribution in sleep–wake disorders following TBI [58,70].

2.4. Inflammation and Neuroinflammation Regulates Sleep

In the healthy brain, experimental studies have shown that inflammatory levels, whether peripheral or within the CNS, affect sleep regulation [71,72]. Cytokines are thought to be among the main effectors linking sleep and inflammation: in fact, IL-1β and TNF-α are sleep regulatory cytokines known to promote longer and deeper sleep. Overexpression of IL-1β and TNF-α following TBI is therefore thought to at least partially contribute to the heightened need for sleep following an injury [73]. Although their effects are smaller, other cytokines and prostaglandins also display sleep regulatory properties [71]. In the daytime, inflammatory levels are associated with fatigue and sleepiness [74]. However, some of these effects seem to be level dependent, where an inverse relation can be observed at higher levels, with high pro-inflammatory cytokines levels being associated with disrupted and fragmented sleep [75]. This observation might partly explain why many chronic inflammatory diseases are associated with sleep disturbances [71]. For instance, in a population with high inflammation and depression, the administration of a TNF blockade significantly improved sleep consolidation [76].

Recent studies show that microglia could play a key mediating role on sleep regulation through their production of sleep regulatory cytokines [77]. Moreover, microglia morphology, phagocytosis activity, and their gene expression were also shown to follow circadian variations [78,79]. Therefore, the normal circadian release of cytokines might contribute to sleep regulation. However, in a study that administered minocycline to attenuate microglial activation in mice that underwent sleep deprivation, a suppression of the normal increase in sleep depth was observed, which did not seem to be mediated by changes in cytokines transcription [80]. These findings suggest that microglial activation play a role in sleep regulation following acute sleep deprivation. Interestingly, animal research has suggested that the duration of post-traumatic sleep is a period that may define vulnerability for a repeated brain injury, which could be more related to glial activation rather than orexin neurons damage [81]. Although it remains unclear as to how exactly neuroinflammation regulates sleep, particularly in clinical populations, current hypotheses include the modulation of synaptic transmission affecting sleep [82,83], and damage to sleep regulatory structures in the brain, such as the thalamus, pituitary, hypothalamus, and brainstem, leading to sleep disturbances and disorders [84]. Alternatively, activated microglia might affect sleep–wake cycles through alterations of hypothalamic neurons that produces hypocretin [77], leading to narcolepsy-like symptoms such as excessive sleepiness, heightened sleep propensity, and disrupted nocturnal sleep. Taken together, current evidence suggest that microglial function regulates sleep, identifying neuroinflammatory processes as potential causes of sleep disturbances in TBI [85]. Furthermore, it seems that the characterization of sleep after TBI is essential to understand better the development of different neuropsychiatric outcomes [86,87].

2.5. Sleep Affects Inflammatory and Neuroinflammatory Processes

Sleep occupies approximately one-third of our lives and plays a central role in maintaining physiological homeostasis. Sleep is also crucial to TBI recovery as it is involved in metabolic and autonomic regulation [72,88–90], synaptic plasticity [91,92], memory consolidation [93] and other cognitive functions [94,95], mood regulation [96], as well as glymphatic clearance of metabolites from the brain [97,98]. In addition, sleep is an important regulator of the immune system [71,72]. It comes as no surprise that disturbed sleep has been shown to affect inflammation [71,72,99]. However, the inflammatory response to sleep loss can change depending on the chronicity: acute sleep deprivation results in lower IL-6, IL-1β, and TNF-α levels, whereas prolonged sleep restriction leads to elevated cytokines levels and increased inflammatory gene expression [71]. Sleep disturbances as well as short sleep duration have been associated with elevated inflammatory markers [100]. In patients with insomnia, the presence of short sleep, sleep fragmentation, and reduced slow-wave sleep were associated with higher inflammasome levels [101]. Sleep loss has also been shown to impact neuroinflammation and microglia. In many animal models, acute and chronic sleep loss generally affects microglial morphology, gene expression, activation [78]. After both chronic sleep loss and/or restriction in mice, microglial activation as well as microglial and astrocytic phagocytosis of synaptic components were observed, which may be a response to higher synaptic activity associated with prolonged wakefulness [102]. The authors suggested that sleep loss promotes "housekeeping" of heavily used synapses to downscale them, but these processes might also result in enhanced susceptibility to brain damage. Furthermore, it has been postulated that stress and poor sleep can trigger glial overactivation and a subsequent low-grade neuroinflammatory state, characterized by high levels of IL-1β and TNF-α, which, in turn, increases the excitability of CNS neurons through mechanisms such as long-term potentiation and increased synaptic efficiency [103].

Peripheral inflammation can also lead to neuroinflammation in the context of poor sleep [104,105]. Chronic sleep loss and sleep disorders such as obstructive sleep apnea have been associated with compromised BBB [106,107], and could result in an increased invasion of peripheral immune cells and cytokines into the CNS, thus contributing to neuroinflammation. One study used a 3-day sleep deprivation protocol in rats, and observed that sleep loss was associated with a cascade of pathological mechanisms, including exacerbated cortisol levels suggestive of a hypothalamic–pituitary–adrenal (HPA) response, altered circadian oscillations of clock genes expression, disrupted BBB integrity and microglial activation with elevated pro-inflammatory cytokines levels (IL-6, IL-1β, and TNF-α) [108].

Overall, sleep disturbances may contribute to poor health outcomes partly through detrimental chronic inflammation that can perpetuate tissue damage [84], which could exacerbate TBI-related inflammation and neuronal damage. Taken together, these recent findings highlight the bidirectional relationship between sleep–wake cycles and neuroinflammation. In the context of TBI, we hypothesize that the occurrence of sleep disturbances could be caused in part by neuroinflammatory processes following the trauma, which then, in turn, could synergically promotes neuroinflammatory-related tissue damage.

2.6. Neuroinflammation and Chronic Pain in the Context of Sleep Disturbances and TBI Chronic Pain

A common consequence of both TBI and poor sleep is chronic pain (i.e., pain lasting longer than 6 months). The interaction between sleep and pain problems is complex and likely bidirectional [109], and the most common pain condition after TBI appears in the form of headache, nowadays named persistent headache attributed to traumatic injury to the head [110,111]. The prevalence of persistent post-traumatic headache is as high as 57.8% (95% confidence interval [CI], 55.5–60.2%) across different time points [112]. In addition to headache, the onset of pain after TBI has also been reported in the neck, in the shoulders, or in the upper limbs [113]. In fact, TBI is accompanied by another pain diagnosis in more than 40% of cases [45], and in moderate-to-severe TBI, musculoskeletal complaints (stiffness and aching in joints) are present in 79% of patients assessed, more than 15 years after trauma [114]. While different potential underlying mechanisms have been identified, a possible underlying mechanism to the sleep and pain interaction relates to inflammatory processes (low grade inflammation or neuroinflammation) [71,115–117]. Accordingly, a recent study highlighted the role of IL-6 in the development of pathological pain, whose receptors seemed to be elevated in the spinal cord and nerve root ganglia in chronic pain states [118]. In addition, prostaglandins, other cytokines such as IL-1 as well as TNF are considered important pronociceptive factors that could mediate the association between sleep loss and increased pain in the context a chronic pain condition, such as post-traumatic headache. Moreover, it seems that melatonin, an endogenous substance produced in the pineal gland that is mainly associated with sleep–wake circadian regulation, is also linked with suppressing pain and inflammation [119]. Indeed, low melatonin has been postulated as a potential moderator for the association between chronic pain, sleep architecture, and immunometabolic traffic, as it can downregulate inflammatory mediators including prostaglandins and cytokines [119]. A recent review also highlighted the lower levels of melatonin on neuroinflammation and oxidative stress resulting from TBI [120], and a pre-clinical study among severe TBI patients found lower serum melatonin levels in the surviving patients [121]. It has also been shown that individuals with pain and mild TBI may need more time to sleep, and the authors concluded that pain could be associated with more pronounced sleep need in these individuals [122].

Additionally, yet not specifically related to trauma populations, other clinical studies have also found peripheral deficiencies compatible with neuroinflammation in pain syndromes such as fibromyalgia [123], where sleep disturbances are present in most of the cases [103]. Hence, the activation of microglia and astrocytes seems to be critical in the development of most chronic pain conditions [103,124].

3. Neuroinflammation and Other Neuropsychiatric Outcomes in the Context of Sleep Disturbances and TBI

3.1. Mood

TBI, sleep and pain are all major risk factors for mental health disorders such as anxiety or depression [125,126]. Interestingly, these frequent long-term consequences of traumatic injuries share neuroinflammation among key pathophysiological mechanisms [58,127–129]. According to a recent systematic review [130], the presence of depressive and/or anxiety symptoms in TBI samples was found to be associated with higher concentrations of serum and CSF, CRP, CSF-derived markers of sVCAM-1, sICAM-1, and sFAS, and IL-10, IL-8, IL-6, and TNF-α. Acute measures of some of these biomarkers predicted the onset of depression at 6 and 12 months post-injury.

Robust animal evidence has linked sleep deprivation to depression and anxiety-like behaviors partly through neuroinflammatory processes [21,108,131,132]. Following sleep deprivation in mice that underwent a TBI, lower corticosterone, enhanced neuroinflammation, exacerbated evidence of neuronal injury, and anxiety-like behaviors were observed as compared to brain-injured mice without sleep deprivation [21].

Taken together, traumatic injuries seem to interact with sleep disturbances in the installation of persistent trauma-related sequelae affecting mood, potentially through shared neuroinflammatory processes.

3.2. Cognitive Dysfunctions and Neurodegeneration

Neuroinflammation is now recognized as a key pathological mechanism to cognitive aging, neurodegeneration and Alzheimer's disease [133]. Meta-analyses have concluded that both sleep disturbances and TBI are risk factors for cognitive decline and incident dementia [7,134,135]. There is increasing evidence suggesting that sleep disturbances interact and/or contributes to peripheral inflammation as well as neuroinflammation to predict cognitive dysfunctions and dementia risk. For instance, inflammatory levels have been shown to moderate the association between sleep disturbances and obstructive sleep apnea with dementia risk [136,137]. In animal models, sleep deprivation or fragmentation lead to cognitive dysfunctions and neurodegenerative processes, at least partly through its effect on neuroinflammation (microglial activation, cytokines production, complement activation) [104,132,138,139]. In mice, one group used a 2-month chronic sleep fragmentation protocol, which resulted in the activation of microglia, endosome-autophagosome-lysosome pathway dysfunction, cortical and hippocampal Aβ accumulation, spatial learning and memory impairments, and anxiety-like behaviors [132]. In sleep deprived rats, inhibiting microglial activation mitigated spatial memory impairments, reduced deleterious effects on neurogenesis and gliosis in the hippocampus, and promoted anti-inflammatory cytokines over pro-inflammatory cytokines [139], supporting the causal role of microglial activation in sleep deprivation-induced cognitive dysfunction. Alternatively, sleep disturbances can also directly promote neurodegenerative processes through other mechanisms, such as a lower metabolic clearance of Aβ via the glymphatic system [97]. Interestingly, convincing evidence indicates that neuroinflammation could effectively modulate neurogenesis at different stages, including proliferation, differentiation, migration, survival of newborn neurons, maturation, synaptogenesis, and neuritogenesis among others [140]. Finally, a recent TBI study concluded that post-injury sleep fragmentation engages the dysfunctional post-injury HPA axis, enhances inflammation, and compromises hippocampal function [141]. The latter study suggested that external stressors that disrupt sleep have an integral role in mediating outcome after brain injury. Thus, both systemic inflammation and neuroinflammation can alter adult hippocampal neurogenesis in neurodegenerative disorders. For a more detailed an extensive review in The Dialogue Between Neuroinflammation and Adult Neurogenesis, please see [140].

Following a TBI, accumulating evidence is showing that neuroinflammation contributes to initial neuronal damage and cognitive dysfunction, but also long-term cognitive impairments, neurodegeneration, and risk of developing dementia [8,84,142]. After a single TBI, patients show evidence of white matter degeneration and persistent neuroinflammation up to 18 years post-injury [143]. In a mouse model of TBI, the neuroinflammatory response was found to drive synaptic degeneration and cognitive decline, which was abolished by complement inhibition, suggesting causality [144]. In humans, concomitant tau aggregation and neuroinflammation was observed using neuroimaging in mild TBI patients [41]. Moreover, it has been reported that TBI can also augment the formation of amyloid-b plaques and tau neurofibrillary tangles (NFTs) through inflammation-dependent gene expression and transcription factor activation, which could, in turn, produce sleep disturbances. Importantly, NFTs are another crucial feature of Alzheimer's disease [84].

Taken together, these findings suggest that the feedback positive loop between TBI, sleep disturbances and neuroinflammation can result in further cognitive dysfunctions and even neurodegeneration.

A summary of the abovementioned interactions and mechanisms can be observed in Figure 1.

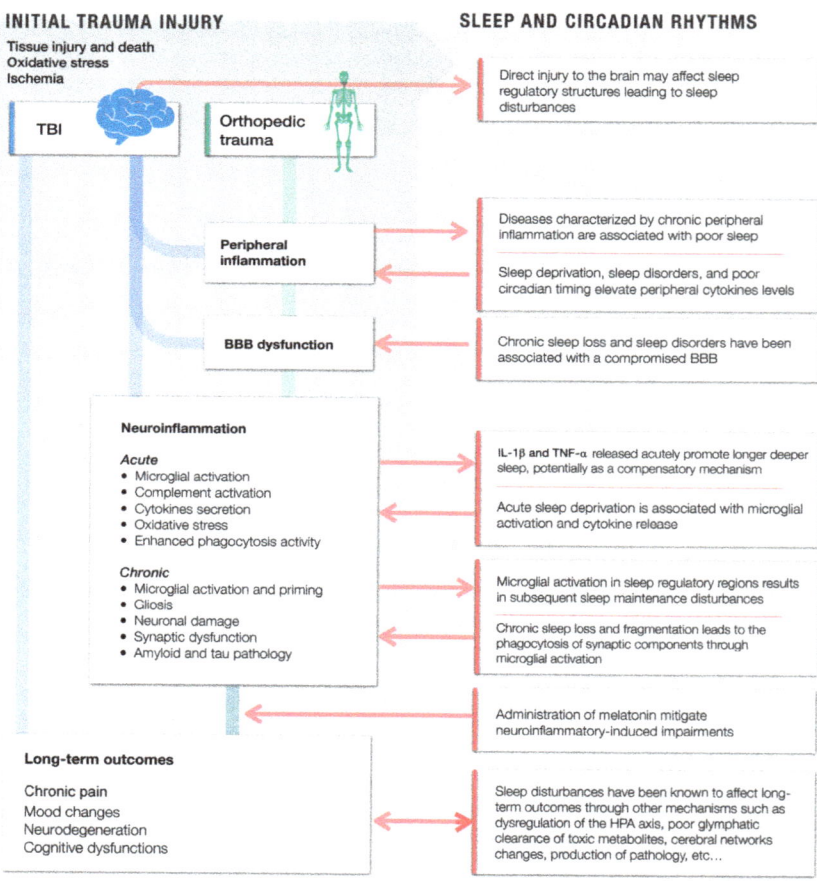

Figure 1. The putative role of neuroinflammation in the acquired traumatic injuries and related sleep disturbances. Traumatic brain injuries (TBI) and orthopedic traumas (OT) both lead to a downstream

pathophysiological cascade that includes peripheral inflammation, blood–brain barrier (BBB) dysfunction, and neuroinflammation. In turn, chronic neuroinflammation plays a role into the development of poor long-term outcomes. At each step of the way, sleep and sleep disturbances interact bidirectionally with traumatic pathological mechanisms and neuroinflammation. Poorer sleep exacerbates peripheral inflammation, BBB dysfunction, neuroinflammation, and worsen long-term outcomes. On the other hand, the trauma itself, its comorbidities, or neuroinflammation affect sleep regulation, which leads to a positive feedback loop, where neuroinflammation and sleep interact together to affect long-term outcomes following an injury.

4. Future Directions for Clinical Practice: Targeting Neuroinflammation

4.1. Sleep as a Therapeutic Target to Inhibit Neuroinflammation

Many sleep disturbances and disorders are treatable, often using non-pharmaceutical therapeutic strategies, thereby make it an appealing treatment target in order to reduce trauma-related neuroinflammation and improve patients' lives [115]. Cognitive behavioral therapy (CBT), the gold-standard treatment for insomnia, has proven to be an efficient way of improving sleep quality and restoring inflammatory levels [145–147]. CBT has also proven effective in TBI patients and show promise for mitigating patients' inflammation-related symptoms such as depression, anxiety and pain [148], along with other non-pharmaceutical strategies such as blue light therapy, problem solving treatment, and combined sleep hygiene interventions [149]. Moreover, in addition to sleep, CBT can also be directed towards pain and other associated disorders such as depression and anxiety in a hybrid approach. Hybrid CBT has shown promising results and it can also be carried out online to improve treatment compliance [150–152].

Although sleep medications, such as benzodiazepines, hypnotics, and sedating antidepressants, could help treat sleep disturbances, especially in the short term, and thereby have the potential to reduce neuroinflammation and TBI's related consequences linked to poor sleep [153], this remains to be investigated thoroughly and cautiously. Although still controversial, usage of sleeping pills has been associated with elevated risk of incident dementia [154,155], Moreover, sleeping medications generally perform worse than behavioral techniques such as CBT in treating sleep disturbances in the long term [156].

Nonetheless, a sleep aid with interesting potential is melatonin, as it has been associated with the inhibition of excessive microglial activation [157]. In addition to its endogenous secretion at night promoting adequate sleep–wake cycles, melatonin is also available as a dietary supplement. Among the proposed mechanisms underlying melatonin's downregulating action on microglial activation is through its role as an antioxidant, therefore reducing ROS [157]. It is also possible that melatonin supplementation could help reduce neuroinflammation through its effect on sleep regulation, although this remains to be confirmed. Interestingly, animal models showed that melatonin administration increased bone fracture healing [158], reduced neuroinflammation and promoted neuroprotection following a TBI [159,160]. In patients that sustained a TBI, a meta-analysis showed that melatonin has a positive effect on pathological findings, neurological status, neurobehavioral outcomes, and cognition [161]. However, it needs to be highlighted that the majority of the included studies were in animal models (i.e., 15 studies in animal models and two in human populations), and that the included human studies were considered to have low quality and were of uncertain significance. Furthermore, a recent randomized clinical trial in a pediatric population with mild TBI (n = 99) showed no significant difference in post-concussive symptoms between the use of melatonin at two different dosages (i.e., 3 and 10 mg) and placebo [162], yet a secondary analysis as per protocol of these data showed some improvements in sleep symptoms with melatonin [163]. Therefore, although there is evidence supporting the use of melatonin treatment after TBI to improve different behavioral and pathological outcomes based on animal models, data remain equivocal in human clinical populations.

4.2. Specifically Targeting Neuroinflammation to Improve Sleep and Trauma-Related Outcomes

Given its relevance and repercussions in different ambits of health, treating neuroinflammation emerges as a critical goal in the management of traumatically injured patients. Whereas peripheral neuroinflammation might be initially targeted with common anti-inflammatory medications, aiming to act on neuroinflammatory processes is much more complex, as some anti-inflammatories can disturb sleep as well, microglia appears as a primary treatment target for novel therapeutics aiming to tackle neuroinflammatory processes, including its selective abolition in animal models [164,165], or being targeted by nanoparticles [166]. Moreover, there are already several inhibitors of TNF-α and IL-1β that are available for clinical use, yet none of them are exempt of potentially serious side effects [167,168]. In addition, the use of psychedelics is receiving again a lot of attention in recent years due to its powerful properties to treat pain and mood disorders, as they have shown potential neuro-restorative effects and anti-neuroinflammatory and pro-immunomodulatory actions [169,170]. Indeed, the effects of some of these compounds is currently being studied in sleep as well [171]. Nonetheless, more development in this line of investigation is needed in the future. For a more detailed summary of pharmacological therapies on TBI, please refer to a recent review of phase 3 clinical trials on this population [172], which highlights key targets for future research.

An important non-pharmacological treatment option is exercise, given that exercise increases astrocytic activation, more specifically glial fibrillary acidic protein expression in hippocampal astrocytes in the stratum radiatum, a region that contains numerous astrocytes and is relevant for learning and memory [103,173]. Exercise is known to become anti-inflammatory or neuroprotective in several neuroinflammatory diseases. It is possible that exercise also reduces gliosis and glial proliferation [103]. Moreover, via its action on CNS glial cells, regular aerobic exercise has been shown to provide an adaptive advantage against perturbations to homeostasis, such as immunological challenge or ageing in animal models [174]. A systematic review and meta-analysis involving 13 RCTs and 514 participants, revealed that physical activity had positive effects on decreasing TNF-α and CRP (pro-inflammatory), while significantly improving BDNF and IGF-1 (neuroprotective) [175]. Furthermore, exercise is a great option for several sleep disorders including insomnia or sleep apnea [176,177], as it can regular cortisol, release endorphins, and decrease fat among others.

Non-pharmacological integrative approaches including mind/body therapies such as yoga, breathing exercises, meditation, all of them being associated with sleep quality improvement as well, have also been demonstrated to reduce pro-inflammatory cytokines and have proved some positive effects on depression, anxiety, cognition, and pain [178]. Moreover, several plant-based interventions (herbs/spices) currently under investigation [179]. While their non-invasiveness and harmless nature make them appealing as supportive therapy, more research is needed before obtaining any firm conclusion regarding their efficacy.

Other emerging techniques that can be used to target pain and sleep disorders, and specifically neuroinflammation, are non-invasive brain stimulation techniques, such as repetitive transcranial magnetic stimulation (rTMS) [180,181]. In different animal studies, rTMS reduced neuroinflammation by modulating astrocytes and microglia activity, reducing TNF-α, and increasing GABA, which can control excitotoxicity [182–185]. Additionally, clinical rTMS studies showed increases in serum GABA and BDNF in patients with chronic insomnia [186]. Thus, rTMS could be used not only to manage chronic pain patients but also to reduce their transition to chronicity by tackling the underlying neuroinflammatory mechanisms [115,185], which becomes especially relevant when applied to traumatically injured patients. While other techniques such as transcranial direct current stimulation, transcranial alternating current stimulation or vagal nerve stimulation hold potential in treating neuroinflammation [181,187], research is still lacking.

5. Conclusions

While the innate immune response following a TBI is necessary for recovery, its often prolonged and excessive nature contributes, paradoxically, to worsen outcomes. In that way, TBI leads to a state of peripheral/central neuroinflammation, which can be associated with sleep disturbances. Additionally, TBI and sleep disturbances also exacerbate the neuroinflammatory state, complicating these deleterious interactions even more, and potentially all leading to mood disorders, pain, cognitive deficits and neurodegeneration states. Importantly, finding treatment strategies, such as treating sleep disturbances or using non-invasive brain stimulation to reduce or modulate pro-inflammatory processes, can be useful in order to help TBI patients' physiological, psychological and cognitive health.

Funding: This work was financially supported by the Foundation Caroline Durand Research Chair in Acute Traumatology of Université de Montréal (LDB) and Canada Research Chairs (GL). The first author (AHB) is funded by a Vanier Scholarship. Additionally, another author (LDB) was also supported by Applied Biomedical Research Program, Research Foundation Flanders (Fonds voor Wetenschappelijk Onderzoek Vlaanderen), Belgium (FWO-TBM project no. TBM2021-T000521N-54252, "Towards PREcision MEdicine for Osteoarthritis: Added value of cognitive behavioural therapy for insomnia (the PREMEO trial)"), and by the Strategic Research Program SRP90 ('Pain Never Sleeps: Unravelling the Sleep-Pain Interaction in Patients with Chronic Pain') funded by the research council of the Vrije Universiteit Brussel, Brussels, Belgium.

Institutional Review Board Statement: Not applicable.

Informed Consent Statement: Not applicable.

Data Availability Statement: Not applicable.

Acknowledgments: We would like to acknowledge Gabrielle Beetz, for her initial contribution to the article and development of the original figure, and specially to the Chaire de recherche de la Fondation Caroline Durand en traumatologie aigue de l'Université de Montréal for their financial support to the project.

Conflicts of Interest: The authors declare no conflict of interest.

References

1. Bramlett, H.M.; Dietrich, W.D. Long-Term Consequences of Traumatic Brain Injury: Current Status of Potential Mechanisms of Injury and Neurological Outcomes. *J. Neurotrauma* **2015**, *32*, 1834–1848. [CrossRef] [PubMed]
2. Wilson, L.; Stewart, W.; Dams-O'Connor, K.; Diaz-Arrastia, R.; Horton, L.; Menon, D.K.; Polinder, S. The chronic and evolving neurological consequences of traumatic brain injury. *Lancet Neurol.* **2017**, *16*, 813–825. [CrossRef] [PubMed]
3. Martins, H.A.L.; Martins, B.B.M.; Ribas, V.R.; Bernardino, S.N.; de Oliveira, D.A.; Silva, L.C.; Sougey, E.B.; Valenca, M.M. Life quality, depression and anxiety symptoms in chronic post-traumatic headache after mild brain injury. *Dement. Neuropsychol.* **2012**, *6*, 53–58. [CrossRef] [PubMed]
4. Leng, Y.; Byers, A.L.; Barnes, D.E.; Peltz, C.B.; Li, Y.; Yaffe, K. Traumatic Brain Injury and Incidence Risk of Sleep Disorders in Nearly 200,000 US Veterans. *Neurology* **2021**, *96*, e1792–e1799. [CrossRef] [PubMed]
5. DiSabato, D.J.; Quan, N.; Godbout, J.P. Neuroinflammation: The devil is in the details. *J. Neurochem.* **2016**, *139* (Suppl. S2), 136–153. [CrossRef] [PubMed]
6. Guzman-Martinez, L.; Maccioni, R.B.; Andrade, V.; Navarrete, L.P.; Pastor, M.G.; Ramos-Escobar, N. Neuroinflammation as a Common Feature of Neurodegenerative Disorders. *Front. Pharmacol.* **2019**, *10*, 1008. [CrossRef] [PubMed]
7. Perry, D.C.; Sturm, V.E.; Peterson, M.J.; Pieper, C.F.; Bullock, T.; Boeve, B.F.; Miller, B.L.; Guskiewicz, K.M.; Berger, M.S.; Kramer, J.H.; et al. Association of traumatic brain injury with subsequent neurological and psychiatric disease: A meta-analysis. *J. Neurosurg.* **2016**, *124*, 511–526. [CrossRef]
8. Collins-Praino, L.E.; Corrigan, F. Does neuroinflammation drive the relationship between tau hyperphosphorylation and dementia development following traumatic brain injury? *Brain Behav. Immun.* **2017**, *60*, 369–382. [CrossRef]
9. Lyman, M.; Lloyd, D.G.; Ji, X.; Vizcaychipi, M.P.; Ma, D. Neuroinflammation: The role and consequences. *Neurosci. Res.* **2014**, *79*, 1–12. [CrossRef]
10. Castriotta, R.J.; Wilde, M.C.; Lai, J.M.; Atanasov, S.; Masel, B.E.; Kuna, S.T. Prevalence and consequences of sleep disorders in traumatic brain injury. *J. Clin. Sleep Med.* **2007**, *3*, 349–356. [CrossRef]
11. Duclos, C.; Dumont, M.; Wiseman-Hakes, C.; Arbour, C.; Mongrain, V.; Gaudreault, P.O.; Khoury, S.; Lavigne, G.; Desautels, A.; Gosselin, N. Sleep and wake disturbances following traumatic brain injury. *Pathol. Biol.* **2014**, *62*, 252–261. [CrossRef] [PubMed]

12. Mollayeva, T.; D'Souza, A.; Mollayeva, S. Sleep and Psychiatric Disorders in Persons With Mild Traumatic Brain Injury. *Curr. Psychiatry Rep.* **2017**, *19*, 47. [CrossRef] [PubMed]
13. Ouellet, M.C.; Beaulieu-Bonneau, S.; Morin, C.M. Insomnia in patients with traumatic brain injury: Frequency, characteristics, and risk factors. *J. Head Trauma Rehabil.* **2006**, *21*, 199–212. [CrossRef] [PubMed]
14. Mathias, J.L.; Alvaro, P.K. Prevalence of sleep disturbances, disorders, and problems following traumatic brain injury: A meta-analysis. *Sleep Med.* **2012**, *13*, 898–905. [CrossRef]
15. Mantua, J.; Grillakis, A.; Mahfouz, S.H.; Taylor, M.R.; Brager, A.J.; Yarnell, A.M.; Balkin, T.J.; Capaldi, V.F.; Simonelli, G. A systematic review and meta-analysis of sleep architecture and chronic traumatic brain injury. *Sleep Med. Rev.* **2018**, *41*, 61–77. [CrossRef]
16. Sandsmark, D.K.; Elliott, J.E.; Lim, M.M. Sleep-Wake Disturbances After Traumatic Brain Injury: Synthesis of Human and Animal Studies. *Sleep* **2017**, *40*. [CrossRef]
17. Yang, H.; Liu, Y.J.; Ye, J.L.; Zhao, L.H.; Li, L.L.; Hou, X.L. Evaluation of sleep disorder in orthopedic trauma patients: A retrospective analysis of 1129 cases. *J. Orthop. Surg. Res.* **2021**, *16*, 344. [CrossRef]
18. Chen, T.Y.; Lee, S.; Buxton, O.M. A Greater Extent of Insomnia Symptoms and Physician-Recommended Sleep Medication Use Predict Fall Risk in Community-Dwelling Older Adults. *Sleep* **2017**, *40*, zsx142. [CrossRef]
19. Wickwire, E.M.; Albrecht, J.S.; Griffin, N.R.; Schnyer, D.M.; Yue, J.K.; Markowitz, A.J.; Okonkwo, D.O.; Valadka, A.B.; Badjatia, N.; Manley, G.T. Sleep disturbances precede depressive symptomatology following traumatic brain injury. *Curr. Neurobiol.* **2019**, *10*, 49–55.
20. Beetz, G.; Babiloni, A.H.; Jodoin, M.; Charlebois-Plante, C.; Lavigne, G.J.; De Beaumont, L.; Rouleau, D.M. Relevance of sleep disturbances to orthopedic surgery: A current concepts narrative and practical review. *J. Bone Jt. Surg. Am.* **2021**, *103*, 2045–2056. [CrossRef]
21. Tapp, Z.M.; Kumar, J.E.; Witcher, K.G.; Atluri, R.R.; Velasquez, J.A.; O'Neil, S.M.; Dziabis, J.E.; Bray, C.E.; Sheridan, J.F.; Godbout, J.P.; et al. Sleep Disruption Exacerbates and Prolongs the Inflammatory Response to Traumatic Brain Injury. *J. Neurotrauma* **2020**, *37*, 1829–1843. [CrossRef] [PubMed]
22. Sulhan, S.; Lyon, K.A.; Shapiro, L.A.; Huang, J.H. Neuroinflammation and blood-brain barrier disruption following traumatic brain injury: Pathophysiology and potential therapeutic targets. *J. Neurosci. Res.* **2020**, *98*, 19–28. [CrossRef] [PubMed]
23. Ellis, A.; Bennett, D.L. Neuroinflammation and the generation of neuropathic pain. *Br. J. Anaesth.* **2013**, *111*, 26–37. [CrossRef] [PubMed]
24. Pape, H.C.; Marcucio, R.; Humphrey, C.; Colnot, C.; Knobe, M.; Harvey, E.J. Trauma-induced inflammation and fracture healing. *J. Orthop. Trauma* **2010**, *24*, 522–525. [CrossRef]
25. Scholz, J.; Woolf, C.J. The neuropathic pain triad: Neurons, immune cells and glia. *Nat. Neurosci.* **2007**, *10*, 1361–1368. [CrossRef]
26. Walker, A.K.; Kavelaars, A.; Heijnen, C.J.; Dantzer, R. Neuroinflammation and comorbidity of pain and depression. *Pharmacol. Rev.* **2014**, *66*, 80–101. [CrossRef]
27. Watkins, L.R.; Milligan, E.D.; Maier, S.F. Glial proinflammatory cytokines mediate exaggerated pain states: Implications for clinical pain. *Adv. Exp. Med. Biol.* **2003**, *521*, 1–21.
28. Shabab, T.; Khanabdali, R.; Moghadamtousi, S.Z.; Kadir, H.A.; Mohan, G. Neuroinflammation pathways: A general review. *Int. J. Neurosci.* **2017**, *127*, 624–633. [CrossRef]
29. Colton, C.A. Heterogeneity of microglial activation in the innate immune response in the brain. *J. Neuroimmune Pharmacol.* **2009**, *4*, 399–418. [CrossRef]
30. Varatharaj, A.; Galea, I. The blood-brain barrier in systemic inflammation. *Brain Behav. Immun.* **2017**, *60*, 1–12. [CrossRef]
31. Yoshiyama, Y.; Higuchi, M.; Zhang, B.; Huang, S.M.; Iwata, N.; Saido, T.C.; Maeda, J.; Suhara, T.; Trojanowski, J.Q.; Lee, V.M. Synapse loss and microglial activation precede tangles in a P301S tauopathy mouse model. *Neuron* **2007**, *53*, 337–351. [CrossRef] [PubMed]
32. Cunningham, C.; Campion, S.; Lunnon, K.; Murray, C.L.; Woods, J.F.; Deacon, R.M.; Rawlins, J.N.; Perry, V.H. Systemic inflammation induces acute behavioral and cognitive changes and accelerates neurodegenerative disease. *Biol. Psychiatry* **2009**, *65*, 304–312. [CrossRef] [PubMed]
33. Witcher, K.G.; Eiferman, D.S.; Godbout, J.P. Priming the inflammatory pump of the CNS after traumatic brain injury. *Trends Neurosci.* **2015**, *38*, 609–620. [CrossRef] [PubMed]
34. Greve, M.W.; Zink, B.J. Pathophysiology of traumatic brain injury. *Mt. Sinai J. Med.* **2009**, *76*, 97–104. [CrossRef]
35. Lozano, D.; Gonzales-Portillo, G.S.; Acosta, S.; de la Pena, I.; Tajiri, N.; Kaneko, Y.; Borlongan, C.V. Neuroinflammatory responses to traumatic brain injury: Etiology, clinical consequences, and therapeutic opportunities. *Neuropsychiatr. Dis. Treat.* **2015**, *11*, 97–106.
36. Morganti-Kossmann, M.C.; Semple, B.D.; Hellewell, S.C.; Bye, N.; Ziebell, J.M. The complexity of neuroinflammation consequent to traumatic brain injury: From research evidence to potential treatments. *Acta Neuropathol.* **2019**, *137*, 731–755. [CrossRef]
37. Wofford, K.L.; Loane, D.J.; Cullen, D.K. Acute drivers of neuroinflammation in traumatic brain injury. *Neural Regen. Res.* **2019**, *14*, 1481–1489.
38. Nimmerjahn, A.; Kirchhoff, F.; Helmchen, F. Resting microglial cells are highly dynamic surveillants of brain parenchyma in vivo. *Science* **2005**, *308*, 1314–1318. [CrossRef]
39. Gao, H.M.; Hong, J.S. Why neurodegenerative diseases are progressive: Uncontrolled inflammation drives disease progression. *Trends Immunol.* **2008**, *29*, 357–365. [CrossRef]
40. Acosta, S.A.; Tajiri, N.; de la Pena, I.; Bastawrous, M.; Sanberg, P.R.; Kaneko, Y.; Borlongan, C.V. Alpha-synuclein as a pathological link between chronic traumatic brain injury and Parkinson's disease. *J. Cell Physiol.* **2015**, *230*, 1024–1032. [CrossRef]

1. Marklund, N.; Vedung, F.; Lubberink, M.; Tegner, Y.; Johansson, J.; Blennow, K.; Zetterberg, H.; Fahlstrom, M.; Haller, S.; Stenson, S.; et al. Tau aggregation and increased neuroinflammation in athletes after sports-related concussions and in traumatic brain injury patients - A PET/MR study. *Neuroimage Clin.* **2021**, *30*, 102665. [CrossRef] [PubMed]

2. Uryu, K.; Chen, X.H.; Martinez, D.; Browne, K.D.; Johnson, V.E.; Graham, D.I.; Lee, V.M.; Trojanowski, J.Q.; Smith, D.H. Multiple proteins implicated in neurodegenerative diseases accumulate in axons after brain trauma in humans. *Exp. Neurol.* **2007**, *208*, 185–192. [CrossRef] [PubMed]

3. Tajiri, N.; Kellogg, S.L.; Shimizu, T.; Arendash, G.W.; Borlongan, C.V. Traumatic brain injury precipitates cognitive impairment and extracellular Aβ aggregation in Alzheimer's disease transgenic mice. *PLoS ONE* **2013**, *8*, e78851. [CrossRef] [PubMed]

4. Gross, T.; Schüepp, M.; Attenberger, C.; Pargger, H.; Amsler, F. Outcome in polytraumatized patients with and without brain injury. *Acta Anaesthesiol. Scand.* **2012**, *56*, 1163–1174. [CrossRef]

5. Jodoin, M.; Rouleau, D.M.; Charlebois-Plante, C.; Benoit, B.; Leduc, S.; Laflamme, G.Y.; Gosselin, N.; Larson-Dupuis, C.; De Beaumont, L. Incidence rate of mild traumatic brain injury among patients who have suffered from an isolated limb fracture: Upper limb fracture patients are more at risk. *Injury* **2016**, *47*, 1835–1840. [CrossRef]

6. Rabinowitz, A.R.; Li, X.; Levin, H.S. Sport and nonsport etiologies of mild traumatic brain injury: Similarities and differences. *Annu. Rev. Psychol.* **2014**, *65*, 301–331. [CrossRef]

7. McDonald, S.J.; Sun, M.; Agoston, D.V.; Shultz, S.R. The effect of concomitant peripheral injury on traumatic brain injury pathobiology and outcome. *J. Neuroinflammation* **2016**, *13*, 90. [CrossRef]

8. Leong, B.K.; Mazlan, M.; Abd Rahim, R.B.; Ganesan, D. Concomitant injuries and its influence on functional outcome after traumatic brain injury. *Disabil. Rehabil.* **2013**, *35*, 1546–1551. [CrossRef]

9. Mayer, C.L.; Huber, B.R.; Peskind, E. Traumatic brain injury, neuroinflammation, and post-traumatic headaches. *Headache* **2013**, *53*, 1523–1530. [CrossRef]

10. Jung, Y.H.; Kim, H.; Jeon, S.Y.; Kwon, J.M.; Lee, W.J.; Kim, Y.C.; Jang, J.H.; Choi, S.H.; Lee, J.Y.; Kang, D.H. Brain Metabolites and Peripheral Biomarkers Associated with Neuroinflammation in Complex Regional Pain Syndrome Using [11C]-(R)-PK11195 Positron Emission Tomography and Magnetic Resonance Spectroscopy: A Pilot Study. *Pain Med.* **2019**, *20*, 504–514. [CrossRef]

11. Prasad Md, A.; Chakravarthy Md, K. Review of complex regional pain syndrome and the role of the neuroimmune axis. *Mol. Pain* **2021**, *17*, 17448069211006617. [CrossRef] [PubMed]

12. Ryan, E.; Bolger, T.; Barrett, M.J.; Blackburn, C.; Okafor, I.; McNamara, R.; Molloy, E.J. Paediatric Head Injury and Traumatic Brain Injury. *Ir. Med. J.* **2020**, *113*, 94. [PubMed]

13. Fraunberger, E.; Esser, M.J. Neuro-Inflammation in Pediatric Traumatic Brain Injury-from Mechanisms to Inflammatory Networks. *Brain Sci.* **2019**, *9*, 319. [CrossRef] [PubMed]

14. Ashwal, S.; Siebold, L.; Krueger, A.C.; Wilson, C.G. Post-traumatic Neuroinflammation: Relevance to Pediatrics. *Pediatr. Neurol.* **2021**, *122*, 50–58. [CrossRef] [PubMed]

15. Rizk, M.; Vu, J.; Zhang, Z. Impact of pediatric traumatic brain injury on hippocampal neurogenesis. *Neural Regen. Res.* **2021**, *16*, 926–933.

16. Zhang, Z.; Ishrat, S.; O'Bryan, M.; Klein, B.; Saraswati, M.; Robertson, C.; Kannan, S. Pediatric Traumatic Brain Injury Causes Long-Term Deficits in Adult Hippocampal Neurogenesis and Cognition. *J. Neurotrauma* **2020**, *37*, 1656–1667. [CrossRef]

17. Ware, A.L.; Yeates, K.O.; Tang, K.; Shukla, A.; Onicas, A.I.; Guo, S.; Goodrich-Hunsaker, N.; Abdeen, N.; Beauchamp, M.H.; Beaulieu, C.; et al. Longitudinal white matter microstructural changes in pediatric mild traumatic brain injury: An A-CAP study. *Hum. Brain Mapp.* **2022**, *43*, 3809–3823. [CrossRef]

18. Lavigne, G.; Khoury, S.; Chauny, J.M.; Desautels, A. Pain and sleep in post-concussion/mild traumatic brain injury. *Pain* **2015**, *156* (Suppl. S1), S75–S85. [CrossRef]

19. Gosselin, N.; Tellier, M. Patients with traumatic brain injury are at high risk of developing chronic sleep-wake disturbances. *J. Neurol. Neurosurg. Psychiatry* **2010**, *81*, 1297. [CrossRef]

20. Imbach, L.L.; Valko, P.O.; Li, T.; Maric, A.; Symeonidou, E.R.; Stover, J.F.; Bassetti, C.L.; Mica, L.; Werth, E.; Baumann, C.R. Increased sleep need and daytime sleepiness 6 months after traumatic brain injury: A prospective controlled clinical trial. *Brain* **2015**, *138 Pt 3*, 726–735. [CrossRef]

21. Baumann, C.R.; Werth, E.; Stocker, R.; Ludwig, S.; Bassetti, C.L. Sleep-wake disturbances 6 months after traumatic brain injury: A prospective study. *Brain* **2007**, *130 Pt 7*, 1873–1883. [CrossRef] [PubMed]

22. Kempf, J.; Werth, E.; Kaiser, P.R.; Bassetti, C.L.; Baumann, C.R. Sleep-wake disturbances 3 years after traumatic brain injury. *J. Neurol. Neurosurg. Psychiatry* **2010**, *81*, 1402–1405. [CrossRef] [PubMed]

23. Saksvik, S.B.; Karaliute, M.; Kallestad, H.; Follestad, T.; Asarnow, R.; Vik, A.; Haberg, A.K.; Skandsen, T.; Olsen, A. The Prevalence and Stability of Sleep-Wake Disturbance and Fatigue throughout the First Year after Mild Traumatic Brain Injury. *J. Neurotrauma* **2020**, *37*, 2528–2541. [CrossRef]

24. Haynes, Z.A.; Collen, J.F.; Poltavskiy, E.A.; Walker, L.E.; Janak, J.; Howard, J.T.; Werner, J.K.; Wickwire, E.M.; Holley, A.B.; Zarzabal, L.A.; et al. Risk factors of persistent insomnia among survivors of traumatic injury: A retrospective cohort study. *J. Clin. Sleep Med.* **2021**, *17*, 1831–1840. [CrossRef] [PubMed]

25. Gosselin, N.; Duclos, C. Insomnia following a mild traumatic brain injury: A missing piece to the work disability puzzle? *Sleep Med.* **2016**, *20*, 155–156. [CrossRef] [PubMed]

66. Mollayeva, T.; Pratt, B.; Mollayeva, S.; Shapiro, C.M.; Cassidy, J.D.; Colantonio, A. The relationship between insomnia and disability in workers with mild traumatic brain injury/concussion: Insomnia and disability in chronic mild traumatic brain injury. *Sleep Med.* **2016**, *20*, 157–166. [CrossRef] [PubMed]
67. Wickwire, E.M.; Albrecht, J.S.; Capaldi, V.F., II; Jain, S.O.; Gardner, R.C.; Werner, J.K.; Mukherjee, P.; McKeon, A.B.; Smith, M.T. Giacino, J.T.; et al. Trajectories of Insomnia in Adults After Traumatic Brain Injury. *JAMA Netw. Open* **2022**, *5*, e2145310. [CrossRef]
68. Baumann, C.R.; Bassetti, C.L.; Valko, P.O.; Haybaeck, J.; Keller, M.; Clark, E.; Stocker, R.; Tolnay, M.; Scammell, T.E. Loss of hypocretin (orexin) neurons with traumatic brain injury. *Ann. Neurol.* **2009**, *66*, 555–559. [CrossRef]
69. Wiseman-Hakes, C.; Duclos, C.; Blais, H.; Dumont, M.; Bernard, F.; Desautels, A.; Menon, D.K.; Gilbert, D.; Carrier, J.; Gosselin, N. Sleep in the Acute Phase of Severe Traumatic Brain Injury: A Snapshot of Polysomnography. *Neurorehabil. Neural Repair* **2016**, *30*, 713–721. [CrossRef]
70. Jahan, A.B.; Tanev, K. Neurobiological Mechanisms Of Depression Following Traumatic Brain Injury. *Brain Inj.* **2023**, *37*, 24–33. [CrossRef]
71. Besedovsky, L.; Lange, T.; Haack, M. The Sleep-Immune Crosstalk in Health and Disease. *Physiol. Rev.* **2019**, *99*, 1325–1380. [CrossRef] [PubMed]
72. Irwin, M.R. Sleep and inflammation: Partners in sickness and in health. *Nat. Rev. Immunol.* **2019**, *19*, 702–715. [CrossRef] [PubMed]
73. Krueger, J.M.; Majde, J.A.; Rector, D.M. Cytokines in immune function and sleep regulation. *Handb. Clin. Neurol.* **2011**, *98*, 229–240. [PubMed]
74. Lasselin, J.; Karshikoff, B.; Axelsson, J.; Åkerstedt, T.; Benson, S.; Engler, H.; Schedlowski, M.; Jones, M.; Lekander, M.; Andreasson, A. Fatigue and sleepiness responses to experimental inflammation and exploratory analysis of the effect of baseline inflammation in healthy humans. *Brain Behav. Immun.* **2020**, *83*, 309–314. [CrossRef]
75. Opp, M.R.; Obal, F., Jr.; Krueger, J.M. Interleukin 1 alters rat sleep: Temporal and dose-related effects. *Am. J. Physiol.* **1991**, *260 Pt 2*, R52–R58. [CrossRef]
76. Weinberger, J.F.; Raison, C.L.; Rye, D.B.; Montague, A.R.; Woolwine, B.J.; Felger, J.C.; Haroon, E.; Miller, A.H. Inhibition of tumor necrosis factor improves sleep continuity in patients with treatment resistant depression and high inflammation. *Brain Behav. Immun.* **2015**, *47*, 193–200. [CrossRef]
77. Nadjar, A.; Wigren, H.M.; Tremblay, M.E. Roles of Microglial Phagocytosis and Inflammatory Mediators in the Pathophysiology of Sleep Disorders. *Front. Cell Neurosci.* **2017**, *11*, 250. [CrossRef]
78. Deurveilher, S.; Golovin, T.; Hall, S.; Semba, K. Microglia dynamics in sleep/wake states and in response to sleep loss. *Neurochem. Int.* **2021**, *143*, 104944. [CrossRef]
79. Fonken, L.K.; Frank, M.G.; Kitt, M.M.; Barrientos, R.M.; Watkins, L.R.; Maier, S.F. Microglia inflammatory responses are controlled by an intrinsic circadian clock. *Brain Behav. Immun.* **2015**, *45*, 171–179. [CrossRef]
80. Wisor, J.P.; Schmidt, M.A.; Clegern, W.C. Evidence for neuroinflammatory and microglial changes in the cerebral response to sleep loss. *Sleep* **2011**, *34*, 261–272. [CrossRef]
81. Rowe, R.K.; Harrison, J.L.; Morrison, H.W.; Subbian, V.; Murphy, S.M.; Lifshitz, J. Acute Post-Traumatic Sleep May Define Vulnerability to a Second Traumatic Brain Injury in Mice. *J. Neurotrauma* **2019**, *36*, 1318–1334. [CrossRef] [PubMed]
82. Krueger, J.M.; Clinton, J.M.; Winters, B.D.; Zielinski, M.R.; Taishi, P.; Jewett, K.A.; Davis, C.J. Involvement of cytokines in slow wave sleep. *Prog. Brain Res.* **2011**, *193*, 39–47.
83. Krueger, J.M.; Obal, F.J.; Fang, J.; Kubota, T.; Taishi, P. The role of cytokines in physiological sleep regulation. *Ann. N. Y. Acad. Sci.* **2001**, *933*, 211–221. [CrossRef] [PubMed]
84. Green, T.R.F.; Ortiz, J.B.; Wonnacott, S.; Williams, R.J.; Rowe, R.K. The Bidirectional Relationship Between Sleep and Inflammation Links Traumatic Brain Injury and Alzheimer's Disease. *Front. Neurosci.* **2020**, *14*, 894. [CrossRef]
85. Rowe, R.K.; Griesbach, G.S. Immune-endocrine interactions in the pathophysiology of sleep-wake disturbances following traumatic brain injury: A narrative review. *Brain Res. Bull.* **2022**, *185*, 117–128. [CrossRef] [PubMed]
86. Saber, M.; Murphy, S.M.; Cho, Y.; Lifshitz, J.; Rowe, R.K. Experimental diffuse brain injury and a model of Alzheimer's disease exhibit disease-specific changes in sleep and incongruous peripheral inflammation. *J. Neurosci. Res.* **2021**, *99*, 1136–1160. [CrossRef]
87. Sanchez, E.; Blais, H.; Duclos, C.; Arbour, C.; Van Der Maren, S.; El-Khatib, H.; Baril, A.A.; Bernard, F.; Carrier, J.; Gosselin, N. Sleep from acute to chronic traumatic brain injury and cognitive outcomes. *Sleep* **2022**, *45*, zsac123. [CrossRef]
88. van Dalfsen, J.H.; Markus, C.R. The influence of sleep on human hypothalamic-pituitary-adrenal (HPA) axis reactivity: A systematic review. *Sleep Med. Rev.* **2018**, *39*, 187–194. [CrossRef]
89. Sauvet, F.; Drogou, C.; Bougard, C.; Arnal, P.J.; Dispersyn, G.; Bourrilhon, C.; Rabat, A.; Van Beers, P.; Gomez-Merino, D.; Faraut, B.; et al. Vascular response to 1 week of sleep restriction in healthy subjects. A metabolic response? *Int. J. Cardiol.* **2015**, *190*, 246–255. [CrossRef]
90. de Zambotti, M.; Trinder, J.; Silvani, A.; Colrain, I.M.; Baker, F.C. Dynamic coupling between the central and autonomic nervous systems during sleep: A review. *Neurosci. Biobehav. Rev.* **2018**, *90*, 84–103. [CrossRef]
91. Frank, M.G.; Cantera, R. Sleep, clocks, and synaptic plasticity. *Trends Neurosci.* **2014**, *37*, 491–501. [CrossRef]
92. Tononi, G.; Cirelli, C. Sleep and synaptic homeostasis: A hypothesis. *Brain Res. Bull.* **2003**, *62*, 143–150. [CrossRef] [PubMed]
93. Rasch, B.; Born, J. About sleep's role in memory. *Physiol. Rev.* **2013**, *93*, 681–766. [CrossRef] [PubMed]
94. Kuula, L.; Pesonen, A.K.; Heinonen, K.; Kajantie, E.; Eriksson, J.G.; Andersson, S.; Lano, A.; Lahti, J.; Wolke, D.; Räikkönen, K. Naturally occurring circadian rhythm and sleep duration are related to executive functions in early adulthood. *J. Sleep Res.* **2018**, *27*, 113–119. [CrossRef] [PubMed]

5. Hudson, A.N.; Van Dongen, H.P.A.; Honn, K.A. Sleep deprivation, vigilant attention, and brain function: A review. *Neuropsychopharmacology* **2020**, *45*, 21–30. [CrossRef] [PubMed]
6. Palagini, L.; Bastien, C.H.; Marazziti, D.; Ellis, J.G.; Riemann, D. The key role of insomnia and sleep loss in the dysregulation of multiple systems involved in mood disorders: A proposed model. *J. Sleep Res.* **2019**, *28*, e12841. [CrossRef] [PubMed]
7. Xie, L.; Kang, H.; Xu, Q.; Chen, M.J.; Liao, Y.; Thiyagarajan, M.; O'Donnell, J.; Christensen, D.J.; Nicholson, C.; Iliff, J.J.; et al. Sleep drives metabolite clearance from the adult brain. *Science* **2013**, *342*, 373–377. [CrossRef] [PubMed]
8. Fultz, N.E.; Bonmassar, G.; Setsompop, K.; Stickgold, R.A.; Rosen, B.R.; Polimeni, J.R.; Lewis, L.D. Coupled electrophysiological, hemodynamic, and cerebrospinal fluid oscillations in human sleep. *Science* **2019**, *366*, 628–631. [CrossRef]
9. Simpson, N.; Dinges, D.F. Sleep and inflammation. *Nutr. Rev.* **2007**, *65 Pt 2*, S244–S252. [CrossRef]
100. Irwin, M.R.; Olmstead, R.; Carroll, J.E. Sleep Disturbance, Sleep Duration, and Inflammation: A Systematic Review and Meta-Analysis of Cohort Studies and Experimental Sleep Deprivation. *Biol. Psychiatry* **2016**, *80*, 40–52. [CrossRef]
101. Wang, J.; Wu, X.; Liang, W.; Chen, M.; Zhao, C.; Wang, X. Objective Short Sleep Duration is Related to the Peripheral Inflammasome Dysregulation in Patients with Chronic Insomnia. *Nat. Sci. Sleep* **2020**, *12*, 759–766. [CrossRef]
102. Bellesi, M.; de Vivo, L.; Chini, M.; Gilli, F.; Tononi, G.; Cirelli, C. Sleep Loss Promotes Astrocytic Phagocytosis and Microglial Activation in Mouse Cerebral Cortex. *J. Neurosci.* **2017**, *37*, 5263–5273. [CrossRef] [PubMed]
103. Nijs, J.; Loggia, M.L.; Polli, A.; Moens, M.; Huysmans, E.; Goudman, L.; Meeus, M.; Vanderweeen, L.; Ickmans, K.; Clauw, D. Sleep disturbances and severe stress as glial activators: Key targets for treating central sensitization in chronic pain patients? *Expert Opin. Ther. Targets* **2017**, *21*, 817–826. [CrossRef] [PubMed]
104. Zhu, B.; Dong, Y.; Xu, Z.; Gompf, H.S.; Ward, S.A.; Xue, Z.; Miao, C.; Zhang, Y.; Chamberlin, N.L.; Xie, Z. Sleep disturbance induces neuroinflammation and impairment of learning and memory. *Neurobiol. Dis.* **2012**, *48*, 348–355. [CrossRef]
105. Zielinski, M.R.; Gibbons, A.J. Neuroinflammation, Sleep, and Circadian Rhythms. *Front. Cell Infect. Microbiol.* **2022**, *12*, 853096. [CrossRef] [PubMed]
106. Lim, D.C.; Pack, A.I. Obstructive sleep apnea and cognitive impairment: Addressing the blood-brain barrier. *Sleep Med. Rev.* **2014**, *18*, 35–48. [CrossRef]
107. Hurtado-Alvarado, G.; Domínguez-Salazar, E.; Pavon, L.; Velázquez-Moctezuma, J.; Gómez-González, B. Blood-Brain Barrier Disruption Induced by Chronic Sleep Loss: Low-Grade Inflammation May Be the Link. *J. Immunol. Res.* **2016**, *2016*, 4576012. [CrossRef]
108. Xing, C.; Zhou, Y.; Xu, H.; Ding, M.; Zhang, Y.; Zhang, M.; Hu, M.; Huang, X.; Song, L. Sleep disturbance induces depressive behaviors and neuroinflammation by altering the circadian oscillations of clock genes in rats. *Neurosci. Res.* **2021**, *171*, 124–132. [CrossRef]
109. Herrero Babiloni, A.; De Koninck, B.P.; Beetz, G.; De Beaumont, L.; Martel, M.O.; Lavigne, G.J. Sleep and pain: Recent insights, mechanisms, and future directions in the investigation of this relationship. *J. Neural Transm.* **2020**, *127*, 647–660. [CrossRef]
110. Irvine, K.A.; Clark, J.D. Chronic Pain After Traumatic Brain Injury: Pathophysiology and Pain Mechanisms. *Pain Med.* **2018**, *19*, 1315–1333. [CrossRef]
111. Headache Classification Committee of the International Headache Society (IHS). The International Classification of Headache Disorders, 3rd edition. *Cephalalgia* **2018**, *38*, 1–211. [CrossRef] [PubMed]
112. Nampiaparampil, D.E. Prevalence of chronic pain after traumatic brain injury: A systematic review. *JAMA* **2008**, *300*, 711–719. [CrossRef] [PubMed]
113. Khoury, S.; Benavides, R. Pain with traumatic brain injury and psychological disorders. *Prog. Neuropsychopharmacol. Biol. Psychiatry* **2018**, *87 Pt B*, 224–233. [CrossRef]
114. Brown, S.; Hawker, G.; Beaton, D.; Colantonio, A. Long-term musculoskeletal complaints after traumatic brain injury. *Brain Inj.* **2011**, *25*, 453–461. [CrossRef]
115. Herrero Babiloni, A.; Beetz, G.; Tang, N.K.Y.; Heinzer, R.; Nijs, J.; Martel, M.O.; Lavigne, G.J. Towards the endotyping of the sleep-pain interaction: A topical review on multitarget strategies based on phenotypic vulnerabilities and putative pathways. *Pain* **2021**, *162*, 1281–1288. [CrossRef] [PubMed]
116. Haack, M.; Simpson, N.; Sethna, N.; Kaur, S.; Mullington, J. Sleep deficiency and chronic pain: Potential underlying mechanisms and clinical implications. *Neuropsychopharmacology* **2020**, *45*, 205–216. [CrossRef] [PubMed]
117. Mullington, J.M.; Simpson, N.S.; Meier-Ewert, H.K.; Haack, M. Sleep loss and inflammation. *Best Pract. Res. Clin. Endocrinol. Metab.* **2010**, *24*, 775–784. [CrossRef]
118. Zhou, Y.Q.; Liu, Z.; Liu, Z.H.; Chen, S.P.; Li, M.; Shahveranov, A.; Ye, D.W.; Tian, Y.K. Interleukin-6: An emerging regulator of pathological pain. *J. Neuroinflammation* **2016**, *13*, 141. [CrossRef]
119. Chaudhry, S.R.; Stadlbauer, A.; Buchfelder, M.; Kinfe, T.M. Melatonin Moderates the Triangle of Chronic Pain, Sleep Architecture and Immunometabolic Traffic. *Biomedicines* **2021**, *9*, 984. [CrossRef]
120. Blum, B.; Kaushal, S.; Khan, S.; Kim, J.H.; Alvarez Villalba, C.L. Melatonin in Traumatic Brain Injury and Cognition. *Cureus* **2021**, *13*, e17776. [CrossRef]
121. Lorente, L.; Martin, M.M.; Ruiz, C.; Abreu-Gonzalez, P.; Ramos-Gomez, L.; Argueso, M.; Sole-Violan, J.; Caceres, J.J.; Jimenez, A. Serum melatonin levels in predicting mortality in patients with severe traumatic brain injury. *Anaesth. Crit. Care Pain Med.* **2021**, *40*, 100966. [CrossRef]
122. Suzuki, Y.; Khoury, S.; El-Khatib, H.; Chauny, J.M.; Paquet, J.; Giguere, J.F.; Denis, R.; Gosselin, N.; Lavigne, G.J.; Arbour, C. Individuals with pain need more sleep in the early stage of mild traumatic brain injury. *Sleep Med.* **2017**, *33*, 36–42. [CrossRef] [PubMed]

123. Uceyler, N.; Zeller, D.; Kahn, A.K.; Kewenig, S.; Kittel-Schneider, S.; Schmid, A.; Casanova-Molla, J.; Reiners, K.; Sommer, C. Small fibre pathology in patients with fibromyalgia syndrome. *Brain* **2013**, *136 Pt 6*, 1857–1867. [CrossRef] [PubMed]
124. Ji, R.R.; Xu, Z.Z.; Gao, Y.J. Emerging targets in neuroinflammation-driven chronic pain. *Nat. Rev. Drug Discov.* **2014**, *13*, 533–548. [CrossRef] [PubMed]
125. Hammond, F.M.; Corrigan, J.D.; Ketchum, J.M.; Malec, J.F.; Dams-O'Connor, K.; Hart, T.; Novack, T.A.; Bogner, J.; Dahdah, M.N.; Whiteneck, G.G. Prevalence of Medical and Psychiatric Comorbidities Following Traumatic Brain Injury. *J. Head Trauma Rehabil.* **2019**, *34*, E1–E10. [CrossRef] [PubMed]
126. Clay, F.J.; Watson, W.L.; Newstead, S.V.; McClure, R.J. A systematic review of early prognostic factors for persisting pain following acute orthopedic trauma. *Pain Res. Manag.* **2012**, *17*, 35–44. [CrossRef] [PubMed]
127. Campos, A.C.P.; Antunes, G.F.; Matsumoto, M.; Pagano, R.L.; Martinez, R.C.R. Neuroinflammation, Pain and Depression: An Overview of the Main Findings. *Front. Psychol.* **2020**, *11*, 1825. [CrossRef]
128. Zhang, L.; Zhang, J.; You, Z. Switching of the Microglial Activation Phenotype Is a Possible Treatment for Depression Disorder. *Front. Cell Neurosci.* **2018**, *12*, 306. [CrossRef]
129. Manchanda, S.; Singh, H.; Kaur, T.; Kaur, G. Low-grade neuroinflammation due to chronic sleep deprivation results in anxiety and learning and memory impairments. *Mol. Cell. Biochem.* **2018**, *449*, 63–72. [CrossRef]
130. Feiger, J.A.; Snyder, R.L.; Walsh, M.J.; Cissne, M.; Cwiek, A.; Al-Momani, S.I.; Chiou, K.S. The Role of Neuroinflammation in Neuropsychiatric Disorders Following Traumatic Brain Injury: A Systematic Review. *J. Head Trauma Rehabil.* **2022**, *37*, E370–E382. [CrossRef]
131. Wadhwa, M.; Chauhan, G.; Roy, K.; Sahu, S.; Deep, S.; Jain, V.; Kishore, K.; Ray, K.; Thakur, L.; Panjwani, U. Caffeine and Modafinil Ameliorate the Neuroinflammation and Anxious Behavior in Rats during Sleep Deprivation by Inhibiting the Microglia Activation. *Front. Cell Neurosci.* **2018**, *12*, 49. [CrossRef] [PubMed]
132. Xie, Y.; Ba, L.; Wang, M.; Deng, S.Y.; Chen, S.M.; Huang, L.F.; Zhang, M.; Wang, W.; Ding, F.F. Chronic sleep fragmentation shares similar pathogenesis with neurodegenerative diseases: Endosome-autophagosome-lysosome pathway dysfunction and microglia-mediated neuroinflammation. *CNS Neurosci. Ther.* **2020**, *26*, 215–227. [CrossRef] [PubMed]
133. Gray, S.C.; Kinghorn, K.J.; Woodling, N.S. Shifting equilibriums in Alzheimer's disease: The complex roles of microglia in neuroinflammation, neuronal survival and neurogenesis. *Neural Regen. Res.* **2020**, *15*, 1208–1219. [PubMed]
134. Bubu, O.M.; Brannick, M.; Mortimer, J.; Umasabor-Bubu, O.; Sebastião, Y.V.; Wen, Y.; Schwartz, S.; Borenstein, A.R.; Wu, Y.; Morgan, D.; et al. Sleep, Cognitive impairment, and Alzheimer's disease: A Systematic Review and Meta-Analysis. *Sleep* **2017**, *40*, zsw032. [CrossRef] [PubMed]
135. Snowden, T.M.; Hinde, A.K.; Reid, H.M.O.; Christie, B.R. Does Mild Traumatic Brain Injury Increase the Risk for Dementia? A Systematic Review and Meta-Analysis. *J. Alzheimers Dis.* **2020**, *78*, 757–775. [CrossRef] [PubMed]
136. Baril, A.A.; Beiser, A.S.; Redline, S.; McGrath, E.R.; Aparicio, H.J.; Gottlieb, D.J.; Seshadri, S.; Pase, M.P.; Himali, J.J. Systemic inflammation as a moderator between sleep and incident dementia. *Sleep* **2021**, *44*, zsaa164. [CrossRef] [PubMed]
137. Baril, A.A.; Beiser, A.S.; Redline, S.; McGrath, E.R.; Gottlieb, D.J.; Aparicio, H.; Seshadri, S.; Himali, J.J.; Pase, M.P. Interleukin-6 Interacts with Sleep Apnea Severity when Predicting Incident Alzheimer's Disease Dementia. *J. Alzheimers Dis.* **2021**, *79*, 1451–1457. [CrossRef]
138. Wadhwa, M.; Prabhakar, A.; Anand, J.P.; Ray, K.; Prasad, D.; Kumar, B.; Panjwani, U. Complement activation sustains neuroinflammation and deteriorates adult neurogenesis and spatial memory impairment in rat hippocampus following sleep deprivation. *Brain Behav. Immun.* **2019**, *82*, 129–144. [CrossRef]
139. Wadhwa, M.; Prabhakar, A.; Ray, K.; Roy, K.; Kumari, P.; Jha, P.K.; Kishore, K.; Kumar, S.; Panjwani, U. Inhibiting the microglia activation improves the spatial memory and adult neurogenesis in rat hippocampus during 48 h of sleep deprivation. *J. Neuroinflammation* **2017**, *14*, 222. [CrossRef]
140. Amanollahi, M.; Jameie, M.; Heidari, A.; Rezaei, N. The Dialogue Between Neuroinflammation and Adult Neurogenesis: Mechanisms Involved and Alterations in Neurological Diseases. *Mol. Neurobiol.* **2022**, *60*, 923–959. [CrossRef]
141. Tapp, Z.M.; Cornelius, S.; Oberster, A.; Kumar, J.E.; Atluri, R.; Witcher, K.G.; Oliver, B.; Bray, C.; Velasquez, J.; Zhao, F.; et al. Sleep fragmentation engages stress-responsive circuitry, enhances inflammation and compromises hippocampal function following traumatic brain injury. *Exp. Neurol.* **2022**, *353*, 114058. [CrossRef] [PubMed]
142. Faden, A.I.; Wu, J.; Stoica, B.A.; Loane, D.J. Progressive inflammation-mediated neurodegeneration after traumatic brain or spinal cord injury. *Br. J. Pharmacol.* **2016**, *173*, 681–691. [CrossRef] [PubMed]
143. Johnson, V.E.; Stewart, J.E.; Begbie, F.D.; Trojanowski, J.Q.; Smith, D.H.; Stewart, W. Inflammation and white matter degeneration persist for years after a single traumatic brain injury. *Brain* **2013**, *136 Pt 1*, 28–42. [CrossRef]
144. Alawieh, A.; Chalhoub, R.M.; Mallah, K.; Langley, E.F.; York, M.; Broome, H.; Couch, C.; Adkins, D.; Tomlinson, S. Complement Drives Synaptic Degeneration and Progressive Cognitive Decline in the Chronic Phase after Traumatic Brain Injury. *J. Neurosci.* **2021**, *41*, 1830–1843. [CrossRef] [PubMed]
145. Irwin, M.R.; Olmstead, R.; Breen, E.C.; Witarama, T.; Carrillo, C.; Sadeghi, N.; Arevalo, J.M.; Ma, J.; Nicassio, P.; Ganz, P.A.; et al. Tai chi, cellular inflammation, and transcriptome dynamics in breast cancer survivors with insomnia: A randomized controlled trial. *J. Natl. Cancer Inst. Monogr.* **2014**, *2014*, 295–301. [CrossRef] [PubMed]

46. Heffner, K.L.; France, C.R.; Ashrafioun, L.; Quiñones, M.; Walsh, P.; Maloney, M.D.; Giordano, B.D.; Pigeon, W.R. Clinical Pain-related Outcomes and Inflammatory Cytokine Response to Pain Following Insomnia Improvement in Adults With Knee Osteoarthritis. *Clin. J. Pain* **2018**, *34*, 1133–1140. [CrossRef] [PubMed]

47. Chen, H.Y.; Cheng, I.C.; Pan, Y.J.; Chiu, Y.L.; Hsu, S.P.; Pai, M.F.; Yang, J.Y.; Peng, Y.S.; Tsai, T.J.; Wu, K.D. Cognitive-behavioral therapy for sleep disturbance decreases inflammatory cytokines and oxidative stress in hemodialysis patients. *Kidney Int.* **2011**, *80*, 415–422. [CrossRef]

48. Nguyen, S.; McKay, A.; Wong, D.; Rajaratnam, S.M.; Spitz, G.; Williams, G.; Mansfield, D.; Ponsford, J.L. Cognitive Behavior Therapy to Treat Sleep Disturbance and Fatigue After Traumatic Brain Injury: A Pilot Randomized Controlled Trial. *Arch. Phys. Med. Rehabil.* **2017**, *98*, 1508–1517.e2. [CrossRef]

49. Bogdanov, S.; Naismith, S.; Lah, S. Sleep outcomes following sleep-hygiene-related interventions for individuals with traumatic brain injury: A systematic review. *Brain Inj.* **2017**, *31*, 422–433. [CrossRef]

50. Tang, N.K.Y.; Moore, C.; Parsons, H.; Sandhu, H.K.; Patel, S.; Ellard, D.R.; Nichols, V.P.; Madan, J.; Collard, V.E.J.; Sharma, U.; et al. Implementing a hybrid cognitive-behavioural therapy for pain-related insomnia in primary care: Lessons learnt from a mixed-methods feasibility study. *BMJ Open* **2020**, *10*, e034764. [CrossRef]

51. Tang, N.K.Y. Cognitive behavioural therapy in pain and psychological disorders: Towards a hybrid future. *Prog. Neuropsychopharmacol. Biol. Psychiatry* **2018**, *87 Pt B*, 281–289. [CrossRef]

52. Finan, P.H.; Buenaver, L.F.; Coryell, V.T.; Smith, M.T. Cognitive-Behavioral Therapy for Comorbid Insomnia and Chronic Pain. *Sleep Med. Clin.* **2014**, *9*, 261–274. [CrossRef] [PubMed]

53. Herrero Babiloni, A.; Beetz, G.; Bruneau, A.; Martel, M.O.; Cistulli, P.A.; Nixdorf, D.R.; Conway, J.M.; Lavigne, G.J. Multitargeting the sleep-pain interaction with pharmacological approaches: A narrative review with suggestions on new avenues of investigation. *Sleep Med. Rev.* **2021**, *59*, 101459. [CrossRef] [PubMed]

54. Chen, P.L.; Lee, W.J.; Sun, W.Z.; Oyang, Y.J.; Fuh, J.L. Risk of dementia in patients with insomnia and long-term use of hypnotics: A population-based retrospective cohort study. *PLoS ONE* **2012**, *7*, e49113. [CrossRef] [PubMed]

55. Desmidt, T.; Delrieu, J.; Lebouvier, T.; Robert, G.; David, R.; Balageas, A.C.; Surget, A.; Belzung, C.; Arlicot, N.; Ribeiro, M.J.; et al. Benzodiazepine use and brain amyloid load in nondemented older individuals: A florbetapir PET study in the Multidomain Alzheimer Preventive Trial cohort. *Neurobiol. Aging* **2019**, *84*, 61–69. [CrossRef] [PubMed]

56. Morin, C.M.; Vallières, A.; Guay, B.; Ivers, H.; Savard, J.; Mérette, C.; Bastien, C.; Baillargeon, L. Cognitive behavioral therapy, singly and combined with medication, for persistent insomnia: A randomized controlled trial. *JAMA* **2009**, *301*, 2005–2015. [CrossRef] [PubMed]

57. Gao, J.; Su, G.; Liu, J.; Zhang, J.; Zhou, J.; Liu, X.; Tian, Y.; Zhang, Z. Mechanisms of Inhibition of Excessive Microglial Activation by Melatonin. *J. Mol. Neurosci.* **2020**, *70*, 1229–1236. [CrossRef]

58. Kose, D.; Kose, A.; Halici, Z.; Gurbuz, M.A.; Aydin, A.; Ugan, R.A.; Karaman, A.; Toktay, E. Do peripheral melatonin agonists improve bone fracture healing? The effects of agomelatine and ramelteon on experimental bone fracture. *Eur. J. Pharmacol.* **2020**, *887*, 173577. [CrossRef]

59. Lin, C.; Chao, H.; Li, Z.; Xu, X.; Liu, Y.; Hou, L.; Liu, N.; Ji, J. Melatonin attenuates traumatic brain injury-induced inflammation: A possible role for mitophagy. *J. Pineal Res.* **2016**, *61*, 177–186. [CrossRef]

60. Babaee, A.; Eftekhar-Vaghefi, S.H.; Asadi-Shekaari, M.; Shahrokhi, N.; Soltani, S.D.; Malekpour-Afshar, R.; Basiri, M. Melatonin treatment reduces astrogliosis and apoptosis in rats with traumatic brain injury. *Iran J. Basic Med. Sci.* **2015**, *18*, 867–872.

61. Barlow, K.M.; Esser, M.J.; Veidt, M.; Boyd, R. Melatonin as a Treatment after Traumatic Brain Injury: A Systematic Review and Meta-Analysis of the Pre-Clinical and Clinical Literature. *J. Neurotrauma* **2019**, *36*, 523–537. [CrossRef]

62. Barlow, K.M.; Brooks, B.L.; Esser, M.J.; Kirton, A.; Mikrogianakis, A.; Zemek, R.L.; MacMaster, F.P.; Nettel-Aguirre, A.; Yeates, K.O.; Kirk, V.; et al. Efficacy of Melatonin in Children With Postconcussive Symptoms: A Randomized Clinical Trial. *Pediatrics* **2020**, *145*, 2812. [CrossRef]

63. Barlow, K.M.; Kirk, V.; Brooks, B.; Esser, M.J.; Yeates, K.O.; Zemek, R.; Kirton, A.; Mikrogianakis, A.; MacMaster, F.; Nettel-Aguirre, A.; et al. Efficacy of Melatonin for Sleep Disturbance in Children with Persistent Post-Concussion Symptoms: Secondary Analysis of a Randomized Controlled Trial. *J. Neurotrauma* **2021**, *38*, 950–959. [CrossRef] [PubMed]

64. Witcher, K.G.; Bray, C.E.; Dziabis, J.E.; McKim, D.B.; Benner, B.N.; Rowe, R.K.; Kokiko-Cochran, O.N.; Popovich, P.G.; Lifshitz, J.; Eiferman, D.S.; et al. Traumatic brain injury-induced neuronal damage in the somatosensory cortex causes formation of rod-shaped microglia that promote astrogliosis and persistent neuroinflammation. *Glia* **2018**, *66*, 2719–2736. [CrossRef] [PubMed]

65. Spangenberg, E.; Severson, P.L.; Hohsfield, L.A.; Crapser, J.; Zhang, J.; Burton, E.A.; Zhang, Y.; Spevak, W.; Lin, J.; Phan, N.Y.; et al. Sustained microglial depletion with CSF1R inhibitor impairs parenchymal plaque development in an Alzheimer's disease model. *Nat. Commun.* **2019**, *10*, 3758. [CrossRef] [PubMed]

66. Cerqueira, S.R.; Ayad, N.G.; Lee, J.K. Neuroinflammation Treatment via Targeted Delivery of Nanoparticles. *Front. Cell Neurosci.* **2020**, *14*, 576037. [CrossRef] [PubMed]

67. Rahimifard, M.; Maqbool, F.; Moeini-Nodeh, S.; Niaz, K.; Abdollahi, M.; Braidy, N.; Nabavi, S.M.; Nabavi, S.F. Targeting the TLR4 signaling pathway by polyphenols: A novel therapeutic strategy for neuroinflammation. *Ageing Res. Rev.* **2017**, *36*, 11–19. [CrossRef] [PubMed]

68. Song, L.; Pei, L.; Yao, S.; Wu, Y.; Shang, Y. NLRP3 Inflammasome in Neurological Diseases, from Functions to Therapies. *Front. Cell Neurosci.* **2017**, *11*, 63. [CrossRef] [PubMed]

169. Elman, I.; Pustilnik, A.; Borsook, D. Beating pain with psychedelics: Matter over mind? *Neurosci. Biobehav. Rev.* **2022**, *134*, 104482. [CrossRef]
170. Calder, A.E.; Hasler, G. Towards an understanding of psychedelic-induced neuroplasticity. *Neuropsychopharmacology* **2023**, *48*, 104–112. [CrossRef]
171. Thomas, C.W.; Blanco-Duque, C.; Breant, B.J.; Goodwin, G.M.; Sharp, T.; Bannerman, D.M.; Vyazovskiy, V.V. Psilocin acutely alters sleep-wake architecture and cortical brain activity in laboratory mice. *Transl. Psychiatry* **2022**, *12*, 77. [CrossRef] [PubMed]
172. Hiskens, M.I. Targets of Neuroprotection and Review of Pharmacological Interventions in Traumatic Brain Injury. *J. Pharmacol. Exp. Ther.* **2022**, *382*, 149–166. [CrossRef]
173. Saur, L.; Baptista, P.P.; de Senna, P.N.; Paim, M.F.; do Nascimento, P.; Ilha, J.; Bagatini, P.B.; Achaval, M.; Xavier, L.L. Physical exercise increases GFAP expression and induces morphological changes in hippocampal astrocytes. *Brain Struct. Funct.* **2014**, *219*, 293–302. [CrossRef]
174. Barad, Z.; Augusto, J.; Kelly, A.M. Exercise-induced modulation of neuroinflammation in ageing. *J. Physiol.* **2022**, *in press* [CrossRef] [PubMed]
175. Ma, C.; Lin, M.; Gao, J.; Xu, S.; Huang, L.; Zhu, J.; Huang, J.; Tao, J.; Chen, L. The impact of physical activity on blood inflammatory cytokines and neuroprotective factors in individuals with mild cognitive impairment: A systematic review and meta-analysis of randomized-controlled trials. *Aging Clin. Exp. Res.* **2022**, *34*, 1471–1484. [CrossRef] [PubMed]
176. De Nys, L.; Anderson, K.; Ofosu, E.F.; Ryde, G.C.; Connelly, J.; Whittaker, A.C. The effects of physical activity on cortisol and sleep: A systematic review and meta-analysis. *Psychoneuroendocrinology* **2022**, *143*, 105843. [CrossRef] [PubMed]
177. Memon, A.R.; Gupta, C.C.; Crowther, M.E.; Ferguson, S.A.; Tuckwell, G.A.; Vincent, G.E. Sleep and physical activity in university students: A systematic review and meta-analysis. *Sleep Med. Rev.* **2021**, *58*, 101482. [CrossRef]
178. Lurie, D.I. An Integrative Approach to Neuroinflammation in Psychiatric disorders and Neuropathic Pain. *J. Exp. Neurosci.* **2018**, *12*, 1179069518793639. [CrossRef]
179. Jacquens, A.; Needham, E.J.; Zanier, E.R.; Degos, V.; Gressens, P.; Menon, D. Neuro-Inflammation Modulation and Post-Traumatic Brain Injury Lesions: From Bench to Bed-Side. *Int. J. Mol. Sci.* **2022**, *23*, 11193. [CrossRef]
180. Lefaucheur, J.P.; Aleman, A.; Baeken, C.; Benninger, D.H.; Brunelin, J.; Di Lazzaro, V.; Filipovic, S.R.; Grefkes, C.; Hasan, A.; Hummel, F.C.; et al. Evidence-based guidelines on the therapeutic use of repetitive transcranial magnetic stimulation (rTMS): An update (2014-2018). *Clin. Neurophysiol.* **2020**, *131*, 474–528. [CrossRef] [PubMed]
181. Herrero Babiloni, A.; Bellemare, A.; Beetz, G.; Vinet, S.A.; Martel, M.O.; Lavigne, G.J.; De Beaumont, L. The effects of non-invasive brain stimulation on sleep disturbances among different neurological and neuropsychiatric conditions: A systematic review. *Sleep Med. Rev.* **2021**, *55*, 101381. [CrossRef] [PubMed]
182. Ljubisavljevic, M.R.; Javid, A.; Oommen, J.; Parekh, K.; Nagelkerke, N.; Shehab, S.; Adrian, T.E. The Effects of Different Repetitive Transcranial Magnetic Stimulation (rTMS) Protocols on Cortical Gene Expression in a Rat Model of Cerebral Ischemic-Reperfusion Injury. *PLoS ONE* **2015**, *10*, e0139892. [CrossRef] [PubMed]
183. Sasso, V.; Bisicchia, E.; Latini, L.; Ghiglieri, V.; Cacace, F.; Carola, V.; Molinari, M.; Viscomi, M.T. Repetitive transcranial magnetic stimulation reduces remote apoptotic cell death and inflammation after focal brain injury. *J. Neuroinflammation* **2016**, *13*, 150. [CrossRef] [PubMed]
184. Crowley, T.; Cryan, J.F.; Downer, E.J.; O'Leary, O.F. Inhibiting neuroinflammation: The role and therapeutic potential of GABA in neuro-immune interactions. *Brain Behav. Immun.* **2016**, *54*, 260–277. [CrossRef] [PubMed]
185. Jodoin, M.; Rouleau, D.; Larson-Dupuis, C.; Gosselin, N.; De Beaumont, L. The clinical utility of repetitive transcranial magnetic stimulation in reducing the risks of transitioning from acute to chronic pain in traumatically injured patients. *Prog. Neuropsychopharmacol. Biol. Psychiatry* **2017**, *87*, 322–331. [CrossRef]
186. Feng, J.; Zhang, Q.; Zhang, C.; Wen, Z.; Zhou, X. The Effect of sequential bilateral low-frequency rTMS over dorsolateral prefrontal cortex on serum level of BDNF and GABA in patients with primary insomnia. *Brain Behav.* **2019**, *9*, e01206. [CrossRef]
187. Regner, G.G.; Torres, I.L.S.; de Oliveira, C.; Pfluger, P.; da Silva, L.S.; Scarabelot, V.L.; Stroher, R.; de Souza, A.; Fregni, F.; Pereira, P. Transcranial direct current stimulation (tDCS) affects neuroinflammation parameters and behavioral seizure activity in pentylenetetrazole-induced kindling in rats. *Neurosci. Lett.* **2020**, *735*, 135162. [CrossRef]

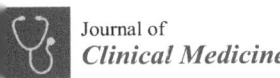

Journal of
Clinical Medicine

MDPI

Review

The Biology of Stress Intolerance in Patients with Chronic Pain—State of the Art and Future Directions

Arne Wyns [1,†], Jolien Hendrix [1,2,3,*,†], Astrid Lahousse [1,3,4,5], Elke De Bruyne [6], Jo Nijs [1,4,7], Lode Godderis [2,8] and Andrea Polli [1,2,3]

1   Pain in Motion Research Group (PAIN), Department of Physiotherapy, Human Physiology and Anatomy, Faculty of Physical Education and Physiotherapy, Vrije Universiteit Brussel, 1090 Brussels, Belgium; arne.wyns@vub.be (A.W.); astrid.lucie.lahousse@vub.be (A.L.); jo.nijs@vub.be (J.N.); andrea.polli@vub.be (A.P.)
2   Department of Public Health and Primary Care, Centre for Environment & Health, KU Leuven, Kapucijnenvoer 35, 3000 Leuven, Belgium; lode.godderis@kuleuven.be
3   Flanders Research Foundation-FWO, 1090 Brussels, Belgium
4   Chronic Pain Rehabilitation, Department of Physical Medicine and Physiotherapy, University Hospital, 1090 Brussels, Belgium
5   Rehabilitation Research (RERE) Research Group, Department of Physiotherapy, Human Physiology and Anatomy, Faculty of Physical Education & Physiotherapy (KIMA), Vrije Universiteit Brussel, 1090 Brussels, Belgium
6   Department of Hematology and Immunology-Myeloma Center Brussels, Vrije Universiteit Brussel, 1090 Brussels, Belgium; elke.de.bruyne@vub.be
7   Unit of Physiotherapy, Department of Health and Rehabilitation, Institute of Neuroscience and Physiology, Sahlgrenska Academy, University of Gothenburg, 405 30 Gothenburg, Sweden
8   External Service for Prevention and Protection at Work, IDEWE, 3001 Heverlee, Belgium
*   Correspondence: jolien.hendrix@vub.be
†   These authors contributed equally to this work.

Abstract: Stress has been consistently linked to negative impacts on physical and mental health. More specifically, patients with chronic pain experience stress intolerance, which is an exacerbation or occurrence of symptoms in response to any type of stress. The pathophysiological mechanisms underlying this phenomenon remain unsolved. In this state-of-the-art paper, we summarised the role of the autonomic nervous system (ANS) and hypothalamus-pituitary-adrenal (HPA) axis, the two major stress response systems in stress intolerance. We provided insights into such mechanisms based on evidence from clinical studies in both patients with chronic pain, showing dysregulated stress systems, and healthy controls supported by preclinical studies, highlighting the link between these systems and symptoms of stress intolerance. Furthermore, we explored the possible regulating role for (epi)genetic mechanisms influencing the ANS and HPA axis. The link between stress and chronic pain has become an important area of research as it has the potential to inform the development of interventions to improve the quality of life for individuals living with chronic pain. As stress has become a prevalent concern in modern society, understanding the connection between stress, HPA axis, ANS, and chronic health conditions such as chronic pain is crucial to improve public health and well-being.

Keywords: chronic pain; stress intolerance; autonomic nervous system; hypothalamus-pituitary-adrenal axis; genetics; epigenetics

Citation: Wyns, A.; Hendrix, J.; Lahousse, A.; De Bruyne, E.; Nijs, J.; Godderis, L.; Polli, A. The Biology of Stress Intolerance in Patients with Chronic Pain—State of the Art and Future Directions. *J. Clin. Med.* **2023**, *12*, 2245. https://doi.org/10.3390/jcm12062245

Academic Editor: Achim Berthele

Received: 9 February 2023
Revised: 7 March 2023
Accepted: 10 March 2023
Published: 14 March 2023

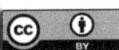
1. Stress Intolerance Plays a Major Role in Chronic Widespread Pain

Chronic pain affects approximately 20% of the global population and is associated with a significant burden for the individual and their significant others [1]. It is moreover influenced by several cognitive, emotional, and social factors [2]. Stress is one such factor that is able to influence pain symptoms and has long been proposed as relevant in the pain experience [3]. The World Health Organization (WHO) defines stress as any type of change

J. Clin. Med. **2023**, *12*, 2245

that causes physical, emotional, or psychological strain [4]. The stress response is the physiological and biological response of the body to any situation causing such strains [5]

Stress is highly subjective. Different individuals might respond differently to the same stressful situation. The stress response, therefore, depends on the perceived amount of stress as well as on the nature, duration, and intensity of the stress stimulus [6–8]. In patients with chronic pain, stress is generally associated with a worsening of pain symptoms and stress-induced hyperalgesia. In fact, stress and pain are highly comorbid, and show significant overlap in both conceptual and biological processes [9]. On the one hand, experiencing stressful events in life puts individuals at risk to develop chronic musculoskeletal pain and patients with symptoms of post-traumatic stress disorder report higher pain severity levels [3,10]. On the other hand, dealing with chronic pain increases the risk to develop stress-related conditions such as depression and anxiety [11]. Furthermore, a recent review showed that a blunted acute stress response predicted chronic pain and poor health at a long-term follow-up (1 year) [12].

However, the impact of stress in patients with chronic pain goes beyond pain modulation. Other symptoms such as fatigue and cognitive symptoms can also be triggered or worsened because of stress [13,14]. Here, we define the exacerbation or occurrence of symptoms in response to stress as stress intolerance.

2. Objectives

This state-of-the-art paper aims to provide an overview of the biological mechanisms that may explain stress intolerance in patients with chronic pain, focussing on the two major stress systems—the autonomic nervous system (ANS) and the hypothalamic pituitary axis (HPA). Although stress intolerance can be induced by physical and mental stress, this state-of-the-art paper focuses on evidence originating from studies investigating mental stress.

Of note, other biological systems should not be ignored when aiming to unravel the pathophysiology of stress intolerance in patients with chronic pain. Considering that stress intolerance comprises various symptoms within different domains, it probably stems from a multisystemic pathophysiology. Other systems showing intricate links with the ANS, the HPA, nociceptive mechanisms, and the stress response are thus likely, collaboratively with the ANS and HPA axis, involved in explaining stress intolerance in chronic pain. The immune system, as well as mechanisms related to the opioid and endocannabinoid system, can all potentially influence and be influenced by pain and stress. We acknowledge the complexity of the aforementioned systems and their interactions. However, a detailed description of such systems is beyond the scope of this review and can be found elsewhere [15–19].

3. Methodology

A search exploring stress system dysregulations in chronic pain was queried on PubMed and Web of Science up to December 2022 using following keywords such as chronic pain, stress physiology, autonomic nervous system, SAM axis, HPA axis, hyperalgesia, (nor)adrenaline, catecholamine, cortisol, glucocorticoids, stress hormone, stress response, (epi)genetics, immunology. Inclusion criteria for relevant articles were: (1) address one of the scopes within this review; (2) describe a rationale for the state-of-the-art aspect; (3) written in English or Dutch; (4) human studies or animal studies if necessary.

4. Two Major Stress Systems: The Autonomic Nervous System and the Hypothala-Mus-Pituitary-Adrenal Axis

The stress response is an evolutionary conserved, complex, and efficient system with modulation in associated neural (CNS), endocrinological, and immunological systems [20]. Perception of a stressor activates several neuronal circuits involving the limbic forebrain, the brainstem, and nuclei of the hypothalamus, which on their part release stress-mediating molecules, initiating a stress response [21]. Physical and psychological stressors activate different neural networks, resulting in a specified stress response [20]. Physiological and behavioural mechanisms simultaneously aim to restore body homeostasis and promote stress adaptation [22]. The two main neural circuits through which our body adapts to stress are the autonomic nervous system (ANS) and the Hypothalamus-Pituitary-Adrenal (HPA) axis (see Figure 1 for a schematic overview). These systems usually work in synchrony and influence each other through mutual, positive feedback loops [23].

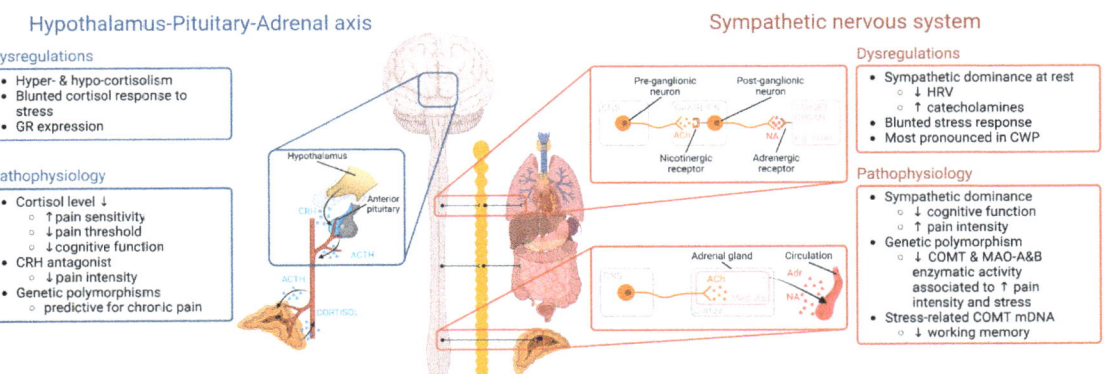

Figure 1. Visual representation of the major stress pathways, together with common dysregulations in chronic pain and their possible pathophysiological implications in stress intolerance. ↑, Increased; ↓, Decreased; ACh, Acetylcholine; Adr, Adrenaline; ACTH, Adrenocorticotropic hormone; COMT, Catechol-O-methyltransferase; CNS, Central nervous system; CWP, Chronic widespread pain; CRH, Corticotropin-releasing hormone; mDNA, DNA methylation; GR, Glucocorticoid receptor; HRV, Heart rate variability; HPA axis, Hypothalamic-pituitary-adrenal axis; MAO-A&B, Monoamine oxidase A&B; NA, Noradrenaline. Created with BioRender.com (Accessed on 9 February 2023).

Under normal circumstances, acute physical or psychological stressors activate the ANS inducing a short-lasting increase in sympathetic nervous system (SNS) activity. Stress activates brainstem catecholaminergic neurons and efferent spinal cord neurons of the dorsal intermediolateral column, which converge in pre-ganglionic sympathetic neurons [24]. These neurons synapse directly to chromaffin cells in the adrenal medulla, which secretes adrenaline and noradrenaline in the circulation. In addition, other pre-ganglionic neurons project to several post-ganglionic sympathetic neurons in paravertebral ganglia, using acetylcholine (ACh) as neurotransmitter. Consequent activation of nicotinic receptors on these post-ganglionic neurons results in noradrenaline secretion at the target tissue [25]. Adrenaline and noradrenaline have diverse physiological functions, depending on the adrenergic receptor (AR) they bind to. ARs are G-protein-coupled receptors and can be divided in α1-, α2- and α1-, β2-, and β3-ARs. The overall effect of α1- and α2-ARs activation is increased heart rate (HR) and blood pressure (BP), and decreased heart rate variability (HRV). Blood flow is increased to the skeletal muscles and decreased towards the abdominal organs, metabolic activity such as glycogenolysis in skeletal muscle and lipolysis in adipocytes are promoted to increase energy availability [24]. On the contrary, β1- and β2-ARs stimulation foster vasodilation, decrease blood pressure and increase HRV, though can either increase or decrease HR [26–28]. Several organs, as well as immune cells, express both α- and β-ARs, allowing fine regulation of their functions. Decreased expression of β-ARs have been associated with several inflammatory conditions such as rheumatic diseases and obesity [29,30]. β2-ARs show potent anti-inflammatory effects [23], and their down-regulation or desensitisation can help explain pain symptoms.

The HPA axis provides a protracted response, yet its activation is delayed compared to the SNS. This response originates when the hypothalamus, the paraventricular nucleus

(PVN) in particular, is triggered by stressors. The PVN releases several neurochemicals such as oxytocin, vasopressin, and corticotrophin-releasing hormone (CRH) [31,32]. CRH reaches the anterior pituitary (adenohypophysis) and stimulates it to synthesise and secrete adrenocorticotrophic hormone (ACTH) [32]. ACTH, on its part, stimulates the cortex of the adrenal gland to produce and release glucocorticoids, mostly cortisol [33]. Cortisol in turn also exerts an effect on the PVN and anterior pituitary, by limiting synaptic plasticity and suppressing neural excitability, thus creating a long and short negative feedback loop [22]. Glucocorticoid secretion in humans follows a general ultradian and circadian rhythm with basal peak cortisol levels around weaking-up time [34]. Cortisol exerts its functions through binding mineralocorticoid receptors (MR) or glucocorticoid receptors (GR), both ligand-activated transcription factors [35]. These receptors are widely expressed throughout the body. Not surprisingly, cortisol affects several organs and systems [36]. The HPA axis regulates blood pressure and vascular tone homeostasis, as well as raises blood glucose levels through gluconeogenesis in the liver during the stress response [37]. Moreover, it is widely known that cortisol signalling in most immune cells generally leads to an immunosuppressive phenotype, which will be discussed later [38].

Both systems convert physical and psychological stressors in the appropriate and situational stress response and are vital for several, if not most, processes in body homeostasis. Dysregulations in these systems may lead to severe disorders, such as a dysfunctional stress response, i.e., stress intolerance. Both the SNS and the HPA axis have been found to be disturbed in several disorders, including chronic pain syndrome [39–42]. In the following parts, we will discuss the role of both systems in stress intolerance in chronic pain disorders. In addition, we briefly touch upon dysregulations in epigenetic modifications and the immune response, in relation to stress intolerance.

5. Sympathetic and Adrenergic Activity Have a Role in Stress Intolerance

Sympathetic dominance as a result of decreased parasympathetic and increased sympathetic activity at baseline has been observed in patients with chronic pain [43–47]. However, the strength of the evidence depends on the clinical aetiology of chronic pain. A meta-analysis by Koenig et al. demonstrated that HRV was consistently decreased only in patients with fibromyalgia and other chronic pain conditions such as pelvic pain, whiplash-associated disorder, and neck-and-shoulder pain [43]. On the contrary, results were conflicting for primary headache or irritable bowel syndrome (IBS) [43]. In addition, the sympathetic stress response in patients with chronic pain is blunted, especially in chronic widespread pain (CWP) syndromes such as fibromyalgia [45,48–53]. In other conditions, such as localised chronic muscle pain and chronic whiplash-associated disorder, hypo-reactivity is less pronounced or absent, respectively [48,54].

Biological measures (e.g., catecholamine levels) point in the same direction. On the one hand, noradrenaline levels at baseline have been found to be elevated in patients with fibromyalgia, which is consistent with an increased sympathetic activity [55–59]. On the other hand, changes in noradrenaline and adrenaline in response to different types of stressors are less pronounced, which is consistent with the blunted stress response [58,60,61]. However, results on catecholamine levels in patients with chronic pain remain conflicting as some studies report no or opposite differences at baseline or in response to stress [61–64].

Autonomic activity has also been associated with various symptoms of stress intolerance [65,66]. Recent systematic reviews concluded that parasympathetic activity was positively associated with self-regulation and pain inhibition capacities, and that cognitive performance is positively associated with HRV [65,66]. Additionally, pain severity showed to be inversely correlated with HRV in an occupational sample comprising people with and without chronic pain. However, this correlation was only significant in the entire sample and in the group without chronic pain, but not in the group with chronic pain, implicating that the autonomic activity of patients with chronic pain relates differently to pain than in those without chronic pain [47]. This is contradicting to the results of Zamunér et al. who demonstrated that pain intensity in fibromyalgia is in fact correlated with sympathetic activity, which is in turn inversely correlated with HRV [67]. Taken together, these results show that sympathetic dominance is associated with symptoms of stress intolerance. Sympathetic dominance might be due to reduced parasympathetic reactivation during recovery from stress, as is the case during recovery from exercise [26].

Preclinical studies also support autonomic involvement in stress intolerance and provide us with deeper insights. Khasar et al. were able to induce hyperalgesia in rats by injection of adrenaline [68]. The hyperalgesia was further enhanced by unexpected sound stress. In addition, removing the adrenal medulla before stress exposure prevented stress-induced enhancement of hyperalgesia [68]. As the adrenal medulla is an important site of adrenaline production, these results indicate that elevated levels of catecholamines are required for the induction of stress-induced hyperalgesia. Their follow-up study later revealed that catecholamines are also pivotal for the maintenance of stress-induced hyperalgesia. Removal of the adrenal medulla after exposure to sound stress reversed the stress-induced hyperalgesia that had occurred in response to stress. Finally, administration of adrenaline in these rats reconstituted the stress-induced hyperalgesia again [69]. These results are in line with another animal study that focussed on the role of α2 ARs, which tightly control noradrenaline release by autoinhibition upon activation. Animals in which the α2 ARs were blocked (through injection of receptor antagonists or knock-out) developed hyperalgesia in response to stress. This stress-induced hyperalgesia was prevented when sympathetic activity was blocked, again showing that sympathetic activity is required for the induction of stress-induced hyperalgesia [70]. Finally, inhibition of the catechol-O-methyltransferase (COMT) enzyme, which prevents the degradation of catecholamines, has been found to increase pain sensitivity through activation of β-ARs [71]. Although some contradictory findings exist [72], accumulating evidence suggests that sympathetic and adrenergic activity may be involved in stress intolerance (see Figure 1).

6. The HPA Axis Is Deregulated in Chronic Pain Syndromes

The HPA axis also plays an important role in stress intolerance (see Figure 1 for a summary of findings). Activation of the HPA axis results in an increased concentration of circulating corticosteroids, especially cortisol. Deregulation of adrenal steroid secretion has been reported in several chronic pathological conditions, including chronic stress and dysfunctional chronic pain conditions [73,74]. Alteration of corticosteroid expression can give rise to two opposite phenomena, namely hyper- and hypocortisolism [75].

Hypercortisolism is characterised by basal hypercortisolism and/or hyper-reactivity. Basal hypercortisolism is defined as a permanently increased cortisol level and decreased negative feedback of the HPA axis, whereas hyperreactivity refers to normal cortisol levels with exaggerated behavioural and cortisol responses to stressful events [76]. Hypercortisolism has been reported in several chronic pain conditions, including myofascial pain and burning mouth syndrome [77,78]. Similarly, hypocortisolism includes basal hypocortisolism and hypo-reactivity to stressful events [74]. Tops et al. found that hypocortisolism occurs after a prolonged period of repetitive stimulation of the HPA axis resulting in excessive cortisol release, suggesting that hypocortisolism chronologically follows hypercortisolism [79]. Hypocortisolism has been reported in patients with myalgic encephalomyelitis/chronic fatigue syndrome (ME/CFS), IBS, and chronic pelvic pain [80–82]. Interestingly, lower cortisol levels have been associated with lowered pain thresholds and increased pain sensitivity, and a blunted cortisol-awakening response with decreased cognitive function [83–86]. In CWP and fibromyalgia, contradicting results have been found. Although most findings report hypocortisolism, several studies also reported increased cortisol levels [87–91]. These contradictory results might be partially explained by the fact that the HPA axis can respond differently depending on previous unknown repetitive stressors that have been present in the lives of the participants [92]. One study by Coppens et al., found a blunted cortisol response and a higher subjective stress rating in response to psychological stress in fibromyalgia patients compared to healthy controls [93]. Concerning these inconsistencies, more research is needed to elucidate whether a true causal link between corticosteroid mechanisms and the pathogenesis of chronic pain exists.

Though research has mostly focused on cortisol as measure of the HPA axis function, other components of the axis have also been investigated. CRH is released from the hypothalamus in response to physical and psychological stressors. It interacts with CRH receptors 1 and 2 [94]. CRH exerts actions in both the periphery and stress-related regions in the brain, i.e., the hypothalamus, amygdala, locus coeruleus, and hippocampus. Preclinical research using rat models demonstrated the involvement of CRH in stress-induced hyperalgesia and stress intolerance [95]. Peripheral administration of a CRH receptor 1 antagonist before water avoidance stress inhibited the development of stress-induced visceral hyperalgesia [96,97]. Additionally, in mice exposed to a forced swim test, administration of the CRH receptor 2 antagonist attenuated the development of stress-induced musculoskeletal hyperalgesia [98]. In patients with IBS, administration of the CRH antagonist alpha-helical CRH reduced electrical stimulation-induced abdominal pain [99,100]. Another study found increased pain intensity and decreased pain thresholds as result of rectal distention in healthy volunteers when CRH was peripherally administered [99,100]. Consistent with the preclinical findings, these results strengthen the evidence that CRH and its receptors are involved in stress-induced hyperalgesia and stress intolerance.

7. A Key Regulatory Role for Genetics and Epigenetics in Stress Intolerance

Despite accumulating evidence implicating the relevance of the abovementioned systems in stress intolerance in patients with chronic pain, stress responses and pain are variable among and within individuals. For instance, the effect of stress on pain (i.e., hypo- or hyperalgesia in response to stress) depends on the magnitude of the individual stress response [101]. Part of the variability in pain and stress among individuals can be explained by genetics. Genetic polymorphisms affecting the activity of COMT or monoamine oxidase A and B (MAO-A/B), which are both catecholamine-degrading enzymes and thus influence catecholamine levels and ANS functioning, have been associated with increased stress responsiveness and pain sensitivity in both animals and humans [102–111]. Typically, polymorphisms that lower enzymatic activity and thus elevate catecholamine levels are associated with higher pain sensitivity [112]. Although some conflicting evidence exists [61–64], these findings are in line with the higher catecholamine levels that have been found in patients with chronic pain.

Genetic polymorphisms of the corticosteroid receptor gene found in chronic pain are also worth mentioning. Macedo et al. found reduced GR expression in combination with the increased prevalence of the MR rs5522 (I180 V) polymorphism in fibromyalgia patients [75]. Other polymorphisms that alter the stress response have also been described. For example, Wüst et al. found that carriers of the GR N363S polymorphism showed increased salivary cortisol response to psychological stimuli, and that the GR *Bcl*I RFLP polymorphism was associated with a diminished cortisol stress response upon psychological stress in healthy individuals [113]. Recently, a study by Linnstaedt et al. found a functional polymorphism in the 3′-UTR of the *FKBP5* gene (rs3800373), a key regulator for glucocorticoid receptor sensitivity, which was associated with a higher chance to develop chronic post-traumatic pain [114]. Finally, the same group found a polymorphism in the corticotropin-releasing hormone binding protein (*CRHBP*) gene (rs7718461) to be highly associated with the *FKBP5* gene, and to be predictive of chronic musculoskeletal pain after a motor vehicle crash [115].

Although genetic polymorphisms can explain at least part of between-subject variability in stress responses and pain [116,117], they cannot explain within-subject variability. Epigenetic changes are strong candidates to explain both variability among individuals and within the same individual as they are dynamic mechanisms, responsive to environmental changes and the context [118]. Only few clinical studies investigated epigenetic changes in relation to chronic pain [119]. The role of epigenetics in the context of stress intolerance in chronic pain has never been investigated in humans, even though epigenetic mechanisms are clearly influenced by acute stress [120,121]. Stress has been reported to influence epigenetic regulation of genes involved in the abovementioned systems. Clinical studies found that DNA methylation—the best-known epigenetic modification—of genes involved in catecholamine degradation (*COMT, MAOA,* and *MAOB*) [122–125] and HPA-axis (*CRHR1, NR3C1*) [126–130] is in fact influenced by early-life stress and altered in patients with stress-related conditions. One study showed that *COMT* DNA methylation associated with lifetime exposure to stress relates to cognitive function in healthy controls [123]. Greater lifetime exposure to stress was associated with reduced *COMT* DNA methylation, which was in turn correlated with reduced working memory accuracy [123]. This study thus supports the involvement of epigenetic mechanisms in stress intolerance as cognitive symptoms, including impaired working memory, may worsen or be triggered in response to stress [13,14].

Genetics and epigenetics are thus both associated with pain and stress. Moreover, genetic polymorphisms can influence DNA methylation in several genes [131–135], as is the case for *COMT* [136,137]. It is thus likely that both genetics and epigenetics underly the role of the ANS and HPA axis in stress intolerance in patients with chronic pain. Of note, the aforementioned studies described stress-related rather than stress-induced epigenetic modifications as all data were obtained from cross-sectional studies. To elucidate a causal and/or regulatory role of epigenetic mechanisms in stress intolerance in chronic pain, future research should investigate the link between acute and chronic stress-induced epigenetic modifications, their downstream effects on the ANS and the HPA axis, and the associated symptoms in both patients with chronic pain and healthy controls.

8. Future Directions for Research

Research suggests that patients suffering from chronic pain conditions react differently to stress. However, the biological and physiological mechanisms linking stress and pain remain vague. We introduced the term "stress intolerance", which refers to the exacerbation or occurrence of symptoms, including but not limited to pain, in response to any type of stress. In this review, we summarised (preliminary) evidence supporting the idea that the two major stress systems, the ANS and the HPA axis, might be able to explain this phenomenon. Furthermore, genetic and epigenetic mechanisms might cover a key regulatory role.

Although evidence indicates that the functionality of the stress systems is deviant in patients with chronic pain, the direction of the link between stress and pain remains unclear. Some studies found that a blunted stress response can predict chronic pain later in life [12,84]. Such results imply that the stress response is already deviant before chronic pain develops. However, other studies could not support this finding [3]. The alternative option is that the stress responses become altered after chronic pain has already developed. This latter option would explain why stress intolerance is common in chronic pain populations. Future studies should thus be designed in a way that would allow us to unravel causal relationships between the two. In a later phase, we can then intervene with the underlying mechanisms and aim to prevent the development of chronic pain and/or the altered stress response.

To date, research on the topic is not only very scarce but the methods and protocols used to measure aspects of the ANS and HPA axis, as well as epigenetic and immune markers, are highly heterogeneous. Consequently, results are often not comparable. Future research methods should be standardised; time of data collection as well as the time between waking up and data collection is crucial and should be clearly reported and standardised. This is especially true when data collection takes place in the morning, due to the cortisol awakening response. We would also suggest employing multiple measurements across several days before and after stress exposure to further control for circadian fluctuations and within-patient variability. Such a design would also allow to investigate the recovery phase after the stressful challenge or event.

Additionally, current research investigated biological outcomes alone, with no link to symptom severity, thus making the available findings less relevant clinically. As stress intolerance is defined by the fluctuations in severity and presence of symptoms after stress exposure, repeated-measure designs investigating solely biological outcomes (without linking them to symptom severity) cannot provide answers on which mechanisms are involved. Future studies should thus also assess symptom severity and biological outcomes at the same time.

Taken together, the current knowledge creates the basis supporting a role for the stress systems in the pathology of chronic pain disorders and specifically stress intolerance. Further studies investigating the stress systems using standardised methods are warranted to obtain a better understanding of the mechanisms at play. A summary of the main future directions for research can be found in Figure 2.

TAKE HOME MESSAGE

Further directions for research:

- Unravel causal mechanisms: what came first, chronic pain or altered stress response?
- Standardise methodology to increase reproducibility
- Expose patients to standardised stressors, physical and mental
- Multiple assessments before and after stress exposure to account for within-individual variability and cover the recovery period
- Increase clinical relevance by including symptomatic assessment

Further directions for clinical practice:

- Biomedical approach alone is not sufficient to treat multidimensional aspects of pain
- Target contributing factors of chronic pain by pain education, and stress and sleep management
- Potential role for epigenetics in preventive medicine

Figure 2. Summary of future directions for research and clinical practice.

9. Future Directions for Clinical Practice

Currently, most physicians provide chronic pain patients with passive and biomedical treatments, which usually consist of medication and surgery. However, this approach often leads to poor benefits and carries a higher risk of adverse events [138]. A biomedical approach to pain omits its multidimensional aspects and disregards the impact of distress, which increases the risk of maintaining the pain experience [139]. Dysfunctional physiological stress response systems add complexity and induce heterogeneity in treatment responses, which emphasises the importance for clinicians of being attentive to stress intolerance.

Several treatment options are available targeting contributing factors to the maintenance of pain and possibly the development of stress intolerance. Educating the patient about pain is relevant in terms of stress management as patients with chronic pain are at higher risk of developing anxiety and depression [139], which in turn have a mediating effect on pain [140,141]. Patient education and reassurance are able to reduce their distress and change their attitudes towards pain [142]. Several systematic reviews with meta-analyses have shown compelling evidence for neuroscience education in reducing pain, perceived disability, and psychosocial factors such as fear-of-movement and catastrophising in patients with chronic pain [142–145]. Cognitive Behavioural therapy (CBT), acceptance and commitment therapy (ACT), and pain education targeting pain interference, stress, and disability, can also be employed, in an attempt to reduce contributing factors to the pain experience [146–149].

Sleep is another important contributing factor to chronic pain that should be addressed during management of chronic pain and stress intolerance [150]. The interplay between sleep, stress, and pain has been demonstrated by numerous chronic pain studies, even though the pathophysiology is not fully understood [151,152]. Disrupted sleep results in a low-grade inflammatory response, which will decrease patients' stress tolerance [153,154]. Clinicians should thus assess sleep problems because sleep deprivation can lead to patients' inability to face daily stressors [153].

Though the aforementioned approaches have been shown to help reduce pain and increase quality of life, research into the pathophysiological mechanisms of chronic pain and stress intolerance is still much needed. Research into the causal mechanisms may highlight the importance of preventive medicine when results show that the physiological stress response is already deviant before chronic pain develops, as is already shown by some studies [12]. In that case, the development of chronic pain may be prevented by targeting mechanisms underlying a dysregulated stress response. Animal studies already demonstrated that several interventions may be of help in targeting a dysregulated stress response. Both physical activity and antidepressant administration have been found to attenuate stress-induced DNA-methylation changes in rats [155,156]. By understanding the effect of various interventions on stress-induced epigenetic changes, we might be able to target key dysregulations underlying stress intolerance.

Author Contributions: Conceptualization, J.N. and A.P.; methodology, A.W., J.H., J.N. and A.P.; investigation, A.W. and J.H.; resources A.W. and J.H.; writing—original draft preparation, A.W., J.H. and A.L.; writing—review and editing, A.L., E.D.B., J.N., L.G. and A.P.; visualization, A.W.; supervision, E.D.B., J.N., L.G. and A.P. All authors have read and agreed to the published version of the manuscript.

Funding: This research was funded by Fonds Wetenschappelijk Onderzoek, grant number FWOTM1051 and FWOTM1069, which are a post-doctoral fellowship of Andrea Polli and a PhD fellowship of Jolien Hendrix, respectively.

Institutional Review Board Statement: Not applicable.

Informed Consent Statement: Not applicable.

Data Availability Statement: Not applicable.

Conflicts of Interest: The authors declare no conflict of interest.

References

1. Treede, R.D.; Rief, W.; Barke, A.; Aziz, Q.; Bennett, M.I.; Benoliel, R.; Cohen, M.; Evers, S.; Finnerup, N.B.; First, M.B.; et al. A classification of chronic pain for ICD-11. *Pain* **2015**, *156*, 1003–1007. [CrossRef] [PubMed]
2. Meints, S.M.; Edwards, R.R. Evaluating psychosocial contributions to chronic pain outcomes. *Prog. Neuropsychopharmacol. Biol. Psychiatry* **2018**, *87*, 168–182. [CrossRef]
3. Generaal, E.; Vogelzangs, N.; Macfarlane, G.J.; Geenen, R.; Smit, J.H.; de Geus, E.J.; Penninx, B.W.; Dekker, J. Biological stress systems, adverse life events and the onset of chronic multisite musculoskeletal pain: A 6-year cohort study. *Ann. Rheum. Dis.* **2016**, *75*, 847–854. [CrossRef]
4. World Health Organization. Stress. 2021. Available online: https://www.who.int/news-room/questions-and-answers/item/stress#:~:text=Stress%20can%20be%20defined%20as,to%20your%20overall%20well%2Dbeing (accessed on 15 January 2023).
5. Selye, H.; Fortier, C. Adaptive reaction to stress. *Psychosom. Med.* **1950**, *12*, 149–157. [CrossRef]
6. Fechir, M.; Breimhorst, M.; Kritzmann, S.; Geber, C.; Schlereth, T.; Baier, B.; Birklein, F. Naloxone inhibits not only stress-induced analgesia but also sympathetic activation and baroreceptor-reflex sensitivity. *Eur. J. Pain* **2012**, *16*, 82–92. [CrossRef]
7. al'Absi, M.; Nakajima, M.; Bruehl, S. Stress and pain: Modality-specific opioid mediation of stress-induced analgesia. *J. Neural. Transm.* **2021**, *128*, 1397–1407. [CrossRef] [PubMed]
8. Ferdousi, M.; Finn, D.P. Chapter 4—Stress-induced modulation of pain: Role of the endogenous opioid system. In *Progress in Brain Research*; O'Mara, S., Ed.; Elsevier: Amsterdam, The Netherlands, 2018; Volume 239, pp. 121–177.
9. Abdallah, C.G.; Geha, P. Chronic Pain and Chronic Stress: Two Sides of the Same Coin? *Chronic. Stress* **2017**, *1*, 2470547017704763. [CrossRef] [PubMed]

10. Åkerblom, S.; Perrin, S.; Rivano Fischer, M.; McCracken, L.M. The Relationship Between Posttraumatic Stress Disorder and Chronic Pain in People Seeking Treatment for Chronic Pain: The Mediating Role of Psychological Flexibility. *Clin. J. Pain* **2018**, *34*, 487–496. [CrossRef]
11. Yalcin, I.; Barrot, M. The anxiodepressive comorbidity in chronic pain. *Curr. Opin. Anesthesiol.* **2014**, *27*, 520–527. [CrossRef] [PubMed]
12. Turner, A.I.; Smyth, N.; Hall, S.J.; Torres, S.J.; Hussein, M.; Jayasinghe, S.U.; Ball, K.; Clow, A.J. Psychological stress reactivity and future health and disease outcomes: A systematic review of prospective evidence. *Psychoneuroendocrinology* **2020**, *114*, 104599. [CrossRef]
13. Dennis, N.L.; Larkin, M.; Derbyshire, S.W.G. 'A giant mess'—Making sense of complexity in the accounts of people with fibromyalgia. *Br. J. Health Psychol.* **2013**, *18*, 763–781. [CrossRef]
14. Alok, R.; Das, S.; Agarwal, G.; Salwahan, L.; Srivastava, R. Relationship of severity of depression, anxiety and stress with severity of fibromyalgia. *Clin. Exp. Rheumatol.-Incl Suppl.* **2011**, *29*, S70.
15. Drolet, G.; Dumont, E.C.; Gosselin, I.; Kinkead, R.; Laforest, S.; Trottier, J.F. Role of endogenous opioid system in the regulation of the stress response. *Prog. Neuropsychopharmacol. Biol. Psychiatry* **2001**, *25*, 729–741. [CrossRef] [PubMed]
16. Malafoglia, V.; Ilari, S.; Vitiello, L.; Tenti, M.; Balzani, E.; Muscoli, C.; Raffaeli, W.; Bonci, A. The Interplay between Chronic Pain, Opioids, and the Immune System. *Neuroscientist* **2022**, *28*, 613–627. [CrossRef]
17. Morena, M.; Patel, S.; Bains, J.S.; Hill, M.N. Neurobiological Interactions Between Stress and the Endocannabinoid System. *Neuropsychopharmacology* **2016**, *41*, 80–102. [CrossRef] [PubMed]
18. Zieglgänsberger, W.; Brenneisen, R.; Berthele, A.; Wotjak, C.T.; Bandelow, B.; Tölle, T.R.; Lutz, B. Chronic Pain and the Endocannabinoid System: Smart Lipids—A Novel Therapeutic Option? *Med. Cannabis. Cannabinoids.* **2022**, *5*, 61–75. [CrossRef] [PubMed]
19. Kenney, M.J.; Ganta, C.K. Autonomic nervous system and immune system interactions. *Compr. Physiol.* **2014**, *4*, 1177–1200. [CrossRef] [PubMed]
20. Godoy, L.; Rossignoli, M.; Delfino-Pereira, P.; Garcia-Cairasco, N.; de Lima Umeoka, E. A Comprehensive Overview on Stress Neurobiology: Basic Concepts and Clinical Implications. *Front. Behav. Neurosci.* **2018**, *12*. [CrossRef] [PubMed]
21. Ulrich-Lai, Y.M.; Herman, J.P. Neural regulation of endocrine and autonomic stress responses. *Nat. Rev. Neurosci.* **2009**, *10*, 397–409. [CrossRef]
22. Joëls, M.; Baram, T.Z. The neuro-symphony of stress. *Nat. Rev. Neurosci.* **2009**, *10*, 459–466. [CrossRef]
23. Elenkov, I.; Wilder, R.; Chrousos, G.; Vizi, E. The sympathetic nerve—An integrative interface between two supersystems: The brain and the immune system. *Pharmacol. Rev.* **2000**, *52*, 595–638. [PubMed]
24. Wehrwein, E.; Orer, H.; Barman, S. Overview of the Anatomy, Physiology, and Pharmacology of the Autonomic Nervous System. *Compr. Physiol.* **2016**, *6*, 1239–1278. [CrossRef] [PubMed]
25. Tank, A.; Lee Wong, D. Peripheral and central effects of circulating catecholamines. *Compr. Physiol.* **2015**, *5*, 1–15. [CrossRef]
26. Van Oosterwijck, J.; Marusic, U.; De Wandele, I.; Meeus, M.; Paul, L.; Lambrecht, L.; Moorkens, G.; Danneels, L.; Nijs, J. Reduced Parasympathetic Reactivation during Recovery from Exercise in Myalgic Encephalomyelitis/Chronic Fatigue Syndrome. *J. Clin. Med.* **2021**, *10*, 4527. [CrossRef]
27. Akgöz, H.; Gürkan, U.; Dayi, S.; Terzi, S.; Akbulut, T.; Torun, A.; Tayyareci, G. The relationship between beta-receptor sensitivity and nocturnal blood pressure and heart rate recovery in normotensive people. *Angiology* **2006**, *57*, 495–500. [CrossRef] [PubMed]
28. Yu, B.-H.; Kang, E.-H.; Ziegler, M.G.; Mills, P.J.; Dimsdale, J.E. Mood states, sympathetic activity, and in vivo β-adrenergic receptor function in a normal population. *Depress. Anxiety* **2008**, *25*, 559–564. [CrossRef] [PubMed]
29. Baerwald, C.; Graefe, C.; Muhl, C.; Von Wichert, P.; Krause, A. Beta 2-adrenergic receptors on peripheral blood mononuclear cells in patients with rheumatic diseases. *Eur. J. Clin. Investig.* **1992**, *22* (Suppl. S1), 42–46.
30. Leite, F.; Lima, M.; Marino, F.; Cosentino, M.; Ribeiro, L. β$_2$ Adrenoceptors are underexpressed in peripheral blood mononuclear cells and associated with a better metabolic profile in central obesity. *Int. J. Med. Sci.* **2017**, *14*, 853–861. [CrossRef] [PubMed]
31. Sawchenko, P.; Brown, E.; Chan, R.; Ericsson, A.; Li, H.; Roland, B.; Kovács, K. The paraventricular nucleus of the hypothalamus and the functional neuroanatomy of visceromotor responses to stress. *Prog. Brain Res.* **1996**, *107*, 201–222. [CrossRef]
32. Vale, W.; Spiess, J.; Rivier, C.; Rivier, J. Characterization of a 41-residue ovine hypothalamic peptide that stimulates secretion of corticotropin and beta-endorphin. *Science* **1981**, *213*, 1394–1397. [CrossRef]
33. Vale, W.; Rivier, C.; Yang, L.; Minick, S.; Guillemin, R. Effects of purified hypothalamic corticotropin-releasing factor and other substances on the secretion of adrenocorticotropin and beta-endorphin-like immunoactivities in vitro. *Endocrinology* **1978**, *103*, 1910–1915. [CrossRef] [PubMed]
34. Spencer, R.L.; Deak, T. A users guide to HPA axis research. *Physiol. Behav.* **2017**, *178*, 43–65. [CrossRef] [PubMed]
35. Mcewen, B.S.; Akil, H. Revisiting the Stress Concept: Implications for Affective Disorders. *J. Neurosci.* **2020**, *40*, 12–21. [CrossRef] [PubMed]
36. Lauren, T.; Jayashree, G.; Sandeep, S. Physiology, Cortisol. 2022. Available online: https://www.ncbi.nlm.nih.gov/books/NBK538239/ (accessed on 22 December 2022).
37. Kadmiel, M.; Cidlowski, J.A. Glucocorticoid receptor signaling in health and disease. *Trends Pharmacol. Sci.* **2013**, *34*, 518–530. [CrossRef]

8. Zen, M.; Canova, M.; Campana, C.; Bettio, S.; Nalotto, L.; Rampudda, M.; Ramonda, R.; Iaccarino, L.; Doria, A. The kaleidoscope of glucocorticoid effects on immune system. *Autoimmun. Rev.* **2011**, *10*, 305–310. [CrossRef]

9. Monaco, A.; Cattaneo, R.; Marci, M.C.; Pietropaoli, D.; Ortu, E. Central Sensitization-Based Classification for Temporomandibular Disorders: A Pathogenetic Hypothesis. *Pain Res. Manag.* **2017**, *2017*, 1–13. [CrossRef]

0. Van Cauwenbergh, D.; Nijs, J.; Kos, D.; Van Weijnen, L.; Struyf, F.; Meeus, M. Malfunctioning of the autonomic nervous system in patients with chronic fatigue syndrome: A systematic literature review. *Eur. J. Clin. Investig.* **2014**, *44*, 516–526. [CrossRef]

1. Ortiz, R.; Gemmill, J.A.L.; Sinaii, N.; Stegmann, B.; Khachikyan, I.; Chrousos, G.; Segars, J.; Stratton, P. Hypothalamic-Pituitary-Adrenal Axis Responses in Women with Endometriosis-Related Chronic Pelvic Pain. *Reprod. Sci.* **2020**, *27*, 1839–1847. [CrossRef]

2. Generaal, E.; Vogelzangs, N.; Macfarlane, G.J.; Geenen, R.; Smit, J.H.; Penninx, B.W.; Dekker, J. Reduced hypothalamic-pituitary-adrenal axis activity in chronic multi-site musculoskeletal pain: Partly masked by depressive and anxiety disorders. *BMC Musculoskelet. Disord.* **2014**, *15*, 227. [CrossRef]

3. Koenig, J.; Falvay, D.; Clamor, A.; Wagner, J.; Jarczok, M.N.; Ellis, R.J.; Weber, C.; Thayer, J.F. Pneumogastric (Vagus) Nerve Activity Indexed by Heart Rate Variability in Chronic Pain Patients Compared to Healthy Controls: A Systematic Review and Meta-Analysis. *Pain. Physician.* **2016**, *19*, E55–E78. [CrossRef]

4. Tracy, L.M.; Ioannou, L.; Baker, K.S.; Gibson, S.J.; Georgiou-Karistianis, N.; Giummarra, M.J. Meta-analytic evidence for decreased heart rate variability in chronic pain implicating parasympathetic nervous system dysregulation. *Pain* **2016**, *157*, 7–29. [CrossRef]

5. Martinez-Lavin, M. Biology and therapy of fibromyalgia. Stress, the stress response system, and fibromyalgia. *Arthritis Res. Ther.* **2007**, *9*, 216. [CrossRef]

6. El-Badawy, M.A.; El Mikkawy, D.M. Sympathetic Dysfunction in Patients with Chronic Low Back Pain and Failed Back Surgery Syndrome. *Clin. J. Pain.* **2016**, *32*, 226–231. [CrossRef]

7. Koenig, J.; Loerbroks, A.; Jarczok, M.N.; Fischer, J.E.; Thayer, J.F. Chronic Pain and Heart Rate Variability in a Cross-Sectional Occupational Sample: Evidence for Impaired Vagal Control. *Clin. J. Pain.* **2016**, *32*, 218–225. [CrossRef]

8. Nilsen, K.B.; Sand, T.; Westgaard, R.H.; Stovner, L.J.; White, L.R.; Leistad, R.B.; Helde, G.; Ro, M. Autonomic activation and pain in response to low-grade mental stress in fibromyalgia and shoulder/neck pain patients. *Eur. J. Pain* **2007**, *11*, 743–755. [CrossRef] [PubMed]

9. Reyes del Paso, G.A.; Garrido, S.; Pulgar, Á.; Duschek, S. Autonomic cardiovascular control and responses to experimental pain stimulation in fibromyalgia syndrome. *J. Psychosom. Res.* **2011**, *70*, 125–134. [CrossRef]

0. Contreras-Merino, A.M.; Davydov, D.M.; Galvez-Sánchez, C.M.; Reyes Del Paso, G.A. Blunted short-term autonomic cardiovascular reactivity to orthostatic and clinostatic challenges in fibromyalgia as an indicator of the severity of chronic pain. *Int. J. Psychophysiol.* **2022**, *175*, 61–70. [CrossRef]

1. Reyes Del Paso, G.A.; Garrido, S.; Pulgar, A.; Martín-Vázquez, M.; Duschek, S. Aberrances in autonomic cardiovascular regulation in fibromyalgia syndrome and their relevance for clinical pain reports. *Psychosom. Med.* **2010**, *72*, 462–470. [CrossRef]

2. López-López, A.; Matías-Pompa, B.; Fernández-Carnero, J.; Gil-Martínez, A.; Alonso-Fernández, M.; Alonso Pérez, J.L.; González Gutierrez, J.L. Blunted Pain Modulation Response to Induced Stress in Women with Fibromyalgia with and without Posttraumatic Stress Disorder Comorbidity: New Evidence of Hypo-Reactivity to Stress in Fibromyalgia? *Behav. Med.* **2021**, *47*, 311–323. [CrossRef] [PubMed]

3. Matías Pompa, B.; López López, A.; Alonso Fernández, M.; Vargas Moreno, E.; González Gutiérrez, J.L. Stress-Recovery State in Fibromyalgia Patients and Healthy People. Relationship with the Cardiovascular Response to Stress in Laboratory Conditions. *Int. J. Environ. Res. Public Health* **2020**, *17*, 3138. [CrossRef] [PubMed]

4. De Kooning, M.; Daenen, L.; Cras, P.; Gidron, Y.; Roussel, N.; Nijs, J. Autonomic response to pain in patients with chronic whiplash associated disorders. *Pain Physician* **2013**, *16*, E277–E285. [PubMed]

5. Rus, A.; Molina, F.; Del Moral, M.L.; Ramírez-Expósito, M.J.; Martínez-Martos, J.M. Catecholamine and Indolamine Pathway: A Case-Control Study in Fibromyalgia. *Biol. Res. Nurs.* **2018**, *20*, 577–586. [CrossRef] [PubMed]

6. Bote, M.E.; García, J.J.; Hinchado, M.D.; Ortega, E. Inflammatory/stress feedback dysregulation in women with fibromyalgia. *Neuroimmunomodulation* **2012**, *19*, 343–351. [CrossRef] [PubMed]

7. Kaufmann, I.; Schelling, G.; Eisner, C.; Richter, H.P.; Krauseneck, T.; Vogeser, M.; Hauer, D.; Campolongo, P.; Chouker, A.; Beyer, A.; et al. Anandamide and neutrophil function in patients with fibromyalgia. *Psychoneuroendocrinology* **2008**, *33*, 676–685. [CrossRef]

8. Bote, M.E.; García, J.J.; Hinchado, M.D.; Ortega, E. Fibromyalgia: Anti-inflammatory and stress responses after acute moderate exercise. *PLoS ONE* **2013**, *8*, e74524. [CrossRef] [PubMed]

9. Harden, R.N.; Rudin, N.J.; Bruehl, S.; Kee, W.; Parikh, D.K.; Kooch, J.; Duc, T.; Gracely, R.H. Increased systemic catecholamines in complex regional pain syndrome and relationship to psychological factors: A pilot study. *Anesth. Analg.* **2004**, *99*, 1478–1485. [CrossRef]

0. Giske, L.; Røe, C.; Knardahl, S.; Vøllestad, N.K. Pain and Sympathoadrenal Responses to Dynamic Exercise in Women with the Fibromyalgia Syndrome. *J. Musculoskelet. Pain* **2007**, *15*, 25–38. [CrossRef]

1. Adler, G.K.; Kinsley, B.T.; Hurwitz, S.; Mossey, C.J.; Goldenberg, D.L. Reduced hypothalamic-pituitary and sympathoadrenal responses to hypoglycemia in women with fibromyalgia syndrome. *Am. J. Med.* **1999**, *106*, 534–543. [CrossRef] [PubMed]

62. Rizzi, M.; Radovanovic, D.; Santus, P.; Airoldi, A.; Frassanito, F.; Vanni, S.; Cristiano, A.; Masala, I.F.; Sarzi-Puttini, P. Influence of autonomic nervous system dysfunction in the genesis of sleep disorders in fibromyalgia patients. *Clin. Exp. Rheumatol.* **2017**, *35* (Suppl. S105), 74–80. [CrossRef]

63. Riva, R.; Mork, P.J.; Westgaard, R.H.; Okkenhaug Johansen, T.; Lundberg, U. Catecholamines and heart rate in female fibromyalgia patients. *J. Psychosom. Res.* **2012**, *72*, 51–57. [CrossRef]

64. Kadetoff, D.; Kosek, E. Evidence of reduced sympatho-adrenal and hypothalamic-pituitary activity during static muscular work in patients with fibromyalgia. *J. Rehabil. Med.* **2010**, *42*, 765–772. [CrossRef]

65. Forte, G.; Favieri, F.; Casagrande, M. Heart Rate Variability and Cognitive Function: A Systematic Review. *Front. Neurosci.* **2019**, *13*, 710. [CrossRef] [PubMed]

66. Forte, G.; Troisi, G.; Pazzaglia, M.; Pascalis, V.; Casagrande, M. Heart Rate Variability and Pain: A Systematic Review. *Brain. Sci.* **2022**, *12*, 153. [CrossRef] [PubMed]

67. Zamunér, A.R.; Barbic, F.; Dipaola, F.; Bulgheroni, M.; Diana, A.; Atzeni, F.; Marchi, A.; Sarzi-Puttini, P.; Porta, A.; Furlan, R. Relationship between sympathetic activity and pain intensity in fibromyalgia. *Clin. Exp. Rheumatol.* **2015**, *33*, S53–S57.

68. Khasar, S.G.; Burkham, J.; Dina, O.A.; Brown, A.S.; Bogen, O.; Alessandri-Haber, N.; Green, P.G.; Reichling, D.B.; Levine, J.D. Stress induces a switch of intracellular signaling in sensory neurons in a model of generalized pain. *J. Neurosci.* **2008**, *28*, 5721–5730. [CrossRef]

69. Khasar, S.G.; Dina, O.A.; Green, P.G.; Levine, J.D. Sound stress-induced long-term enhancement of mechanical hyperalgesia in rats is maintained by sympathoadrenal catecholamines. *J. Pain.* **2009**, *10*, 1073–1077. [CrossRef] [PubMed]

70. Donello, J.E.; Guan, Y.; Tian, M.; Cheevers, C.V.; Alcantara, M.; Cabrera, S.; Raja, S.N.; Gil, D.W. A peripheral adrenoceptor-mediated sympathetic mechanism can transform stress-induced analgesia into hyperalgesia. *Anesthesiology* **2011**, *114*, 1403–1416. [CrossRef] [PubMed]

71. Nackley, A.G.; Tan, K.S.; Fecho, K.; Flood, P.; Diatchenko, L.; Maixner, W. Catechol-O-methyltransferase inhibition increases pain sensitivity through activation of both beta2- and beta3-adrenergic receptors. *Pain* **2007**, *128*, 199–208. [CrossRef]

72. Oyadeyi, A.; Ajao, F.; Ibironke, G.; Afolabi, A. Acute restraint stress induces hyperalgesia via non-adrenergic mechanisms in rats. *Afr. J. Biomed. Res.* **2005**, *8*, 123–125. [CrossRef]

73. Biondi, M.; Picardi, A. Psychological stress and neuroendocrine function in humans: The last two decades of research. *Psychother. Psychosom.* **1999**, *68*, 114–150. [CrossRef]

74. Heuser, I.; Lammers, C. Stress and the brain. *Neurobiol. Aging* **2003**, *24* (Suppl. S1), S69–S76. [CrossRef]

75. Woda, A.; Picard, P.; Dutheil, F. Dysfunctional stress responses in chronic pain. *Psychoneuroendocrinology* **2016**, *71*, 127–135. [CrossRef] [PubMed]

76. Essex, M.; Klein, M.; Cho, E.; Kalin, N. Maternal stress beginning in infancy may sensitize children to later stress exposure: Effects on cortisol and behavior. *Biol. Psychiatry* **2002**, *52*, 776–784. [CrossRef] [PubMed]

77. Tosato, J.D.P.; Caria, P.H.F.; Gomes, C.A.F.D.P.; Berzin, F.; Politti, F.; Gonzalez, T.D.O.; Biasotto-Gonzalez, D.A. Correlation of stress and muscle activity of patients with different degrees of temporomandibular disorder. *J. Phys. Ther. Sci.* **2015**, *27*, 1227–1231. [CrossRef]

78. Kim, H.-I.; Kim, Y.-Y.; Chang, J.-Y.; Ko, J.-Y.; Kho, H.-S. Salivary cortisol, 17β-estradiol, progesterone, dehydroepiandrosterone, and α-amylase in patients with burning mouth syndrome. *Oral Dis.* **2012**, *18*, 613–620. [CrossRef]

79. Tops, M.; Riese, H.; Oldehinkel, A.J.; Rijsdijk, F.V.; Ormel, J. Rejection sensitivity relates to hypocortisolism and depressed mood state in young women. *Psychoneuroendocrinology* **2008**, *33*, 551–559. [CrossRef] [PubMed]

80. Nijhof, S.; Rutten, J.; Uiterwaal, C.; Bleijenberg, G.; Kimpen, J.; Putte, E. The role of hypocortisolism in chronic fatigue syndrome. *Psychoneuroendocrinology* **2014**, *42*, 119–206. [CrossRef]

81. Chang, L.; Sundaresh, S.; Elliott, J.; Anton, P.A.; Baldi, P.; Licudine, A.; Mayer, M.; Vuong, T.; Hirano, M.; Naliboff, B.D.; et al. Dysregulation of the hypothalamic-pituitary-adrenal (HPA) axis in irritable bowel syndrome. *Neurogastroenterol. Motil.* **2009**, *21*, 149–159. [CrossRef]

82. Heim, C.; Ehlert, U.; Hanker, J.; Hellhammer, D. Abuse-related posttraumatic stress disorder and alterations of the hypothalamic-pituitary-adrenal axis in women with chronic pelvic pain. *Psychosom. Med.* **1998**, *60*, 309–318. [CrossRef]

83. Bagnato, G.; Cordova, F.; Sciortino, D.; Miceli, G.; Bruno, A.; Ferrera, A.; Sangari, D.; Coppolino, G.; Muscatello, M.R.A.; Pandolfo, G.; et al. Association between cortisol levels and pain threshold in systemic sclerosis and major depression. *Rheumatol. Int.* **2018**, *38*, 433–441. [CrossRef]

84. Paananen, M.; O'Sullivan, P.; Straker, L.; Beales, D.; Coenen, P.; Karppinen, J.; Pennell, C.; Smith, A. A low cortisol response to stress is associated with musculoskeletal pain combined with increased pain sensitivity in young adults: A longitudinal cohort study. *Arthritis. Res.* **2015**, *17*, 355. [CrossRef]

85. Trevino, C.; Geier, T.; Morris, R.; Cronn, S.; deRoon-Cassini, T. Relationship Between Decreased Cortisol and Development of Chronic Pain in Traumatically Injured. *J. Surg. Res.* **2022**, *270*, 286–292. [CrossRef] [PubMed]

86. Ennis, G.E.; Moffat, S.D.; Hertzog, C. The cortisol awakening response and cognition across the adult lifespan. *Brain. Cogn.* **2016**, *105*, 66–77. [CrossRef]

87. Riva, R.; Mork, P.; Westgaard, R.; Rø, M.; Lundberg, U. Fibromyalgia syndrome is associated with hypocortisolism. *Int. J. Behav. Med.* **2010**, *17*, 223–233. [CrossRef] [PubMed]

8.	Torgrimson-Ojerio, B.; Ross, R.L.; Dieckmann, N.F.; Avery, S.; Bennett, R.M.; Jones, K.D.; Guarino, A.J.; Wood, L.J. Preliminary evidence of a blunted anti-inflammatory response to exhaustive exercise in fibromyalgia. *J. Neuroimmunol.* **2014**, *277*, 160–167. [CrossRef] [PubMed]

9.	Pereira Pernambuco, A.; De Souza Cota Carvalho, L.; Pereira Leite Schetino, L.; Cunha Polese, J.; De Souza Viana, R.; D' Ávila Reis, D. Effects of a health education program on cytokines and cortisol levels in fibromyalgia patients: A randomized controlled trial. *Adv. Rheumatol.* **2018**, *58*. [CrossRef]

0.	Tak, L.; Cleare, A.; Ormel, J.; Manoharan, A.; Kok, I.; Wessely, S.; Rosmalen, J. Meta-analysis and meta-regression of hypothalamic-pituitary-adrenal axis activity in functional somatic disorders. *Biol. Psychol.* **2011**, *87*, 183–194. [CrossRef] [PubMed]

1.	Úbeda-D'Ocasar, E.; Jiménez Díaz-Benito, V.; Gallego-Sendarrubias, G.M.; Valera-Calero, J.A.; Vicario-Merino, Á.; Hervás-Pérez, J.P. Pain and Cortisol in Patients with Fibromyalgia: Systematic Review and Meta-Analysis. *Diagnostics* **2020**, *10*, 922. [CrossRef]

2.	McEwen, B.S. Physiology and Neurobiology of Stress and Adaptation: Central Role of the Brain. *Physiol. Rev.* **2007**, *87*, 873–904. [CrossRef]

3.	Coppens, E.; Kempke, S.; Van Wambeke, P.; Claes, S.; Morlion, B.; Luyten, P.; Van Oudenhove, L. Cortisol and Subjective Stress Responses to Acute Psychosocial Stress in Fibromyalgia Patients and Control Participants. *Psychosom. Med.* **2018**, *80*, 317–326. [CrossRef]

4.	Bale, T.; Vale, W. CRF and CRF receptors: Role in stress responsivity and other behaviors. *Annu. Rev. Pharmacol. Toxicol.* **2004**, *44*, 525–557. [CrossRef]

5.	Olango, W.M.; Finn, D.P. Neurobiology of Stress-Induced Hyperalgesia. In *Behavioral Neurobiology of Chronic Pain*; Taylor, B.K., Finn, D.P., Eds.; Springer: Berlin/Heidelberg, Germany, 2014; pp. 251–280. [CrossRef]

6.	Schwetz, I.; Bradesi, S.; McRoberts, J.; Sablad, M.; Miller, J.; Zhou, H.; Ohning, G.; Mayer, E. Delayed stress-induced colonic hypersensitivity in male Wistar rats: Role of neurokinin-1 and corticotropin-releasing factor-1 receptors. *Am. J. Physiol. Gastrointest. Liver Physiol.* **2004**, *286*, G683–G691. [CrossRef]

7.	Million, M.; Grigoriadis, D.; Sullivan, S.; Crowe, P.; McRoberts, J.; Zhou, H.; Saunders, P.; Maillot, C.; Mayer, E.; Taché, Y. A novel water-soluble selective CRF1 receptor antagonist, NBI 35965, blunts stress-induced visceral hyperalgesia and colonic motor function in rats. *Brain Res.* **2003**, *985*, 32–42. [CrossRef] [PubMed]

8.	Abdelhamid, R.E.; Kovacs, K.J.; Pasley, J.D.; Nunez, M.G.; Larson, A.A. Forced swim-induced musculoskeletal hyperalgesia is mediated by CRF2 receptors but not by TRPV1 receptors. *Neuropharmacology* **2013**, *72*, 29–37. [CrossRef] [PubMed]

9.	Sagami, Y. Effect of a corticotropin releasing hormone receptor antagonist on colonic sensory and motor function in patients with irritable bowel syndrome. *Gut* **2004**, *53*, 958–964. [CrossRef] [PubMed]

100.	Schwetz, I.; Naliboff, B.; Munakata, J.; Lembo, T.; Chang, L.; Matin, K.; Ohning, G.; Mayer, E. Anti-hyperalgesic effect of octreotide in patients with irritable bowel syndrome. *Aliment. Pharmacol. Ther.* **2004**, *19*, 123–131. [CrossRef]

101.	Geva, N.; Defrin, R. Opposite Effects of Stress on Pain Modulation Depend on the Magnitude of Individual Stress Response. *J. Pain* **2018**, *19*, 360–371. [CrossRef] [PubMed]

102.	Bouma, E.M.C.; Riese, H.; Doornbos, B.; Ormel, J.; Oldehinkel, A.J. Genetically based reduced MAOA and COMT functioning is associated with the cortisol stress response: A replication study. *Mol. Psychiatry* **2012**, *17*, 119–121. [CrossRef]

103.	Hernaus, D.; Collip, D.; Lataster, J.; Ceccarini, J.; Kenis, G.; Booij, L.; Pruessner, J.; Van Laere, K.; van Winkel, R.; van Os, J.; et al. COMT Val158Met genotype selectively alters prefrontal [18F]fallypride displacement and subjective feelings of stress in response to a psychosocial stress challenge. *PLoS ONE* **2013**, *8*, e65662. [CrossRef]

104.	Papaleo, F.; Crawley, J.N.; Song, J.; Lipska, B.K.; Pickel, J.; Weinberger, D.R.; Chen, J. Genetic dissection of the role of catechol-O-methyltransferase in cognition and stress reactivity in mice. *J. Neurosci.* **2008**, *28*, 8709–8723. [CrossRef]

105.	Tammimäki, A.; Männistö, P.T. Catechol-O-methyltransferase gene polymorphism and chronic human pain: A systematic review and meta-analysis. *Pharm. Genom.* **2012**, *22*, 673–691. [CrossRef] [PubMed]

106.	Antypa, N.; Giegling, I.; Calati, R.; Schneider, B.; Hartmann, A.M.; Friedl, M.; Konte, B.; Lia, L.; De Ronchi, D.; Serretti, A.; et al. MAOA and MAOB polymorphisms and anger-related traits in suicidal participants and controls. *Eur. Arch. Psychiatry Clin. Neurosci.* **2013**, *263*, 393–403. [CrossRef]

107.	Melas, P.A.; Wei, Y.; Wong, C.C.Y.; Sjöholm, L.K.; Åberg, E.; Mill, J.; Schalling, M.; Forsell, Y.; Lavebratt, C. Genetic and epigenetic associations of MAOA and NR3C1 with depression and childhood adversities. *Int. J. Neuropsychopharmacol.* **2013**, *16*, 1513–1528. [CrossRef]

108.	Kim, H.; Lee, H.; Rowan, J.; Brahim, J.; Dionne, R.A. Genetic polymorphisms in monoamine neurotransmitter systems show only weak association with acute post-surgical pain in humans. *Mol. Pain* **2006**, *2*, 24. [CrossRef]

109.	Serý, O.; Hrazdilová, O.; Didden, W.; Klenerová, V.; Staif, R.; Znojil, V.; Sevcík, P. The association of monoamine oxidase B functional polymorphism with postoperative pain intensity. *Neuro Endocrinol. Lett.* **2006**, *27*, 333–337.

110.	Treister, R.; Pud, D.; Ebstein, R.P.; Laiba, E.; Gershon, E.; Haddad, M.; Eisenberg, E. Associations between polymorphisms in dopamine neurotransmitter pathway genes and pain response in healthy humans. *Pain* **2009**, *147*, 187–193. [CrossRef] [PubMed]

111.	Buhck, M.; Achenbach, J.; Wiese, B.; Tran, A.T.; Stuhrmann, M.; Jaeger, B.; Bernateck, M.; Schneider, N.; Karst, M. The interplay of chronic stress and genetic traits discriminates between patients suffering from multisomatoform disorder with pain as the leading symptom and matched controls. *J. Affect. Disord.* **2022**, *308*, 466–472. [CrossRef]

112. Diatchenko, L.; Slade, G.D.; Nackley, A.G.; Bhalang, K.; Sigurdsson, A.; Belfer, I.; Goldman, D.; Xu, K.; Shabalina, S.A.; Shagin, D.; et al. Genetic basis for individual variations in pain perception and the development of a chronic pain condition. *Hum. Mol. Genet.* **2004**, *14*, 135–143. [CrossRef]
113. Wüst, S.; Van Rossum, E.; Federenko, I.; Koper, J.; Kumsta, R.; Hellhammer, D. Common polymorphisms in the glucocorticoid receptor gene are associated with adrenocortical responses to psychosocial stress. *J. Clin. Endocrinol. Metab.* **2004**, *89*, 565–573 [CrossRef]
114. Linnstaedt, S.D.; Riker, K.D.; Rueckeis, C.A.; Kutchko, K.M.; Lackey, L.; Mccarthy, K.R.; Tsai, Y.-H.; Parker, J.S.; Kurz, M.C.; Hendry, P.L.; et al. A Functional riboSNitch in the 3' Untranslated Region of *FKBP5* Alters MicroRNA-320a Binding Efficiency and Mediates Vulnerability to Chronic Post-Traumatic Pain. *J. Neurosci.* **2018**, *38*, 8407–8420. [CrossRef] [PubMed]
115. Linnstaedt, S.D.; Bortsov, A.V.; Soward, A.C.; Swor, R.; Peak, D.A.; Jones, J.; Rathlev, N.; Lee, D.C.; Domeier, R.; Hendry, P.L.; et al. CRHBP polymorphisms predict chronic pain development following motor vehicle collision. *Pain* **2016**, *157*, 273–279. [CrossRef]
116. Mogil, J.S. Pain genetics: Past, present and future. *Trends. Genet.* **2012**, *28*, 258–266. [CrossRef] [PubMed]
117. Mueller, A.; Strahler, J.; Armbruster, D.; Lesch, K.-P.; Brocke, B.; Kirschbaum, C. Genetic contributions to acute autonomic stress responsiveness in children. *Int. J. Psychophysiol.* **2012**, *83*, 302–308. [CrossRef]
118. Gutierrez-Arcelus, M.; Lappalainen, T.; Montgomery, S.B.; Buil, A.; Ongen, H.; Yurovsky, A.; Bryois, J.; Giger, T.; Romano, L.; Planchon, A.; et al. Passive and active DNA methylation and the interplay with genetic variation in gene regulation. *Elife* **2013**, *2*, e00523. [CrossRef]
119. Polli, A.; Godderis, L.; Ghosh, M.; Ickmans, K.; Nijs, J. Epigenetic and miRNA Expression Changes in People with Pain: A Systematic Review. *J. Pain* **2020**, *21*, 763–780. [CrossRef]
120. Unternaehrer, E.; Luers, P.; Mill, J.; Dempster, E.; Meyer, A.H.; Staehli, S.; Lieb, R.; Hellhammer, D.H.; Meinlschmidt, G. Dynamic changes in DNA methylation of stress-associated genes (OXTR, BDNF) after acute psychosocial stress. *Transl. Psychiatry* **2012**, *2*, e150. [CrossRef] [PubMed]
121. Wiegand, A.; Blickle, A.; Brückmann, C.; Weller, S.; Nieratschker, V.; Plewnia, C. Dynamic DNA Methylation Changes in the COMT Gene Promoter Region in Response to Mental Stress and Its Modulation by Transcranial Direct Current Stimulation. *Biomolecules* **2021**, *11*, 1726. [CrossRef] [PubMed]
122. Ziegler, C.; Richter, J.; Mahr, M.; Gajewska, A.; Schiele, M.A.; Gehrmann, A.; Schmidt, B.; Lesch, K.P.; Lang, T.; Helbig-Lang, S.; et al. MAOA gene hypomethylation in panic disorder—Reversibility of an epigenetic risk pattern by psychotherapy. *Transl. Psychiatry* **2016**, *6*, e773. [CrossRef]
123. Ursini, G.; Bollati, V.; Fazio, L.; Porcelli, A.; Iacovelli, L.; Catalani, A.; Sinibaldi, L.; Gelao, B.; Romano, R.; Rampino, A.; et al. Stress-related methylation of the catechol-O-methyltransferase Val 158 allele predicts human prefrontal cognition and activity. *J. Neurosci.* **2011**, *31*, 6692–6698. [CrossRef]
124. Peng, H.; Zhu, Y.; Strachan, E.; Fowler, E.; Bacus, T.; Roy-Byrne, P.; Goldberg, J.; Vaccarino, V.; Zhao, J. Childhood Trauma, DNA Methylation of Stress-Related Genes, and Depression: Findings From Two Monozygotic Twin Studies. *Psychosom. Med.* **2018**, *80*, 599–608. [CrossRef]
125. Xu, Q.; Jiang, M.; Gu, S.; Wang, F.; Yuan, B. Early Life Stress Induced DNA Methylation of Monoamine Oxidases Leads to Depressive-Like Behavior. *Front. Cell Dev. Biol.* **2020**, *8*, 582247. [CrossRef] [PubMed]
126. Bakusic, J.; Vrieze, E.; Ghosh, M.; Bekaert, B.; Claes, S.; Godderis, L. Increased methylation of NR3C1 and SLC6A4 is associated with blunted cortisol reactivity to stress in major depression. *Neurobiol. Stress* **2020**, *13*, 100272. [CrossRef] [PubMed]
127. Schartner, C.; Ziegler, C.; Schiele, M.A.; Kollert, L.; Weber, H.; Zwanzger, P.; Arolt, V.; Pauli, P.; Deckert, J.; Reif, A.; et al. CRHR1 promoter hypomethylation: An epigenetic readout of panic disorder? *Eur. Neuropsychopharmacol.* **2017**, *27*, 360–371. [CrossRef] [PubMed]
128. Oberlander, T.F.; Weinberg, J.; Papsdorf, M.; Grunau, R.; Misri, S.; Devlin, A.M. Prenatal exposure to maternal depression, neonatal methylation of human glucocorticoid receptor gene (NR3C1) and infant cortisol stress responses. *Epigenetics* **2008**, *3*, 97–106. [CrossRef]
129. Radtke, K.M.; Ruf, M.; Gunter, H.M.; Dohrmann, K.; Schauer, M.; Meyer, A.; Elbert, T. Transgenerational impact of intimate partner violence on methylation in the promoter of the glucocorticoid receptor. *Transl. Psychiatry* **2011**, *1*, e21. [CrossRef]
130. McGowan, P.O.; Sasaki, A.; D'Alessio, A.C.; Dymov, S.; Labonté, B.; Szyf, M.; Turecki, G.; Meaney, M.J. Epigenetic regulation of the glucocorticoid receptor in human brain associates with childhood abuse. *Nat. Neurosci.* **2009**, *12*, 342–348. [CrossRef]
131. Hawe, J.S.; Wilson, R.; Schmid, K.T.; Zhou, L.; Lakshmanan, L.N.; Lehne, B.C.; Kühnel, B.; Scott, W.R.; Wielscher, M.; Yew, Y.W.; et al. Genetic variation influencing DNA methylation provides insights into molecular mechanisms regulating genomic function. *Nat. Genet.* **2022**, *54*, 18–29. [CrossRef] [PubMed]
132. Gaunt, T.R.; Shihab, H.A.; Hemani, G.; Min, J.L.; Woodward, G.; Lyttleton, O.; Zheng, J.; Duggirala, A.; McArdle, W.L.; Ho, K.; et al. Systematic identification of genetic influences on methylation across the human life course. *Genome Biol.* **2016**, *17*, 61. [CrossRef]
133. Hannon, E.; Gorrie-Stone, T.J.; Smart, M.C.; Burrage, J.; Hughes, A.; Bao, Y.; Kumari, M.; Schalkwyk, L.C.; Mill, J. Leveraging DNA-Methylation Quantitative-Trait Loci to Characterize the Relationship between Methylomic Variation, Gene Expression, and Complex Traits. *Am. J. Hum. Genet.* **2018**, *103*, 654–665. [CrossRef]
134. Bonder, M.J.; Luijk, R.; Zhernakova, D.V.; Moed, M.; Deelen, P.; Vermaat, M.; van Iterson, M.; van Dijk, F.; van Galen, M.; Bot, J.; et al. Disease variants alter transcription factor levels and methylation of their binding sites. *Nat. Genet.* **2017**, *49*, 131–138. [CrossRef]

35. Bonder, M.J.; Kasela, S.; Kals, M.; Tamm, R.; Lokk, K.; Barragan, I.; Buurman, W.A.; Deelen, P.; Greve, J.-W.; Ivanov, M.; et al. Genetic and epigenetic regulation of gene expression in fetal and adult human livers. *BMC Genom.* **2014**, *15*, 860. [CrossRef] [PubMed]

36. Polli, A.; Hendrix, J.; Ickmans, K.; Bakusic, J.; Ghosh, M.; Monteyne, D.; Velkeniers, B.; Bekaert, B.; Nijs, J.; Godderis, L. Genetic and epigenetic regulation of Catechol-O-methyltransferase in relation to inflammation in chronic fatigue syndrome and Fibromyalgia. *J. Transl. Med.* **2022**, *20*, 487. [CrossRef] [PubMed]

37. Schreiner, F.; El-Maarri, O.; Gohlke, B.; Stutte, S.; Nuesgen, N.; Mattheisen, M.; Fimmers, R.; Bartmann, P.; Oldenburg, J.; Woelfle, J. Association of COMT genotypes with S-COMT promoter methylation in growth-discordant monozygotic twins and healthy adults. *BMC Med. Genet.* **2011**, *12*, 115. [CrossRef]

38. Crofford, L.J. Adverse effects of chronic opioid therapy for chronic musculoskeletal pain. *Nat. Rev. Rheumatol.* **2010**, *6*, 191–197. [CrossRef]

39. Crofford, L.J. Chronic Pain: Where the Body Meets the Brain. *Trans. Am. Clin. Clim. Assoc.* **2015**, *126*, 167–183.

40. Michaelides, A.; Zis, P. Depression, anxiety and acute pain: Links and management challenges. *Postgrad Med.* **2019**, *131*, 438–444. [CrossRef]

41. Marshall, P.W.M.; Schabrun, S.; Knox, M.F. Physical activity and the mediating effect of fear, depression, anxiety, and catastrophizing on pain related disability in people with chronic low back pain. *PLoS ONE* **2017**, *12*, e0180788. [CrossRef] [PubMed]

42. Louw, A.; Diener, I.; Butler, D.S.; Puentedura, E.J. The Effect of Neuroscience Education on Pain, Disability, Anxiety, and Stress in Chronic Musculoskeletal Pain. *Arch. Phys. Med. Rehabil.* **2011**, *92*, 2041–2056. [CrossRef] [PubMed]

43. Watson, J.A.; Ryan, C.G.; Cooper, L.; Ellington, D.; Whittle, R.; Lavender, M.; Dixon, J.; Atkinson, G.; Cooper, K.; Martin, D.J. Pain Neuroscience Education for Adults With Chronic Musculoskeletal Pain: A Mixed-Methods Systematic Review and Meta-Analysis. *J. Pain.* **2019**, *20*, 1140.e1–1140.e22. [CrossRef] [PubMed]

44. Tegner, H.; Frederiksen, P.; Esbensen, B.A.; Juhl, C. Neurophysiological Pain Education for Patients With Chronic Low Back Pain: A Systematic Review and Meta-Analysis. *Clin. J. Pain.* **2018**, *34*, 778–786. [CrossRef] [PubMed]

45. O'Keeffe, M.; O'Sullivan, P.; Purtill, H.; Bargary, N.; O'Sullivan, K. Cognitive functional therapy compared with a group-based exercise and education intervention for chronic low back pain: A multicentre randomised controlled trial (RCT). *Br. J. Sport. Med.* **2020**, *54*, 782–789. [CrossRef] [PubMed]

46. Veehof, M.M.; Trompetter, H.R.; Bohlmeijer, E.T.; Schreurs, K.M. Acceptance- and mindfulness-based interventions for the treatment of chronic pain: A meta-analytic review. *Cogn. Behav.* **2016**, *45*, 5–31. [CrossRef] [PubMed]

47. Soundararajan, K.; Prem, V.; Kishen, T.J. The effectiveness of mindfulness-based stress reduction intervention on physical function in individuals with chronic low back pain: Systematic review and meta-analysis of randomized controlled trials. *Complement. Clin. Pr.* **2022**, *49*, 101623. [CrossRef]

48. Haugmark, T.; Hagen, K.B.; Smedslund, G.; Zangi, H.A. Mindfulness- and acceptance-based interventions for patients with fibromyalgia—A systematic review and meta-analyses. *PLoS ONE* **2019**, *14*, e0221897. [CrossRef] [PubMed]

49. Hajihasani, A.; Rouhani, M.; Salavati, M.; Hedayati, R.; Kahlaee, A.H. The Influence of Cognitive Behavioral Therapy on Pain, Quality of Life, and Depression in Patients Receiving Physical Therapy for Chronic Low Back Pain: A Systematic Review. *Pm. R.* **2019**, *11*, 167–176. [CrossRef] [PubMed]

50. Nijs, J.; D'Hondt, E.; Clarys, P.; Deliens, T.; Polli, A.; Malfliet, A.; Coppieters, I.; Willaert, W.; Tumkaya Yilmaz, S.; Elma, Ö.; et al. Lifestyle and Chronic Pain across the Lifespan: An Inconvenient Truth? *Pm. R.* **2020**, *12*, 410–419. [CrossRef]

51. Denis, D.; Akhtar, R.; Holding, B.C.; Murray, C.; Panatti, J.; Claridge, G.; Sadeh, A.; Barclay, N.L.; O'Leary, R.; Maughan, B.; et al. Externalizing Behaviors and Callous-Unemotional Traits: Different Associations with Sleep Quality. *Sleep* **2017**, *40*. [CrossRef]

52. Nakamura, M.; Nagamine, T. Neuroendocrine, Autonomic, and Metabolic Responses to an Orexin Antagonist, Suvorexant, in Psychiatric Patients with Insomnia. *Innov. Clin. Neurosci.* **2017**, *14*, 30–37.

53. Nijs, J.; Loggia, M.L.; Polli, A.; Moens, M.; Huysmans, E.; Goudman, L.; Meeus, M.; Vanderweeën, L.; Ickmans, K.; Clauw, D. Sleep disturbances and severe stress as glial activators: Key targets for treating central sensitization in chronic pain patients? *Expert Opin. Targets* **2017**, *21*, 817–826. [CrossRef]

54. Haack, M.; Simpson, N.; Sethna, N.; Kaur, S.; Mullington, J. Sleep deficiency and chronic pain: Potential underlying mechanisms and clinical implications. *Neuropsychopharmacology* **2020**, *45*, 205–216. [CrossRef] [PubMed]

55. Rodrigues, G.M., Jr.; Toffoli, L.V.; Manfredo, M.H.; Francis-Oliveira, J.; Silva, A.S.; Raquel, H.A.; Martins-Pinge, M.C.; Moreira, E.G.; Fernandes, K.B.; Pelosi, G.G.; et al. Acute stress affects the global DNA methylation profile in rat brain: Modulation by physical exercise. *Behav. Brain Res.* **2015**, *279*, 123–128. [CrossRef] [PubMed]

56. Sales, A.J.; Joca, S.R.L. Antidepressant administration modulates stress-induced DNA methylation and DNA methyltransferase expression in rat prefrontal cortex and hippocampus. *Behav. Brain Res.* **2018**, *343*, 8–15. [CrossRef] [PubMed]

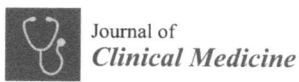

Journal of
Clinical Medicine

MDPI

Review

The Biology of Placebo and Nocebo Effects on Experimental and Chronic Pain: State of the Art

Giacomo Rossettini [1,†], Francesco Campaci [2,†], Joel Bialosky [3,4], Eva Huysmans [5,6], Lene Vase [7] and Elisa Carlino [2,*]

1 School of physiotherapy, University of Verona, 37129 Verona, Italy
2 Department of Neuroscience "Rita Levi Montalcini", University of Turin, 10124 Turin, Italy
3 Department of Physical Therapy, University of Florida, Gainesville, FL 32611, USA
4 Clinical Research Center, Brooks Rehabilitation, Jacksonville, FL 32211, USA
5 Pain in Motion Research Group (PAIN), Department of Physiotherapy, Human Physiology and Anatomy, Faculty of Physical Education & Physiotherapy, Vrije Universiteit Brussel, Laarbeeklaan 103, 1090 Brussels, Belgium
6 Department of Physical Medicine and Physiotherapy, Universitair Ziekenhuis Brussel, Laarbeeklaan 101, 1090 Brussels, Belgium
7 Department of Psychology and Behavioural Sciences, School of Business and Social Sciences, Aarhus University, 8000 Aarhus, Denmark
* Correspondence: elisa.carlino@unito.it; Tel.: +39-011-6708491
† These authors contributed equally to this work.

Abstract: (1) Background: In recent years, placebo and nocebo effects have been extensively documented in different medical conditions, including pain. The scientific literature has provided strong evidence of how the psychosocial context accompanying the treatment administration can influence the therapeutic outcome positively (placebo effects) or negatively (nocebo effects). (2) Methods: This state-of-the-art paper aims to provide an updated overview of placebo and nocebo effects on pain. (3) Results: The most common study designs, the psychological mechanisms, and neurobiological/genetic determinants of these phenomena are discussed, focusing on the differences between positive and negative context effects on pain in experimental settings on healthy volunteers and in clinical settings on chronic pain patients. Finally, the last section describes the implications for clinical and research practice to maximize the medical and scientific routine and correctly interpret the results of research studies on placebo and nocebo effects. (4) Conclusions: While studies on healthy participants seem consistent and provide a clear picture of how the brain reacts to the context, there are no unique results of the occurrence and magnitude of placebo and nocebo effects in chronic pain patients, mainly due to the heterogeneity of pain. This opens up the need for future studies on the topic.

Keywords: placebo effect; nocebo effect; expectation; conditioning; pain; contextual factor

Citation: Rossettini, G.; Campaci, F.; Bialosky, J.; Huysmans, E.; Vase, L.; Carlino, E. The Biology of Placebo and Nocebo Effects on Experimental and Chronic Pain: State of the Art. *J. Clin. Med.* **2023**, *12*, 4113. https://doi.org/10.3390/jcm12124113

Academic Editor: Guy Hans

Received: 22 May 2023
Revised: 13 June 2023
Accepted: 15 June 2023
Published: 18 June 2023

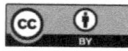
1. Introduction

In recent years, placebo and nocebo effects have strongly influenced pain studies, which fostered the interest in this topic and encouraged debate among scholars, researchers, and clinicians worldwide [1–3].

From their earliest days, placebos have been identified as inert substances (e.g., sugar pills, saline injections) used in clinical trials to control the efficacy of new treatments [3]. Today, neuroscientists and clinicians recognize that placebos are more than inert substances, introducing the concept of "context surrounding a treatment" [4]. Accordingly, placebo and nocebo effects are now defined as, respectively, the positive or negative effects due to the administration of a treatment (be it real or simulated) in a therapeutic context [5]. The context that triggers these effects comprises symbols, rituals, and cues (e.g., provider's words, patient's expectations and previous experiences, physical aspects of the treatment) that accompany patients during their healthcare experiences [6,7]. In the field of pain, the administration of an inert treatment in a positive context can induce a reduction of pain (as reported by subjective pain reports) as well as a modulation of specific brain circuits involved in pain processing. On the contrary, when an inert treatment is administered in a negative context, participants/patients can experience pain exacerbation as well as increased activation of pain-related brain regions [8]. Similarly, it has been documented that administering treatments without a proper context (e.g., when patients are unaware that a medication/drug has been delivered) strongly reduced the efficacy of the medication [9].

Thus, from this perspective, analyzing how the therapeutic context can influence treatment efficacy represents an opportunity for both clinicians and researchers. This state-of-the-art paper aims to provide an updated overview of placebo and nocebo studies on pain, showing how treatments (active or inert) administered in positive or negative contexts trigger different outcomes. Thus, this paper will serve to help clinicians to be more aware of the use of context in their medical routine. Moreover, it will serve to help researchers to build upon the best evidence for designing future trials and implementing new studies to increase our knowledge on the biological determinants of placebo and nocebo effects on pain. The first section provides the reader with a solid background of the mechanisms and the neurobiological determinants of placebo and nocebo effects on pain. The second section describes the future implications for clinical practice to maximize the medical routine. Moreover, implications for research are discussed to help researchers design future trials and develop new innovative studies on pain.

This state-of-the-art paper has been prepared and developed following methodological guidelines for narrative reviews (Table 1) [10]. The articles included in this state-of-the-art overview needed to (1) be scientific works (experimental studies, systematic or narrative reviews (including meta-analyses), or RTCs) published in peer-reviewed journals; (2) be primarily focused on the analgesia/hyperalgesia manifestation of placebo/nocebo effects and/or on the psychological and neurobiological mechanisms involved; (3) provide significant data for a comprehensive, descriptive, and state-of-the-art overview; and (4) provide a detailed description of the methodological approaches used (only in the case of experimental articles). Additionally, the articles presented in Section 3 needed to focus on chronic pain conditions, specifically. Overall, 80 experimental studies and RCTs on placebo and nocebo effects on healthy volunteers and chronic pain patients have been reviewed. Study characteristics of these experimental studies are summarized in Table A1 (Appendix A), including the sample size, population involved, pain type or pain type induction, investigated outcome, objective measures, and level of significance reported by the authors. Furthermore, 31 reviews and 24 meta-analyses and systematic reviews have been included in order to provide a clear and broad overview of the literature concerning placebo/nocebo phenomena in healthy volunteers and chronic pain patients.

Table 1. Narrative review methodology used for research and analysis [10].

Typology	Details
Sources accessed	• *Database*: Cumulative Index to Nursing and Allied Health Literature—CINAHL, Excerpta Medica database—EMBASE, MEDLINE through PubMed, Web of Science. • *Other*: bibliographic lists of relevant articles.
Search terms	• *Key-words*: placebo, nocebo, effects, pain, acute, chronic, analgesia, hyperalgesia. • *Boolean operators*: AND, OR.
Limits	• *Time*: from inception of databases to 1st of January 2023. • *Language*: English.

Table 1. *Cont.*

Typology	Details
Studies included	• *Design*: primary quantitative studies (e.g., experimental research, clinical trials) and secondary (e.g., narrative review, systematic review, metanalysis). • *Target*: healthy participants, patients with acute and chronic pain of different origins (e.g., musculoskeletal, surgical). • *Topic*: placebo and nocebo effects in acute and chronic pain.
Steps for writing	• *Analysis*: collection, analysis, and organization of findings, grouping of findings with similar content. • *Reporting*: organization of the main text into subsections, synthesis of findings into tables and figures, definition of key points for future research and practice, summary of new, evidence-based points.

Abbreviations: CINAHL, Cumulative Index to Nursing and Allied Health Literature; EMBASE, Excerpta Medica database.

2. State of the Art

2.1. Experimental Approaches to Study Placebo and Nocebo Effects

Placebo and nocebo effects on pain have been extensively studied using experimental research designs [6,11–15]. Different approaches have been used to trigger pain amelioration or exacerbation: the two most common procedures are (1) the use of positive or negative expectations and (2) the use of conditioning approaches [11,12]. In the first case, inert treatments are administered along with verbal information that a real treatment is delivered: using this approach, participants or patients are made to believe that a treatment is administered and a positive or negative effect is expected [16–19]. In the second case, using conditioning protocols, a real treatment is administered for different trials and subsequently replaced by an inert treatment: using this approach, participants or patients experience a positive effect when the active treatment is administered, and they expect the same effect when the inert treatment is delivered unbeknownst to them [20–22]. Studies in healthy volunteers showed that conditioning protocols produce more robust [23,24] and long-lasting placebo effects that cannot be attributable to carryover effects of the active treatment. On the contrary, nocebos seem to result in a great worsening of pain even without a conditioning procedure [25]. Interestingly, the conditioned placebo effect seems to be transferable from one modality (analgesia conditioning) to another (motor performance) [26].

Besides expectation and conditioning studies, context effects have been extensively documented using the so-called "open-hidden" design, in which participants or patients receive a real analgesic drug in two different conditions: in the open condition, they are aware that the drug is administered (presence of the context), in the hidden one, they are unaware of receiving it (absence of the context) [27]. Studies consistently find pain relieving medication of established effectiveness to be significantly more effective when administered in an open fashion as compared to when individuals are unaware of receiving the medication [28]. Thus, the difference between the two conditions shows how exposure to a context influences the effectiveness of a treatment which is in fact proven to be active. Recently, another approach has been used is the open–label nondeceptive approach, whereby participants are informed that an inert treatment will be administered, and that this treatment can be effective [11,12,29,30]. These two approaches (open–hidden and open–label) offer the possibility to study placebo effects in clinical settings without the ethical controversies of deception: indeed, in the first case, a real drug is administered, and the effect of the context is studied without using an inert treatment. In the second case, the use of a placebo is fully disclosed.

2.2. Neurobiology

Over the last few decades, different studies and projects have been conducted, using different approaches ranging from pharmacology to neuroimaging [31–33], to describe the brain circuitry and neurotransmitter systems that trigger or block placebo and nocebo effects. The study of the neurobiological determinants of these phenomena is crucial for different reasons: (1) it provides solid knowledge of the objective effects of the context on our brain, (2) it demonstrates that placebo/nocebo and drugs share common biochemical pathways and activate the same receptor pathways, which suggests possible interference between the context and rituals that surround a treatment on the one hand and pharmacological agents on the other. Major studies on healthy participants exposed to experimental pain will be discussed in the next sections. Subsequently, a focus on patients with chronic pain will be presented.

2.2.1. Pharmacological Evidence

Pharmacological studies demonstrated that inert treatments activate the endogenous opioid and endocannabinoid systems (Figure 1A). In these studies, conducted on healthy volunteers, a conditioning protocol was induced, in which opioids (e.g., morphine) or cannabinoids (e.g., ketorolac) were administered and subsequently replaced by a placebo. After morphine administration, μ-opioid antagonists (e.g., naloxone) block placebo analgesia [20,34,35]. The same effect has been discovered using CB1-antagonist (e.g., rimonabant) after cannabinoid administration [36]. Interestingly, naloxone has also been seen to block open–label nondeceptive placebo analgesia, indicating that the same mechanisms may mediate nondeceptive and deceptive placebo analgesia [37]. Indirect confirmations of the involvement of the opioid system have been reported investigating the role of cholecystokinin (CCK), an anti-opioid peptide, and in particular, the role of CCK antagonists (e.g., proglumide) and CCK agonists (e.g., pentagastrin). Proglumide enhances placebo analgesic effects while pentagastrin disrupts them [38–42]. Furthermore, nocebo hyperalgesia seems to be modulated by the activation of the opioid system, as CCK antagonists can reverse it [38]. Scott et al. (2008) [43] found a deactivation of the μ-opioid receptor system during nocebo hyperalgesia (Figure 1B).

Beside opioid and cannabinoid systems, the dopamine system has been explored in this context [32,33]. Some studies indicate that dopamine may be involved in placebo analgesia influencing the activity of pain-related areas, such as the thalamus, insula, anterior cingulate cortex [44,45], and the ventrolateral prefrontal cortex [46]. These data are controversial. Indeed, it is likely that dopamine may not be fundamental for placebo analgesia itself [47,48], but it may be more generally involved in placebo responsiveness [46,49]. In particular, dopamine may affect patients' expectations and desire for improvement [47] and the recalled efficacy of a placebo [46].

Other neurotransmitters, e.g., oxytocin and vasopressin, may be involved in expectancy-induced analgesia [50,51]. Interestingly, the administration of vasopressin has been observed to be associated with increased placebo analgesia, but the effect was restricted to women [50]. The hypothesis behind the involvement of these neurotransmitters takes into account their role in social behavior [52,53], but the results are still preliminary, as other studies do not support the facilitating effect of oxytocin on placebo analgesia [50]. Finally, placebos and nocebos modulate the synthesis of prostaglandins, being important targets of analgesic drugs [54], and the plasma level of pro-inflammatory cytokine (IL-18) during pain experience [55]. It is crucial to consider that the mechanisms addressed above were studied in healthy volunteers exposed to experimental pain protocols. As will be discussed below, fewer studies investigated placebo and nocebo effects in patients with chronic pain, and it has been suggested that the knowledge derived from studies on healthy volunteers may not be entirely transferrable to chronic pain populations [56].

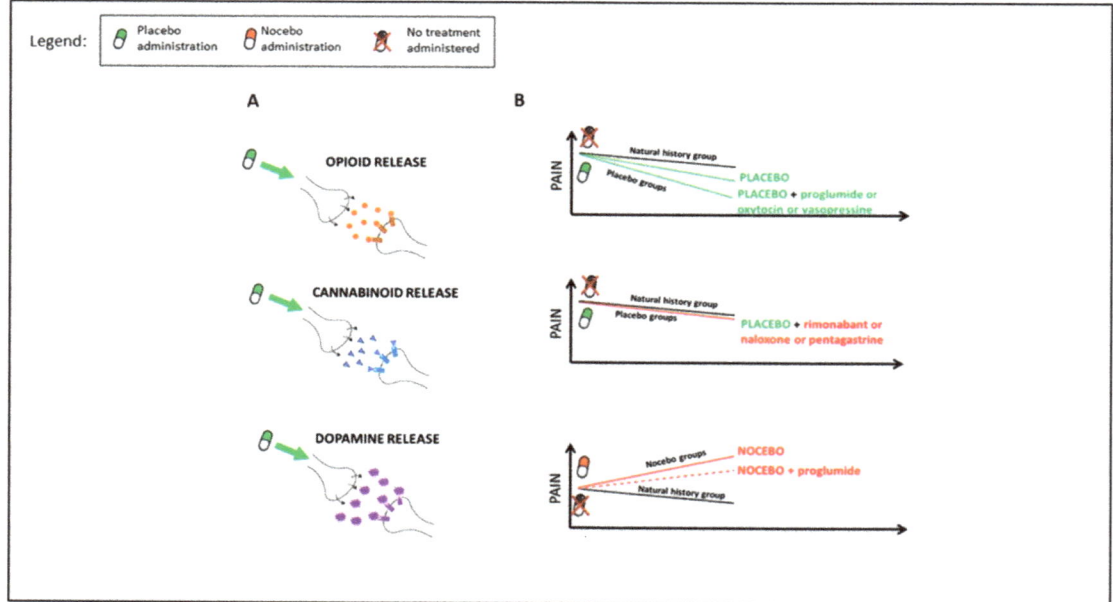

Figure 1. Pharmacological evidences. As reported by different pharmacological studies, placebo administration activates endogenous opioid, cannabinoid, and dopamine systems (**A**). Participants in the placebo groups experienced analgesic effects, namely pain reduction, compared to participants that received no treatments (natural history group). This analgesic effect is enhanced by proglumide, oxytocin, and vasopressine ((**B**), upper graph) while it is disrupted by rimonabant, naloxone, and pentagastrin ((**B**), middle graph). Nocebo effects exacerbate pain perception compared no treatment groups (natural history group). This effect is partially reversed by CCK antagonist proglumide ((**B**), bottom graph).

2.2.2. Neuroimaging Studies

Neuroimaging studies have provided crucial insights into how exposure to a context can positively change pain perception at different temporal phases and high and low levels of the central nervous system [57–65].

Temporal Aspects

Considering the temporal aspects, pain can be studied during the expectation phase (e.g., when pain is anticipated) and during the perception phase (e.g., when pain is experienced) (Figure 2). During the expectation phase, activation of the anterior cingulate cortex, precentral and lateral prefrontal cortex, and periaqueductal gray has been documented; during the perception phase, deactivation has been found in different brain regions such as the mid- and posterior cingulate cortex, superior temporal and precentral gyri, the anterior and posterior insula, the claustrum and putamen, and the thalamus and caudate body [66] (Figure 2A). As for nocebo effects, where hyperalgesia is expected, increased activity in different brain regions involved in nociceptive processing and emotion regulation (such as the prefrontal cortex, anterior cingulate cortex and insula, primary somatosensory cortex, cerebellum, superior temporal gyrus, and operculum) has been documented [67–70]. During the perception phase, an enhanced activation has been found in regions such as the prefrontal cortex, anterior cingulate cortex, middle frontal gyrus, insula, claustrum, putamen, superior parietal lobule, amygdala, hippocampus, middle temporal gyrus, and periaqueductal gray [71,72] (Figure 2B). These findings concerning the temporal component of pain are confirmed by electroencephalographic (EEG) studies. Interestingly, placebos and nocebos can change EEG brain activity during both the expectation and perception phases [23,73,74]. For example, the expectation of receiving a nonpainful or painful stimulus respectively decreases or increases the amplitude of the contingent negative variation, i.e., an EEG slow negative wave that represents an objective measure of expectation of a specific incoming event (e.g., the expectation of analgesia or hyperalgesia) [23]. Considering the "perception phase", placebo treatments produce decreased laser-evoked potentials, which represents an early measure of nociceptive processes, since it occurs 200–250 ms after painful stimulation [73]. The source of both these evoked potentials has been evaluated and the supplementary motor area, anterior cingulate cortex, middle cingulate cortex, and insula seem fundamental for contingent negative variation, and anterior cingulate cortex, operculum, and secondary sensorial cortex for laser-evoked potentials [75,76]. Moreover, placebo analgesia treatments significantly reduce the amplitude of the N1, P2, and P3 event-related potential components elicited by painful stimulation [77] (Figure 2C).

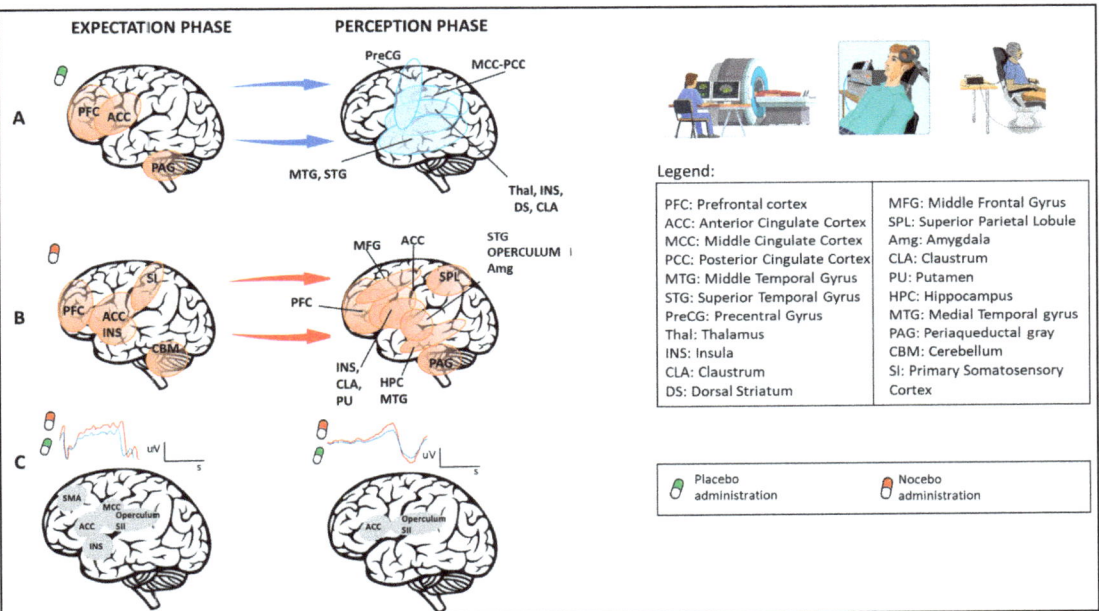

Figure 2. Neuroimaging studies: temporal aspects (expectation and perception phases) related to brain area activity after placebo or nocebo administration. As reported by different neuroimaging studies, expectations of pain relief, triggered by placebos, activate brain areas such as PFC, ACC, and PAG (P1); in the perception phase, deactivation has been found in different brain regions, including MCC, PCC, MTG, STG, PreCG, Thal, INS, CLA, and DS (**A**). On the contrary, expectations of pain worsening, triggered by nocebos, enhance activity in brain regions that include PFC, ACC, INS, SI, and CBM; in the perception phase, increased activity in PFC, ACC, MFG, INS, CLA, PU, HPC, MTG, SPL, STG, OPERCULUM, and INS has been found (**B**). Electroencephalographic (EEG) studies report that placebos and nocebos change EEG brain activity. In particular, the expectation of receiving no painful or painful stimuli respectively decreases (green line) or increases (red line) the amplitude of the contingent negative variation (CNV). Considering the "perception phase", placebo treatments produce a decrease (blue line) in laser-evoked potential (LEP), an EEG wave that represents an early measure of nociceptive processes (**C**).

Central Nervous System

Placebos and nocebos can affect the activity and the connectivity of cortical, subcortical, and spinal areas (Figure 3).

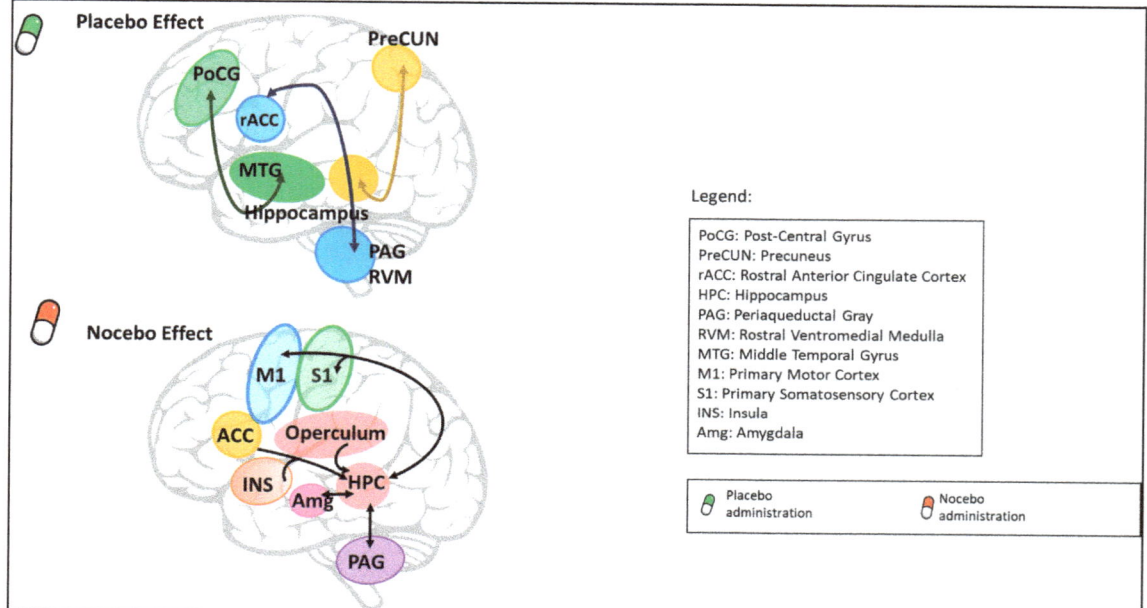

Figure 3. Connectivity analysis data. Connectivity studies have documented changes in functional connectivity in the placebo analgesic effect between PreCUN-HPC, MTG–PoCG, and rACC–PAG–RVM). In the nocebo hyperalgesic effect, functional connectivity changes have been observed among HPC/Operculum and many brain areas, namely ACC, INS, M1, and S1. In addition, functional connectivity between HPC and PAG and Amg has been suggested to play a role in the nocebo hyperalgesic effect.

High Central Nervous System Levels

Starting from the cortical and subcortical levels in placebo expectation studies where inert treatments were delivered along with a verbal suggestion of symptom amelioration, an increase in µ opioid neurotransmission has been observed in different brain areas, such as the pre- and subgenual rostral anterior cingulate cortex [78–82], dorsolateral prefrontal cortex [79–81], orbitofrontal cortex [80,82], anterior insular cortex [79–82], nucleus accumbens [79,81,82], amygdala [79,80,82], thalamus [79,80], and periaqueductal gray [79,82]. On the contrary, when pain exacerbation is expected, a subjective increase in pain ratings has been reported along with increased activity in different brain regions involved in pain processing and emotion regulation, such as the prefrontal cortex, anterior cingulate cortex, and insula [70,71,83,84].

Similar results have been observed in open–hidden studies, where the open (placebo) condition, which maximizes the context effects, produced a behavioral analgesic effect along with deactivation of pain matrix areas, such as the mid and posterior cingulate cortex, insula, and thalamus, and activation of the dorsolateral prefrontal cortex and rostral anterior cingulate cortex [85]. On the contrary, in the hidden (nocebo) condition, which is a condition that significantly reduces the context effects, no changes in pain perception and no pain matrix deactivation were observed. Interestingly, expectations of drug interruption, e.g., expecting the analgesic effect to end, were followed by a blockage of drug analgesia and enhanced activity in the hippocampus [85].

Among all these areas, the dorsolateral prefrontal cortex and intraparietal sulcus seem to play a pivotal role in placebo responsiveness [31]. Studies supporting these conclusions are on healthy volunteers and patients with impairment in frontal regions. In

Alzheimer's patients who show compromised frontal lobes, the placebo analgesia negatively correlates with prefrontal activity impairment [86]. In healthy subjects, the prefrontal inactivation with repetitive transcranial magnetic stimulation results in a blockade of the placebo response [87], while active transcranial direct current stimulation, compared with sham transcranial direct current stimulation, boosts the placebo and blunts the nocebo effects [88]. Frontal activity seems to be crucial for placebo and nocebo responsiveness as researchers found a correlation between frontal activity and placebo effect magnitude; for example, placebo analgesia has been found to correlate with (1) fronto-parietal activity in regions associated with emotion regulation [63], (2) dorsolateral prefrontal cortex connectivity [89–91], and (3) opioid binding in the prefrontal cortex [45,65].

Low Central Nervous System Levels

Besides the study of high-level regions, recent studies have shown that placebo analgesia also involves nociception inhibition at the spinal level [92] and modulation of thalamocortical pathways related to nociception and pain [93,94]. At the same time, connectivity studies have documented changes in functional connectivity between precuneus-hippocampus and middle temporal gyrus-postcentral gyrus [95], and between the rostral anterior cingulate cortex and brain stem [63,90,96]. In particular, significant results suggest the involvement of the descending rostral anterior cingulate cortex-periaqueductal gray-rostral ventromedial medulla pain-modulating pathway, which in concert with other brainstem sites, such as the parabrachial nucleus, substantia nigra, and locus coeruleus, can influence the experience of pain by modulating activity at the level of the dorsal horn [97]. Interestingly, reductions in brain activity in areas that are not often considered, such as the habenula and the cerebellum, have been found [98]. Moreover, neural interactions between the prefrontal areas, brainstem, and spinal cord seem to regulate the nocebo effect. In particular, cognition interacts with the pain pathway through the rostral anterior cingulate cortex-periaqueductal gray-spinal axis, influencing nociceptive processing at the spinal level [99]. When nocebo hyperalgesia occurs, functional connectivity changes have been observed among hippocampus-operculum and other brain areas, including the anterior cingulate cortex, insula, primary motor cortex, and primary somatosensory cortex [71]. In addition, a recent study suggests a relevant role of the hippocampus and its functional connectivity with brain regions involved in the processing of sensory-discriminative aspects of pain, such as the periaqueductal gray and amygdala, in nocebo hyperalgesia [100].

Despite placebo analgesia and nocebo hyperalgesia interfering in pain perception and changing activity in different areas involved in nociceptive processing, it is still unclear if there is a strong correlation between the magnitude of the subjective placebo analgesia and objective changes in the latter areas. Given that the available literature suggests only a small subjective–objective correlation, it is likely that other mechanisms beyond the bottom-up nociceptive processing are involved in placebo analgesia [101]. Indeed, brain regions that are not associated with nociception but with self-regulation and high-level action selection, particularly the supplementary motor area, exhibit reduced activity during placebo analgesia. These effects may reflect a shift in motivation and decision making in the context of pain [31].

2.3. Genetics

Finally, a crucial and novel aspect of placebo and nocebo responsiveness is related to the role of genetic factors that can substantially contribute to these phenomena. The research in this field is in its early years, but it is plausible that placebo effects are determined by a complex network of genetic factors, individual medical experiences, and environmental factors [102]. The study of polymorphisms associated with placebo responsiveness has been focused on the systems involved in the placebo response, e.g., dopamine, opioid, and endocannabinoid systems [103–105]. For example, the polymorphism of the μ-opioid receptor gene (OPRM1) seems to be involved in the individual differences in placebo responsiveness [105,106]. Due to the high incidence of placebo effects in randomized controlled trials (RCTs) of treatments for mood diseases, an interplay with placebo-effect-related genes may also be present in the serotonergic system [103]. Several genes have been suggested to be involved in the serotoninergic system related to placebo remission [79,102]. Hall and colleagues coined the term "placebome" [103] to define the plausible genetic factors that influence the responsiveness to placebos [107]. The former created a placebome module consisting of 54 proteins and evaluated the proximity of the module to modules related to diseases or symptoms known to have a high or low-to-no placebo response by utilizing a seed connector algorithm. Results showed that the placebome was located proximate to the module for diseases or symptoms known to have a high placebo response and distal to conditions known to have a low-to-no placebo response [104]. It is worth noticing that, despite the role played by genetic factors in placebo responsiveness, results from a recent pilot twin study suggest that individual learning experiences are more important than genetic influences, at least in placebo analgesia induced through a conditioning paradigm [108].

2.4. Placebo and Nocebo Effects in Chronic Pain

The study of placebo and nocebo effects in chronic pain patients is extremely complicated. Patients with chronic pain are usually exposed to different long-lasting painful conditions, generally longer than three months, with different levels of pain experience [109]. Indeed, chronic pain is used as an "umbrella term" that incorporates a wide range of clinical conditions, ranging from fibromyalgia, migraine, musculoskeletal pain, or long-standing pain states with or without actual known causes [109]. Therefore, there are no consistent results for the occurrence and magnitude of placebo analgesia in chronic pain disorders [3]. Different studies report that placebo treatments successfully induce analgesia in chronic pain patients [90,110–112], and the effect seems to be stronger in women than in men [113]. RCTs point out that some of the common therapies for low back pain were no better than placebo [114] or only minimally better [115], suggesting that placebo responses can be large and clinically significant [116,117]. Other studies report mixed results. For example, in the meta-analysis of Morozov et al. (2022), placebo demonstrated a significant efficacy on subjective parameters (e.g., visual analogic scale and McGill pain questionnaire) [14]. Generally, a positive patient–clinician communication atmosphere seems a relevant aspect that triggers placebo analgesic effects; for instance, Kaptchuk et al. (2008) compared two placebo acupuncture treatments in patients with irritable bowel syndrome and showed that, while both treatments were superior to a natural history group, the positive therapeutic relationship further increased the efficacy of placebo acupuncture [111].

Overall, even if different studies have confirmed the occurrence of placebo analgesia in patients with chronic pain, it remains unclear if the mechanisms underlying these effects are different or similar to those observed in response to experimental pain protocols in healthy participants [13]. One crucial point is that, due to their personal medical experiences, both populations show completely different pain and treatment efficacy expectations [118,119]. These experiences would likely change the responsiveness to placebo or nocebo contexts. For example, the meta-analysis of Peerdman et al. (2016) indicates that expectations of patients may largely influence experimental and acute pain, whereas they have small effects on chronic pain [120]. Moreover, Muller et al. (2016) observed that, even if placebo analgesia was found to be large for both acute experimental and chronic pain, the two placebo responses were not related [118]. The main role of prior therapeutic experiences is supported by the results of Colloca et al. (2020) that showed a similar placebo analgesia magnitude in both healthy participants and chronic pain patients, which was directly linked to prior therapeutic experiences (conditioning procedure) [121].

Also, from a neurobiological point of view, there seem to be differences between patients and healthy controls in terms of placebo responsiveness, starting with the observation that naloxone appears not to block placebo analgesia in chronic pain states [110,122]. The results suggest that, in chronic pain patients, the opioid system may not be involved in placebo analgesia as in healthy subjects. From one perspective, it is surprising since pharmacological opioids are often used to treat chronic pain [123–125], but it is still true that the efficacy of opioids on chronic pain is debated, especially for long-term treatment [126]. A possible explanation for these results lays in the altered functioning of the opioid system as reported in chronic pain animal models [127] and human patients [128–130]. Different theories try to explain the persistence of pain in chronic conditions. For example, pain perception can be viewed as an inferential process in which top-down expectations and priors interact with bottom-up sensorial data. After administering a treatment, when bottom-up sensorial data changes, priors can be updated following bottom-up changes or maintained. In the case of chronic pain patients, there could be a bias in the interpretation of bottom-up information along with the use of immunization strategies that prevent the update of priors and expectations [131]. In line with this, chronic pain patients tend to explain ambiguous stimuli as pain- or condition-related without positively updating their previous expectations and cognitions [132–135]. An inability to update expectations based on outcomes (e.g., when the pain experience is less than anticipated) would result in a system that is poorly attuned to the external environment [135], and patients with chronic pain seem to lack this ability: studies show that patients are less capable of improving their performance on reward-dependent learning tasks [136–139] and showed an altered loss aversion in a monetary gambling task [140]. In line with this, it is suggested that the reward-related processes in the inability to update expectations are playing a role in the development of prolonged pain [141]. One hypothesis takes into account the possible absence of reward signaling related to endogenous opioid transmission [125], as supported by the studies on the altered opioid system in chronic pain patients [128–130].

Beyond the role of the opioid system, differences in the dopamine system, described both in animals and humans with chronic pain [142], may contribute to the development and maintenance of a chronic pain condition [143]. For example, a single-blinded-placebo trial in chronic pain patients showed that placebo responders had higher functional connectivity enriched by the dopamine transporter than nonresponders. This result suggests that those patients with the strongest dopamine-related neurotransmission might benefit the most from expectancy/placebo effects [125].

Differences in placebo responsiveness in chronic pain patients have also been related to other brain structures and function characteristics. In particular, (functional) Magnetic Resonance Imaging ((f)MRI) research demonstrated that subcortical limbic volume asymmetry, sensorimotor cortical thickness, and functional coupling of prefrontal regions, anterior cingulate cortex, and periaqueductal gray were predictive of placebo responses [90]. It is worth noting that these brain traits were present before administrating a placebo treatment, which provides evidence for a placebo responsiveness propensity and, as demonstrated using a machine learning algorithm, a biosignature to predict the placebo response at group level [90,144].

Despite these differences between healthy controls and chronic pain patients, close correspondence in mechanisms underlying placebo responses in these populations has also been found. For example, levels of activation in the dorsolateral prefrontal cortex and orbitofrontal cortex, as well as the coupling of the dorsolateral prefrontal cortex and rostral anterior cingulate cortex with antinociceptive circuitry [89,90], are believed to be part of both placebo responses [90].

Overall, it remains debatable whether the mechanisms underlying placebo responses in patients really differ from the ones in healthy controls, as well as whether there are true differences in these mechanisms in response to either acute or chronic pain. However, it seems plausible that the results of placebo research in experimental settings on healthy volunteers may not be totally transferable to placebo responses in chronic pain populations.

3. Future Directions for Clinical Practice

As documented in the previous section, the mechanistic placebo literature suggests that inert interventions provided within a specific context can relieve pain [5]. Translation of these findings into clinical practice requires the acknowledgement that positive clinical outcomes in patients seeking care for different painful conditions (e.g., musculoskeletal pain) are related to many factors [131]. Generally, an intervention's effectiveness for a given patient may be attributable to a combined effect of: (1) factors such as natural history and regression to the mean: the natural history of many musculoskeletal disorders is favorable, and patients tend to seek care when their symptoms are at their worst, resulting in regression to the mean with repeated assessment over time; (2) the specific effects of the intervention resulting in improved outcomes regardless of the context of administration; and (3) factors related to the context of the intervention such as whether the patient expects the intervention to be effective and the relationship between the patient and the provider [145,146]. Positive and negative contexts influence the effectiveness of all pain management interventions [147–149]. For example, contextual effects accounted for more than 75% of the improvements observed in RCTs of interventions for osteoarthritis [150] and following surgical interventions for pain [151]. In patients with painful conditions, individual interventions often fail to show added value when directly compared to other interventions with modest treatment effects at best [152,153]. Observing only small differences in effects across multiple interventions that are different based on their theoretical working mechanisms suggests a significant role for contextual factors that these interventions have in common [131]. For instance, consciously seeking to maximize the contextual effects in clinical practice offers an intriguing opportunity to enhance treatment effects by maximizing the specific mechanisms of interventions as well as the context surrounding intervention administration [6,7].

Previously highlighted factors known to influence placebo analgesia also influence clinical outcomes in patients with different chronic pain conditions. For example, recovery expectations [154–156] and the relationship between the patient and provider [157] are known influential factors for the clinical outcome of patients experiencing musculoskeletal pain. Expectations mediating placebo analgesia appear to be depending on social learning [21,22,158–160]. Specifically, expectations may be formed and manipulated through verbal instruction, observation, and conditioning [158,160]. Experimental studies suggest that providing a placebo intervention with the following instruction: "the agent you have just received is known to powerfully reduce pain in some patients" [110], having a participant watch someone else experience pain relief in response to a placebo [161], or undergoing a conditioning protocol [162] are all approaches to enhance expectations which can result in increased placebo analgesia. Similar approaches in the clinic, such as educating patients on the effectiveness of a chosen intervention, making patients aware of the provider's own personal observations of success, the use of patient testimonials, or providing interventions to which a patient has previously had positive experiences, may all be ways to maximize the contextual benefits of interventions for pain through the maximizing of expectations [62,120].

Therapeutic alliance is characterized in psychotherapy as the bond including trust and attachment between the patient and provider and includes consideration of agreement on the goals of therapy and assignment of tasks [163]. The literature on placebos suggests that therapeutic alliance can be enhanced and placebo analgesia increased when a sham intervention is administered by a provider who is warm and friendly, practices active listening, expresses empathy, and expresses confidence in the intervention [111,164,165]. These clinical results support the findings from the literature on experimental placebos [166]. Consequently, outcomes of patients presenting with pain may be improved when a strong therapeutic alliance is established between the patient and the provider [1,2].

In summary, patients with chronic pain may experience improved outcomes in response to an intervention for a variety of reasons beyond the specific effect of the intervention [6,7]. Contextual effects are a component of all interventions for pain that clinicians should implement in their clinical practice (Table 2). The literature on mechanistic placebos provides insight into how these effects can be successfully utilized in clinical practice.

Table 2. Key points for clinical practice and research.

Area	Actions
Clinical Practice	• Considering the patient's previous positive and negative experiences when drawing up the treatment plan. • Evaluate the patient's positive and negative expectations prior to the administration of therapy. • Pay attention to the relationship and therapeutic alliance between the patient and provider during the care continuum. • Emphasizing the clinical improvements that have occurred as a result of therapy. • Consciously and conscientiously use contextual effects to enhance the specific effect of therapy.
Research	• Ensuring the blinding of patients, evaluating and reporting it in placebo-controlled trials. • Using comparators in sham groups that are similar in characteristics to the real treatments in placebo-controlled trials. • Assess patient expectations in placebo-controlled trials. • Recognize that a nontreatment control group to exclude confounders (e.g., the natural history of the disease) in placebo-controlled trials is necessary to establish the magnitude of the placebo effect size. • Assess patient's belief in having participated in the control or active group once placebo-controlled trials have ended.

4. Future Directions for Research and Clinical Trials

High-quality RCTs are the gold standard for treatment effectiveness. The traditional interpretation of null findings in placebo RCTs is considering the experimental intervention as ineffective. Specific to pain as an outcome, this assumption neglects the potential analgesic response to a placebo [145,146]. Consequently, a studied intervention providing no greater pain relief than a placebo comparator may suggest two equally effective interventions, potentially with differing mechanisms behind their effectiveness [167]. Different factors need to be considered for designing and interpreting placebo-controlled studies on interventions for pain [145,146]. The blinding of both patients and providers is an important consideration in placebo-controlled trials given that participants are made aware during the consent process of a 50% chance of receiving a placebo [146]. Blinding may be compromised due to poorly designed placebos which are not credible. Furthermore, blinding may be lost in placebo-controlled medication studies due to sensations unique to the studied intervention [168] or side effects in the active arm [169]. Based on a literature review of sham-controlled trials concerning back pain interventions, it appeared that a higher percentage of participants in active trial arms correctly identified their intervention, e.g., active and not sham, while blinding was successful in the sham arms of the studies [170]. Importantly, larger treatment effect sizes were observed in response to both the studied intervention and sham intervention when participants believed they received the active intervention [170]. Therefore, blinding should be carefully considered in placebo-controlled trials of pain management interventions and care should be taken to design sham or placebo comparators which are effective in maintaining blinding. Furthermore, blinding success should be assessed and reported in such trials [145,146].

Moreover, expectations are a primary mechanism of placebo analgesia [147]. Discrepancies between participant expectations concerning the success of a provided intervention between the active and placebo arms of a study could influence the observed outcomes [171]. Consequently, when designing placebo comparators for interventions for pain, care should be taken to assess expectations and ensure that the expectations for each arm of the study are similar [160].

Then, the true effect size of contextual effects on clinical outcomes requires additional consideration beyond the traditional two-arm placebo RCT. First, attributing changes in outcomes in a placebo treatment arm of a study to the placebo effect is temping; however, such an approach can be misleading [145,146]. Changes in the placebo arm should be considered as the placebo response; however, accurately measuring the placebo effect requires a no-treatment control group to account for influences such as natural history and regression to the mean [8].

Participants in an RCT are aware through the consent process of having a 50% chance of receiving a placebo. Consequently, individuals volunteering to participate in an RCT may differ from those presenting for clinical care, where expectations for improvement tend to be high [172,173]. Placebo mechanism studies differ from placebo-controlled studies given that participants are provided a placebo but instructed that they are receiving an effective intervention [147,148]. This study design is more consistent with clinical care in which interventions are generally provided by enthusiastic practitioners who instruct the patient of the likely effectiveness of the chosen intervention [147,148]. Placebo responses are greater in placebo mechanism studies than in placebo control studies [147] and similar approaches may result in a more accurate representation of the magnitude of contextual effect sizes in clinical practice. Furthermore, placebo-controlled studies may underestimate the effect of interventions. A literature review of studies on antidepressants observed significantly greater responses to treatment in terms of depression in studies with active comparators as compared to placebo-controlled studies [174]. Participants in studies with an active comparator were twice as likely to respond and one and a half times as likely to experience remission compared to participants in a traditional placebo-controlled study on antidepressants [174]. Such findings may be attributable to the expectations of participants in the active arm of the placebo-controlled studies who are also aware of the possibility that their intervention is a placebo [171]. Collectively, these findings suggest RCTs may underestimate both the placebo and treatment effects due to differences in expectations from those observed in clinical care [171]. Carefully designed studies may be necessary to account for the true magnitude of the influence of these factors on outcomes and provide a more accurate indication of their role in the effectiveness of interventions, offering opportunity for future research (Table 2).

5. Conclusions and Limitations

In summary, while studies on healthy participants seem consistent and provide a clear picture of how the brain reacts to different contexts at biological, neurophysiological, and genetical levels, there are no consistent results for the occurrence and magnitude of placebo and nocebo effects in chronic pain patients, mainly due to the heterogeneity of painful conditions. Thus, while it is a common experience that the same therapy offered in different contexts may influence the patient's outcome in care settings representing an opportunity for clinicians, future studies on placebo and nocebo effects on patients with chronic pain are urgently needed, calling researchers and trialists to action worldwide.

This state-of-the-art paper presents some limitations. First, given that this paper comprises a narrative overview of the current state of the art, the included studies and data were not selected by adopting a systematic review approach. However, recommendations for performing a narrative biomedical review have been followed [10]. Second, the paper is mainly focused on the neurobiological and clinical aspects of placebo and nocebo effects, without describing the psychological mechanisms and determinants of these phenomena in detail. Third, the paper is limited to the specific topic of pain, even if it is well documented that there is not one sole placebo/nocebo effect, and instead many effects are mediated by a variety of psychological and biological mechanisms.

Author Contributions: Conceptualization, G.R. and E.C.; writing—original draft preparation, G.R., F.C., J.B., L.V. and E.C.; writing—review and editing, G.R., F.C., J.B., E.H., L.V. and E.C.; visualization, G.R., F.C., J.B., E.H., L.V. and E.C.; supervision, E.C.; project administration, E.C. All authors have read and agreed to the published version of the manuscript.

Funding: This research received no external funding.

Institutional Review Board Statement: Not applicable.

Informed Consent Statement: Not applicable.

Data Availability Statement: Being a state of the art review, this study does not contain original data.

Conflicts of Interest: GR leads educational programs on placebo, nocebo effects, and contextual factors in healthcare to under- and postgraduate students along with private CPD courses. The remaining authors declare that the research was conducted in the absence of any commercial or financial relationships that could be construed as a potential conflicts of interest.

Abbreviations

RCT	Randomized Controlled Trial
fMRI	functional Magnetic Resonance Imaging
PET	Positron Emission Tomography
EEG	electroencephalography
VAS	Visual Analogue Scale
NRS	Numerical Rating Scale
CI	Confidence Interval
rTMS	repetitive Transcranial Magnetic Stimulation
ROI	Regions of Interest
M	Male
F	Female

Appendix A

Table A1. Characteristics of the experimental placebo–nocebo studies included in this paper.

Paper ID	Sample Size (M, F, Not Analysed) *	Population Type	Pain Type/Pain Induction	Investigated Outcome	Outcome Measure	Level of Significance
Amanzio and Benedetti, 1999 [20]	229 (132, 97)	Healthy subjects	Experimental ischemic pain	Behavioral (Pharmacological)	Pain tolerance (min)	$p < 0.05$
Amanzio et al., 2001 [21]	364 (278 patients; 86 healthy controls)	Patients (thoracic surgery) and healthy controls	Postoperative pain; experimental ischemic arm pain	Behavioral (Pharmacological)	NRS (0–10)	$p < 0.05$
Benedetti et al., 1995 [40]	93 (52, 41)	Patients (thoracotomy for lung surgery)	Post-surgery pain	Behavioral (Pharmacological)	NRS (0–10)	$p < 0.02$
Benedetti et al., 1996 [39]	340 (154, 186)	Healthy subjects	Experimental ischemic pain	Behavioral (Pharmacological)	NRS (0–10)	$p < 0.05$
Benedetti et al., 1997 [38]	180 (119, 61)	Patients (video-assisted thoracoscopy)	Post-surgery pain	Behavioral (Pharmacological)	NRS (0–10)	$p < 0.05$
Benedetti et al., 2006 [42]	49 (23, 26)	Healthy subjects	Experimental ischemic pain	Behavioral (Pharmacological)	NRS (0–10)	$p < 0.05$
Benedetti et al., 2006 [86]	44 (28 patients (11, 17), 16 controls)	Patients (Alzheimer's disease) and healthy subjects	Burning pain after venipuncture	Electrophysiological (EEG)	NRS (0–10)	$p < 0.05$
Benedetti et al., 2010 [41]	40 (20, 20)	Healthy subjects	Experimental ischemic pain	Behavioral (Pharmacological)	Tolerance time	$p < 0.05$
Benedetti et al., 2011 [36]	82 (41, 41)	Healthy subjects	Experimental ischemic pain	Behavioral (Pharmacological)	Tolerance time	95%CI
Benedetti et al., 2014 [54]	74 (30, 44)	Healthy subjects	Hypobaric hypoxia headache	Behavioral (Pharmacological)	NRS (0–10)	95%CI
Benedetti et al., 2022 [37]	149 (82, 67)	Healthy subjects	Experimental ischemic pain	Behavioral (Pharmacological)	0–10 rating scale	$p < 0.05$

Table A1. *Cont.*

Paper ID	Sample Size (M, F, Not Analysed) *	Population Type	Pain Type/Pain Induction	Investigated Outcome	Outcome Measure	Level of Significance
Bingel et al. 2011 [85]	22 (15, 7)	Healthy subjects	Heat pain	Neuroimaging (fMRI)	VAS (0–100)	$p < 0.05$
Bingel et al., 2022 [100]	22 (15, 7)	Healthy subjects	Heat pain	Neuroimaging; functional connectivity (fMRI)	VAS (0–100)	$p < 0.05$
Bush et al., 2021 [95]	37 (12, 25)	Healthy subjects	Heat pain	Neuroimaging; functional connectivity (fMRI)	VAS (0–100)	$p < 0.05$
Camerone et al., 2021 [16]	166 (78, 88, 9)	Healthy subjects	Electrical stimuli	Behavioral	NRS (0–10)	$p < 0.05$
Camerone et al., 2021 [17]	77 (24, 24, 29)	Healthy subjects	Cold pressor test (CPT)	Behavioral	Numerical Pain Intensity (0–100)	$p < 0.05$
Camerone et al., 2022 [18]	51 (24, 27, 10)	Healthy subjects	Cold pressor test (CPT)	Behavioral	NRS (0–10)	$p < 0.05$
Carlino et al., 2015 [73]	34 (20, 14)	Healthy subjects	Laser stimulation	Electrophysiology (EEG)	NRS (0–10)	$p < 0.05$
Carlino et al., 2016 [26]	80 (34, 46)	Healthy subjects	Electrical stimuli	Behavioral	NRS (0–10)	$p < 0.05$
Colloca et al., 2006 [24]	30 (5, 25)	Healthy subjects	Electrical stimuli	Behavioral	NRS (0–10)	$p < 0.05$
Colloca et al., 2008 [21]	116 (0, 116)	Healthy subjects	Electrical stimuli	Behavioral	NRS (0–10)	$p < 0.05$
Colloca et al., 2010 [25]	46 (16, 30)	Healthy subjects	Electrical stimuli	Behavioral	VAS (0–10	$p < 0.05$
Colloca et al., 2016 [50]	109 (55, 54, 1)	Healthy subjects	Electrical stimuli	Behavioral	VAS (0–10)	$p < 0.05$
Colloca et al., 2019 [105]	160 (58, 102)	Healthy subjects	Electrical and heat stimuli	DNA genotyping; epistasis	VAS (0–10)	$p < 0.001$
Colloca et al., 2020 [121]	763 (363 patients (85, 278); 400 healthy controls (162; 238)	Patients (chronic orofacial pain) and healthy subjects	Heat stimuli	Behavioral	VAS	$p < 0.05$
Disley et al., 2021 [30]	104 (10, 65, 29)	Healthy subjects	Cold pressor test (CPT)	Behavioral	VAS (0–100)	$p = 0.05$
Eippert et al., 2009 [34]	48 (48, -, 8)	Healthy subjects	Heat pain	Neuroimaging (fMRI)	VAS (0–100)	$p \leq 0.05$
Eippert et al., 2009 [92]	15 (15, 0)	Healthy subjects	Heat pain	Neuroimaging (fMRI)	VAS (0–100)	$p < 0.05$
Ellerbrock et al., 2015 [35]	40 (20, 20, 1)	Healthy subjects	Heat pain	Neuroimaging; functional connectivity (fMRI)	VAS (0–100)	$p < 0.05$
Fuentes et al., 2014 [164]	117	Patients (chronic low back pain)	-	Behavioral	NRS (0–10)	$p < 0.05$
Hashmi et al., 2014 [91]	42	Patients (chronic knee osteoarthritis)	Heat pain	Neuroimaging (fMRI)	Gracely Sensory Scale (0–20)	$p < 0.05$
Jarcho et al., 2016 [46]	15 (0, 15)	Healthy subjects	Heat pain	Neuroimaging (PET; fMRI)	VAS (0–100)	$p < 0.005$

Table A1. *Cont.*

Paper ID	Sample Size (M, F, Not Analysed) *	Population Type	Pain Type/Pain Induction	Investigated Outcome	Outcome Measure	Level of Significance
Kaptchuk et al., 2008 [111]	262 (63, 199)	Patients (irritable bowel syndrome)	-	Behavioral	Global improvement scale (range 1–7); adequate relief of symptoms; symptom severity	$p < 0.01$
Kelley et al., 2009 [165]	189	Patients (irritable bowel syndrome)	-	Behavioral	Combined outcome (IBS Symptom Severity Scale; IBS Quality of Like Scale; IBS Global Improvement Scale; IBS Adequate Relief)	$p < 0.05$
Kessner et al., 2013 [51]	80 (80, 0)	Healthy subjects	Heat pain	Behavioral (Pharmacological)	Visual Analogue Scale (0–100)	$p < 0.05$
Klinger et al., 2017 [112]	48 (12, 36)	Patients (chronic back pain)	Electrical stimuli	Behavioral	NRS (0–10)	95% CI
Kong et al., 2006 [57]	24 (13, 11)	Healthy subjects	Heat pain	Neuroimaging (fMRI)	0–20 Sensory Box Scale	$p < 0.0001$ for ROI $p = 0.05$
Kong et al., 2008 [71]	20 (5, 8, 7)	Healthy subjects	Heat pain	Neuroimaging (fMRI)	Gracely Sensory and Affective Scales	$p < 0.05$
Koyama et al., 2005 [70]	10 (8, 2)	Healthy subjects	Heat pain	Neuroimaging (fMRI)	VAS	$p < 0.01$
Krummenacher et al., 2010 [87]	40 (40, 0)	Healthy subjects	Heat pain	rTMS	VAS (0–10)	$p \leq 0.05$
Kube et al., 2020 [29]	117 (48, 53, 16)	Healthy subjects	Heat pain	Behavioral	Pain tolerance	$p < 0.05$
Lieberman et al., 2004 [58]	52 (29 active drug; 23 placebo condition)	Patients (irritable bowel syndrome)	-	Neuroimaging (PET)	Symptom diary (4 weeks)	$p < 0.005$
Malfiet et al., 2019 [79]	83	Patients (chronic neck pain)	-	Behavioral	VAS (0–100)	$p = 0.05$
Martins et al., 2022 [125]	56	Patients (chronic knee osteoarthritis)	-	Neuroimaging; functional connectivity (fMRI)	VAS (0–10)	$p < 0.05$
Morton et al., 2010 [74]	67 (21, 35, 11)	Healthy subjects	Laser stimulation	Electrophysiological (EEG)	0–10 scale	$p = 0.05$
Müller et al., 2016 [118]	50 (27, 32, 1)	Patients (chronic pain)	Pressure-pain stimuli	Behavioral	VAS (0–100)	$p < 0.05$
Olson et al., 2021 [113]	280 (65, 215)	Patients (chronic orofacial pain)	Heat pain	Behavioral	VAS (0–100)	$p < 0.05$
Peciña et al., 2015 [106]	50 (21, 29)	Healthy subjects	5% hypertonic saline	DNA genotyping; Neuroimaging (PET)	VAS (0–100)	$p < 0.05$
Petrovic et al., 2002 [60]	9	Healthy subjects	Heat stimuli	Neuroimaging (PET)	VAS (0–100)	$p = 0.005$
Petrovic et al., 2010 [59]	24 (9, 15)	Healthy subjects	Heat stimuli	Neuroimaging (PET; fMRI)	VAS (0–100)	$p < 0.05$
Piedimonte et al., 2017 [23]	34 (16, 18, -)	Healthy subject	Electrical stimuli	Electrophysiological (EEG)	NRS (0–10)	$p < 0.05$

Table A1. *Cont.*

Paper ID	Sample Size (M, F, Not Analysed) *	Population Type	Pain Type/Pain Induction	Investigated Outcome	Outcome Measure	Level of Significance
Ploghaus et al., 1999 [67]	12 (7, 5)	Healthy subjects	Heat stimuli	Neuroimaging (fMRI)	VAS (0–10)	$p < 0.05$
Pollo et al., 2001 [81]	38	Patients (thoracotomized patients)	-	Behavioral	NRS (0–10)	$p < 0.01$
Porro et al., 2002 [69]	30 (10, 16, 4)	Healthy subjects	Acid solution injection	Neuroimaging (fMRI)	0–100 scale rating	$p < 0.05$
Price et al., 1999 [162]	40 (16, 24)	Healthy subjects	Heat pain	Behavioral	VAS (0–10)	$p < 0.05$
Price et al., 2007 [61]	9	Patients (irritable bowel syndrome)	Barostat balloon distension—pressure stimuli	Neuroimaging (fMRI)	100-unit rating scale	$p < 0.05$
Prossin et al., 2022 [55]	37 (12, 25)	Healthy subjects	Hypertonic saline injection	Neuroimaging (PET, MRI)	VAS (0–100)	$p < 0.05$
Rief et al., 2012 [168]	144 (50, 904)	Healthy participants	Heat pain	Behavioral	Pain threshold change in °C	$p < 0.05$
Ruscheweyh et al., 2014 [98]	60 (30 patients, 30 controls)	Patients (cerebellum infarction) and healthy subjects	Heat; pressure; pinprick pain	Behavioral	NRS (0–10)	$p < 0.05$
Sawamoto et al., 2000 [83]	10 (10, 0)	Healthy subjects	Laser thermal stimulation	Neuroimaging (fMRI)	0–100 scale	$p < 0.05$
Schmid et al., 2015 [84]	44 (22, 22)	Healthy subjects	Rectal distension	Neuroimaging (fMRI)	VAS (0–100)	$p < 0.05$
Schwartz et al., 2022 [161]	44 (18, 26)	Patients (chronic low back pain)	-	Behavioral	NRS (0–10)	$p < 0.05$
Scott et al., 2007 [49]	48 (30 Study1; 16 Study2; 18 Male controls)	Healthy subjects	5% hypertonic saline injection	Neuroimaging (Study1—PET, fMRI Study2—fMRI)	VAS (0–100)	$p < 0.05$
Scott et al., 2008 [43]	20 (9, 11); 18 (18, 0)	Healthy subjects	Sustained muscle pain challenge	Neuroimaging (PET, MRI)	VAS (0–100)	$p < 0.0001$ for ROI $p = 0.05$
Skyt et al., 2018 [47]	19 (10, 9)	Patients (neuropathic pain)	Pinprick-evoked pain; wind-up-like pain	Behavioral	VAS (0–10; 0–100)	$p < 0.05$
Tétreault et al., 2016 [89]	98 (17 Study1; 39 Study2; 42 Study3)	Patients (chronic knee osteoarthritis pain)	-	Neuroimaging (fMRI)	VAS (0–10); Western Ontario and McMaster Universities Osteoarthritis Index	$p < 0.05$
Tinnermann et al., 2017 [99]	57 (27, 22, 8)	Healthy subjects	Heat stimuli	Neuroimaging (fMRI)	VAS (0–100)	$p < 0.05$
Tu et al., 2021 [88]	81 (44, 37)	Healthy subjects	Heat stimuli	Neuroimaging (fMRI); tDCS	Gracely Sensory Scale (0–20)	$p < 0.05$
Vachon-Presseau et al., 2018 [90]	129 (43 placebo group, 20 controls, 66 excluded)	Patients (chronic back pain)	Back pain intensity	Neuroimaging (MRI, fMRI)	VAS (0–10)	$p < 0.05$
Vachon-Presseau et al., 2022 [144]	181 (94 randomized to 3 arms, 87 excluded)	Patients (chronic low back pain)	Back pain intensity	Neuroimaging (fMRI)	Likert Scale (twice a day)	$p < 0.05$

Table A1. *Cont.*

Paper ID	Sample Size (M, F, Not Analysed) *	Population Type	Pain Type/Pain Induction	Investigated Outcome	Outcome Measure	Level of Significance
Van der Meulen et al., 2017 [72]	30 (13, 17)	Healthy subjects	Heat stimuli	Neuroimaging (fMRI)	VAS (0–100)	$p < 0.05$
Vase et al., 2003 [82]	13	Patients (irritable bowel syndrome)	Evoked rectal distension; heat pain	Behavioral	VAS (0–10)	$p < 0.05$
Vase et al., 2005 [110]	26 (0, 26)	Patients (irritable bowel syndrome)	Rectal distension	Behavioral (Pharmacological)	VAS (0–10)	$p < 0.05$
Vecchio et al., 2021 [77]	63 (31, 32)	Healthy subjects	Electrical stimuli	Electrophysiological (EEG)	7 point Likert scale	$p = 0.05$
Wager et al., 2004 [64]	47	Healthy subjects	Shock pain; heat pain	Neuroimaging (fMRI)	10 point scale	$p < 0.05$
Wager et al., 2007 [65]	15 (15, 0)	Healthy subjects	Heat stimuli	Neuroimaging (PET)	VAS (0–10)	$p < 0.05$
Wager et al., 2011 [63]	47	Healthy subjects	Shock pain; heat pain	Neuroimaging (fMRI)	10 point scale	$p < 0.001$
Wanigasekera et al., 2018 [96]	16	Patients (Post-traumatic neuropathic pain)	-	Neuroimaging (MRI)	NRS (0–10)	$p = 0.05$
Weimer et al., 2019 [108]	39 (25 monozygotic; 14 dizygotic twin pairs)	Healthy subjects	Heat pain	Behavioral	NRS (0–10)	$p < 0.05$
Wrobel et al., 2014 [48]	50 (28, 32, 12)	Healthy subjects	Heat pain	Neuroimaging (fMRI); Pharmacological	VAS (0–100)	$p < 0.05$

* If not differently specified.

References

1. Hohenschurz-Schmidt, D.; Thomson, O.P.; Rossettini, G.; Miciak, M.; Newell, D.; Roberts, L.; Vase, L.; Draper-Rodi, J. Avoiding nocebo and other undesirable effects in chiropractic, osteopathy and physiotherapy: An invitation to reflect. *Musculoskelet. Sci. Pract.* **2022**, *62*, 102677. [CrossRef] [PubMed]
2. Palese, A.; Rossettini, G.; Colloca, L.; Testa, M. The impact of contextual factors on nursing outcomes and the role of placebo/nocebo effects: A discussion paper. *Pain Rep.* **2019**, *4*, e716. [CrossRef] [PubMed]
3. Colloca, L. Placebo effects in pain. *Int. Rev. Neurobiol.* **2020**, *153*, 167–185. [CrossRef] [PubMed]
4. Ongaro, G.; Kaptchuk, T.J. Symptom perception, placebo effects, and the Bayesian brain. *Pain* **2019**, *160*, 1–4. [CrossRef] [PubMed]
5. Benedetti, F.; Frisaldi, E.; Shaibani, A. Thirty Years of Neuroscientific Investigation of Placebo and Nocebo: The Interesting, the Good, and the Bad. *Annu. Rev. Pharmacol. Toxicol.* **2022**, *62*, 323–340. [CrossRef]
6. Carlino, E.; Frisaldi, E.; Benedetti, F. Pain and the context. *Nat. Rev. Rheumatol.* **2014**, *10*, 348–355. [CrossRef]
7. Carlino, E.; Benedetti, F. Different contexts, different pains, different experiences. *Neuroscience* **2016**, *338*, 19–26. [CrossRef]
8. Benedetti, F. Placebo and the new physiology of the doctor-patient relationship. *Physiol. Rev.* **2013**, *93*, 1207–1246. [CrossRef]
9. Colloca, L.; Lopiano, L.; Lanotte, M.; Benedetti, F. Overt versus covert treatment for pain, anxiety, and Parkinson's disease. *Lancet Neurol.* **2004**, *3*, 679–684. [CrossRef]
10. Gasparyan, A.Y.; Ayvazyan, L.; Blackmore, H.; Kitas, G.D. Writing a narrative biomedical review: Considerations for authors, peer reviewers, and editors. *Rheumatol. Int.* **2011**, *31*, 1409–1417. [CrossRef]
11. Benedetti, F.; Piedimonte, A. The neurobiological underpinnings of placebo and nocebo effects. *Semin. Arthritis Rheum.* **2019**, *49*, S18–S21. [CrossRef]
12. Carlino, E.; Piedimonte, A.; Benedetti, F. Chapter 48—Nature of the placebo and nocebo effect in relation to functional neurologic disorders. In *Handbook of Clinical Neurology*; Hallett, M., Stone, J., Carson, A., Eds.; Elsevier: Amsterdam, The Netherlands, 2016; Volume 139, pp. 597–606.
13. Klinger, R.; Stuhlreyer, J.; Schwartz, M.; Schmitz, J.; Colloca, L. Clinical Use of Placebo Effects in Patients with Pain Disorders. *Int. Rev. Neurobiol.* **2018**, *139*, 107–128. [CrossRef]
14. Morozov, A.; Bazarkin, A.; Babaevskaya, D.; Taratkin, M.; Kozlov, V.; Suvorov, A.; Spivak, L.; McFarland, J.; Russo, G.I.; Enikeev, D. A systematic review and meta-analysis of placebo effect in clinical trials on chronic prostatitis/chronic pelvic pain syndrome. *Prostate* **2022**, *82*, 633–656. [CrossRef]

15. Colagiuri, B.; Schenk, L.A.; Kessler, M.D.; Dorsey, S.G.; Colloca, L. The placebo effect: From concepts to genes. *Neuroscience* **2015**, *307*, 171–190. [CrossRef]
16. Camerone, E.M.; Piedimonte, A.; Testa, M.; Wiech, K.; Vase, L.; Zamfira, D.A.; Benedetti, F.; Carlino, E. The Effect of Temporal Information on Placebo Analgesia and Nocebo Hyperalgesia. *Psychosom. Med.* **2021**, *83*, 43–50. [CrossRef] [PubMed]
17. Camerone, E.M.; Wiech, K.; Benedetti, F.; Carlino, E.; Job, M.; Scafoglieri, A.; Testa, M. 'External timing' of placebo analgesia in an experimental model of sustained pain. *Eur. J. Pain* **2021**, *25*, 1303–1315. [CrossRef] [PubMed]
18. Camerone, E.M.; Battista, S.; Benedetti, F.; Carlino, E.; Sansone, L.G.; Buzzatti, L.; Scafoglieri, A.; Testa, M. The Temporal Modulation of Nocebo Hyperalgesia in a Model of Sustained Pain. *Front. Psychiatry* **2022**, *13*, 807138. [CrossRef] [PubMed]
19. Rosenkjær, S.; Lunde, S.J.; Kirsch, I.; Vase, L. Expectations: How and when do they contribute to placebo analgesia? *Front. Psychiatry* **2022**, *13*, 817179. [CrossRef]
20. Amanzio, M.; Benedetti, F. Neuropharmacological dissection of placebo analgesia: Expectation-activated opioid systems versus conditioning-activated specific subsystems. *J. Neurosci.* **1999**, *19*, 484–494. [CrossRef]
21. Colloca, L.; Sigaudo, M.; Benedetti, F. The role of learning in nocebo and placebo effects. *PAIN®* **2008**, *136*, 211–218. [CrossRef]
22. Colloca, L.; Miller, F.G. How placebo responses are formed: A learning perspective. *Philos. Trans. R. Soc. Lond. B. Biol. Sci.* **2011**, *366*, 1859–1869. [CrossRef] [PubMed]
23. Piedimonte, A.; Guerra, G.; Vighetti, S.; Carlino, E. Measuring expectation of pain: Contingent negative variation in placebo and nocebo effects. *Eur. J. Pain* **2017**, *21*, 874–885. [CrossRef] [PubMed]
24. Colloca, L.; Benedetti, F. How prior experience shapes placebo analgesia. *Pain* **2006**, *124*, 126–133. [CrossRef]
25. Colloca, L.; Petrovic, P.; Wager, T.D.; Ingvar, M.; Benedetti, F. How the number of learning trials affects placebo and nocebo responses. *Pain* **2010**, *151*, 430–439. [CrossRef]
26. Carlino, E.; Guerra, G.; Piedimonte, A. Placebo effects: From pain to motor performance. *Neurosci. Lett.* **2016**, *632*, 224–230. [CrossRef]
27. Benedetti, F.; Carlino, E.; Pollo, A. Hidden administration of drugs. *Clin. Pharmacol. Ther.* **2011**, *90*, 651–661. [CrossRef]
28. Amanzio, M.; Pollo, A.; Maggi, G.; Benedetti, F. Response variability to analgesics: A role for non-specific activation of endogenous opioids. *Pain* **2001**, *90*, 205–215. [CrossRef]
29. Kube, T.; Rief, W.; Vivell, M.B.; Schäfer, N.L.; Vermillion, T.; Körfer, K.; Glombiewski, J.A. Deceptive and Nondeceptive Placebos to Reduce Pain: An Experimental Study in Healthy Individuals. *Clin. J. Pain* **2020**, *36*, 68–79. [CrossRef]
30. Disley, N.; Kola-Palmer, S.; Retzler, C. A comparison of open-label and deceptive placebo analgesia in a healthy sample. *J. Psychosom. Res.* **2021**, *140*, 110298. [CrossRef] [PubMed]
31. Zunhammer, M.; Spisák, T.; Wager, T.D.; Bingel, U. Meta-analysis of neural systems underlying placebo analgesia from individual participant fMRI data. *Nat. Commun.* **2021**, *12*, 1391. [CrossRef] [PubMed]
32. Frisaldi, E.; Shaibani, A.; Benedetti, F. Understanding the mechanisms of placebo and nocebo effects. *Swiss Med. Wkly.* **2020**, *150*, w20340. [CrossRef]
33. Ortega, Á.; Salazar, J.; Galban, N.; Rojas, M.; Ariza, D.; Chávez-Castillo, M.; Nava, M.; Riaño-Garzón, M.E.; Díaz-Camargo, E.A.; Medina-Ortiz, O.; et al. Psycho-Neuro-Endocrine-Immunological Basis of the Placebo Effect: Potential Applications beyond Pain Therapy. *Int. J. Mol. Sci.* **2022**, *23*, 4196. [CrossRef]
34. Eippert, F.; Bingel, U.; Schoell, E.D.; Yacubian, J.; Klinger, R.; Lorenz, J.; Büchel, C. Activation of the opioidergic descending pain control system underlies placebo analgesia. *Neuron* **2009**, *63*, 533–543. [CrossRef] [PubMed]
35. Ellerbrock, I.; Wiehler, A.; Arndt, M.; May, A. Nocebo context modulates long-term habituation to heat pain and influences functional connectivity of the operculum. *Pain* **2015**, *156*, 2222–2233. [CrossRef]
36. Benedetti, F.; Amanzio, M.; Rosato, R.; Blanchard, C. Nonopioid placebo analgesia is mediated by CB1 cannabinoid receptors. *Nat. Med.* **2011**, *17*, 1228–1230. [CrossRef]
37. Benedetti, F.; Shaibani, A.; Arduino, C.; Thoen, W. Open-label nondeceptive placebo analgesia is blocked by the opioid antagonist naloxone. *Pain* **2022**, *164*, 984–990. [CrossRef]
38. Benedetti, F.; Amanzio, M.; Casadio, C.; Oliaro, A.; Maggi, G. Blockade of nocebo hyperalgesia by the cholecystokinin antagonist proglumide. *Pain* **1997**, *71*, 135–140. [CrossRef]
39. Benedetti, F. The opposite effects of the opiate antagonist naloxone and the cholecystokinin antagonist proglumide on placebo analgesia. *Pain* **1996**, *64*, 535–543. [CrossRef] [PubMed]
40. Benedetti, F.; Amanzio, M.; Maggi, G. Potentiation of placebo analgesia by proglumide. *Lancet* **1995**, *346*, 1231. [CrossRef] [PubMed]
41. Benedetti, F.; Amanzio, M.; Thoen, W. Disruption of opioid-induced placebo responses by activation of cholecystokinin type-2 receptors. *Psychopharmacology* **2011**, *213*, 791–797. [CrossRef]
42. Benedetti, F.; Amanzio, M.; Vighetti, S.; Asteggiano, G. The biochemical and neuroendocrine bases of the hyperalgesic nocebo effect. *J. Neurosci.* **2006**, *26*, 12014–12022. [CrossRef]
43. Scott, D.J.; Stohler, C.S.; Egnatuk, C.M.; Wang, H.; Koeppe, R.A.; Zubieta, J.K. Placebo and nocebo effects are defined by opposite opioid and dopaminergic responses. *Arch. Gen. Psychiatry* **2008**, *65*, 220–231. [CrossRef] [PubMed]
44. Irizarry, K.J.; Licinio, J. An explanation for the placebo effect? *Science* **2005**, *307*, 1411–1412. [CrossRef] [PubMed]
45. Peciña, M.; Zubieta, J.K. Molecular mechanisms of placebo responses in humans. *Mol. Psychiatry* **2015**, *20*, 416–423. [CrossRef]

5. Jarcho, J.M.; Feier, N.A.; Labus, J.S.; Naliboff, B.; Smith, S.R.; Hong, J.Y.; Colloca, L.; Tillisch, K.; Mandelkern, M.A.; Mayer, E.A.; et al. Placebo analgesia: Self-report measures and preliminary evidence of cortical dopamine release associated with placebo response. *NeuroImage Clin.* **2016**, *10*, 107–114. [CrossRef] [PubMed]

7. Skyt, I.; Moslemi, K.; Baastrup, C.; Grosen, K.; Benedetti, F.; Petersen, G.L.; Price, D.D.; Hall, K.T.; Kaptchuk, T.J.; Svensson, P.; et al. Dopaminergic tone does not influence pain levels during placebo interventions in patients with chronic neuropathic pain. *Pain* **2018**, *159*, 261–272. [CrossRef]

8. Wrobel, N.; Wiech, K.; Forkmann, K.; Ritter, C.; Bingel, U. Haloperidol blocks dorsal striatum activity but not analgesia in a placebo paradigm. *Cortex* **2014**, *57*, 60–73. [CrossRef]

9. Scott, D.J.; Stohler, C.S.; Egnatuk, C.M.; Wang, H.; Koeppe, R.A.; Zubieta, J.K. Individual differences in reward responding explain placebo-induced expectations and effects. *Neuron* **2007**, *55*, 325–336. [CrossRef]

10. Colloca, L.; Pine, D.S.; Ernst, M.; Miller, F.G.; Grillon, C. Vasopressin Boosts Placebo Analgesic Effects in Women: A Randomized Trial. *Biol. Psychiatry* **2016**, *79*, 794–802. [CrossRef]

11. Kessner, S.; Sprenger, C.; Wrobel, N.; Wiech, K.; Bingel, U. Effect of oxytocin on placebo analgesia: A randomized study. *JAMA* **2013**, *310*, 1733–1735. [CrossRef] [PubMed]

12. Feng, C.; Hackett, P.D.; DeMarco, A.C.; Chen, X.; Stair, S.; Haroon, E.; Ditzen, B.; Pagnoni, G.; Rilling, J.K. Oxytocin and vasopressin effects on the neural response to social cooperation are modulated by sex in humans. *Brain Imaging Behav.* **2015**, *9*, 754–764. [CrossRef]

13. Thompson, R.; Gupta, S.; Miller, K.; Mills, S.; Orr, S. The effects of vasopressin on human facial responses related to social communication. *Psychoneuroendocrinology* **2004**, *29*, 35–48. [CrossRef] [PubMed]

14. Benedetti, F.; Durando, J.; Vighetti, S. Nocebo and placebo modulation of hypobaric hypoxia headache involves the cyclooxygenase-prostaglandins pathway. *Pain* **2014**, *155*, 921–928. [CrossRef] [PubMed]

15. Prossin, A.; Koch, A.; Campbell, P.; Laumet, G.; Stohler, C.S.; Dantzer, R.; Zubieta, J.K. Effects of placebo administration on immune mechanisms and relationships with central endogenous opioid neurotransmission. *Mol. Psychiatry* **2022**, *27*, 831–839. [CrossRef] [PubMed]

16. Skyt, I.; Lunde, S.J.; Baastrup, C.; Svensson, P.; Jensen, T.S.; Vase, L. Neurotransmitter systems involved in placebo and nocebo effects in healthy participants and patients with chronic pain: A systematic review. *Pain* **2020**, *161*, 11–23. [CrossRef]

17. Kong, J.; Gollub, R.L.; Rosman, I.S.; Webb, J.M.; Vangel, M.G.; Kirsch, I.; Kaptchuk, T.J. Brain activity associated with expectancy-enhanced placebo analgesia as measured by functional magnetic resonance imaging. *J. Neurosci.* **2006**, *26*, 381–388. [CrossRef]

18. Lieberman, M.D.; Jarcho, J.M.; Berman, S.; Naliboff, B.D.; Suyenobu, B.Y.; Mandelkern, M.; Mayer, E.A. The neural correlates of placebo effects: A disruption account. *NeuroImage* **2004**, *22*, 447–455. [CrossRef]

19. Petrovic, P.; Kalso, E.; Petersson, K.M.; Andersson, J.; Fransson, P.; Ingvar, M. A prefrontal non-opioid mechanism in placebo analgesia. *Pain* **2010**, *150*, 59–65. [CrossRef]

20. Petrovic, P.; Kalso, E.; Petersson, K.M.; Ingvar, M. Placebo and opioid analgesia—Imaging a shared neuronal network. *Science* **2002**, *295*, 1737–1740. [CrossRef]

51. Price, D.D.; Craggs, J.; Verne, G.N.; Perlstein, W.M.; Robinson, M.E. Placebo analgesia is accompanied by large reductions in pain-related brain activity in irritable bowel syndrome patients. *Pain* **2007**, *127*, 63–72. [CrossRef]

52. Tracey, I. Getting the pain you expect: Mechanisms of placebo, nocebo and reappraisal effects in humans. *Nat. Med.* **2010**, *16*, 1277–1283. [CrossRef]

53. Wager, T.D.; Atlas, L.Y.; Leotti, L.A.; Rilling, J.K. Predicting individual differences in placebo analgesia: Contributions of brain activity during anticipation and pain experience. *J. Neurosci.* **2011**, *31*, 439–452. [CrossRef]

54. Wager, T.D.; Rilling, J.K.; Smith, E.E.; Sokolik, A.; Casey, K.L.; Davidson, R.J.; Kosslyn, S.M.; Rose, R.M.; Cohen, J.D. Placebo-induced changes in FMRI in the anticipation and experience of pain. *Science* **2004**, *303*, 1162–1167. [CrossRef]

55. Wager, T.D.; Scott, D.J.; Zubieta, J.K. Placebo effects on human mu-opioid activity during pain. *Proc. Natl. Acad. Sci. USA* **2007**, *104*, 11056–11061. [CrossRef]

56. Palermo, S.; Benedetti, F.; Costa, T.; Amanzio, M. Pain anticipation: An activation likelihood estimation meta-analysis of brain imaging studies. *Hum. Brain Mapp.* **2015**, *36*, 1648–1661. [CrossRef]

57. Ploghaus, A.; Tracey, I.; Gati, J.S.; Clare, S.; Menon, R.S.; Matthews, P.M.; Rawlins, J.N. Dissociating pain from its anticipation in the human brain. *Science* **1999**, *284*, 1979–1981. [CrossRef] [PubMed]

58. Koyama, T.; Tanaka, Y.Z.; Mikami, A. Nociceptive neurons in the macaque anterior cingulate activate during anticipation of pain. *NeuroReport* **1998**, *9*, 2663–2667. [CrossRef] [PubMed]

59. Porro, C.A.; Baraldi, P.; Pagnoni, G.; Serafini, M.; Facchin, P.; Maieron, M.; Nichelli, P. Does anticipation of pain affect cortical nociceptive systems? *J. Neurosci.* **2002**, *22*, 3206–3214. [CrossRef] [PubMed]

70. Koyama, T.; McHaffie, J.G.; Laurienti, P.J.; Coghill, R.C. The subjective experience of pain: Where expectations be come reality. *Proc. Natl. Acad. Sci. USA* **2005**, *102*, 12950–12955. [CrossRef]

71. Kong, J.; Gollub, R.L.; Polich, G.; Kirsch, I.; Laviolette, P.; Vangel, M.; Rosen, B.; Kaptchuk, T.J. A functional magnetic resonance imaging study on the neural mechanisms of hyperalgesic nocebo effect. *J. Neurosci.* **2008**, *28*, 13354–13362. [CrossRef]

72. Van der Meulen, M.; Kamping, S.; Anton, F. The role of cognitive reappraisal in placebo analgesia: An fMRI study. *Soc. Cogn. Affect. Neurosci.* **2017**, *12*, 1128–1137. [CrossRef] [PubMed]

73. Carlino, E.; Torta, D.M.; Piedimonte, A.; Frisaldi, E.; Vighetti, S.; Benedetti, F. Role of explicit verbal information in conditioned analgesia. *Eur. J. Pain* **2015**, *19*, 546–553. [CrossRef] [PubMed]
74. Morton, D.L.; Brown, C.A.; Watson, A.; El-Deredy, W.; Jones, A.K. Cognitive changes as a result of a single exposure to placebo. *Neuropsychologia* **2010**, *48*, 1958–1964. [CrossRef] [PubMed]
75. Nagai, Y.; Critchley, H.D.; Featherstone, E.; Fenwick, P.B.; Trimble, M.R.; Dolan, R.J. Brain activity relating to the contingent negative variation: An fMRI investigation. *NeuroImage* **2004**, *21*, 1232–1241. [CrossRef]
76. Garcia-Larrea, L.; Frot, M.; Valeriani, M. Brain generators of laser-evoked potentials: From dipoles to functional significance. *Neurophysiol. Clin.* **2003**, *33*, 279–292. [CrossRef]
77. Vecchio, A.; De Pascalis, V. ERP Indicators of Self-Pain and Other Pain Reductions due to Placebo Analgesia Responding: The Moderating Role of the Fight-Flight-Freeze System. *Brain Sci.* **2021**, *11*, 1192. [CrossRef]
78. Linde, K.; Atmann, O.; Meissner, K.; Schneider, A.; Meister, R.; Kriston, L.; Werner, C. How often do general practitioners use placebos and non-specific interventions? Systematic review and meta-analysis of surveys. *PLoS ONE* **2018**, *13*, e0202211 [CrossRef]
79. Malfliet, A.; Lluch Girbés, E.; Pecos-Martin, D.; Gallego-Izquierdo, T.; Valera-Calero, A. The Influence of Treatment Expectations on Clinical Outcomes and Cortisol Levels in Patients With Chronic Neck Pain: An Experimental Study. *Pain Pract.* **2019** *19*, 370–381. [CrossRef]
80. Pavlov, I.; Thompson, W. *The Work of the Digestive Glands*; C. Griffin: London, UK, 1902.
81. Pollo, A.; Amanzio, M.; Arslanian, A.; Casadio, C.; Maggi, G.; Benedetti, F. Response expectancies in placebo analgesia and their clinical relevance. *Pain* **2001**, *93*, 77–84. [CrossRef]
82. Vase, L.; Robinson, M.E.; Verne, G.N.; Price, D.D. The contributions of suggestion, desire, and expectation to placebo effects in irritable bowel syndrome patients. An empirical investigation. *Pain* **2003**, *105*, 17–25. [CrossRef] [PubMed]
83. Sawamoto, N.; Honda, M.; Okada, T.; Hanakawa, T.; Kanda, M.; Fukuyama, H.; Konishi, J.; Shibasaki, H. Expectation of pain enhances responses to nonpainful somatosensory stimulation in the anterior cingulate cortex and parietal operculum/posterior insula: An event-related functional magnetic resonance imaging study. *J. Neurosci.* **2000**, *20*, 7438–7445. [CrossRef]
84. Schmid, J.; Bingel, U.; Ritter, C.; Benson, S.; Schedlowski, M.; Gramsch, C.; Forsting, M.; Elsenbruch, S. Neural underpinnings of nocebo hyperalgesia in visceral pain: A fMRI study in healthy volunteers. *NeuroImage* **2015**, *120*, 114–122. [CrossRef] [PubMed]
85. Bingel, U.; Wanigasekera, V.; Wiech, K.; Ni Mhuircheartaigh, R.; Lee, M.C.; Ploner, M.; Tracey, I. The effect of treatment expectation on drug efficacy: Imaging the analgesic benefit of the opioid remifentanil. *Sci. Transl. Med.* **2011**, *3*, 70ra14. [CrossRef] [PubMed]
86. Benedetti, F.; Arduino, C.; Costa, S.; Vighetti, S.; Tarenzi, L.; Rainero, I.; Asteggiano, G. Loss of expectation-related mechanisms in Alzheimer's disease makes analgesic therapies less effective. *Pain* **2006**, *121*, 133–144. [CrossRef] [PubMed]
87. Krummenacher, P.; Candia, V.; Folkers, G.; Schedlowski, M.; Schönbächler, G. Prefrontal cortex modulates placebo analgesia. *Pain* **2010**, *148*, 368–374. [CrossRef]
88. Tu, Y.; Wilson, G.; Camprodon, J.; Dougherty, D.D.; Vangel, M.; Benedetti, F.; Kaptchuk, T.J.; Gollub, R.L.; Kong, J. Manipulating placebo analgesia and nocebo hyperalgesia by changing brain excitability. *Proc. Natl. Acad. Sci. USA* **2021**, *118*. [CrossRef]
89. Tétreault, P.; Mansour, A.; Vachon-Presseau, E.; Schnitzer, T.J.; Apkarian, A.V.; Baliki, M.N. Brain Connectivity Predicts Placebo Response across Chronic Pain Clinical Trials. *PLoS Biol.* **2016**, *14*, e1002570. [CrossRef]
90. Vachon-Presseau, E.; Berger, S.E.; Abdullah, T.B.; Huang, L.; Cecchi, G.A.; Griffith, J.W.; Schnitzer, T.J.; Apkarian, A.V. Brain and psychological determinants of placebo pill response in chronic pain patients. *Nat. Commun.* **2018**, *9*, 3397. [CrossRef]
91. Hashmi, J.A.; Kong, J.; Spaeth, R.; Khan, S.; Kaptchuk, T.J.; Gollub, R.L. Functional network architecture predicts psychologically mediated analgesia related to treatment in chronic knee pain patients. *J. Neurosci.* **2014**, *34*, 3924–3936. [CrossRef]
92. Eippert, F.; Finsterbusch, J.; Bingel, U.; Büchel, C. Direct evidence for spinal cord involvement in placebo analgesia. *Science* **2009**, *326*, 404. [CrossRef]
93. Duerden, E.G.; Albanese, M.C. Localization of pain-related brain activation: A meta-analysis of neuroimaging data. *Hum. Brain Mapp.* **2013**, *34*, 109–149. [CrossRef]
94. Segerdahl, A.R.; Mezue, M.; Okell, T.W.; Farrar, J.T.; Tracey, I. The dorsal posterior insula subserves a fundamental role in human pain. *Nat. Neurosci.* **2015**, *18*, 499–500. [CrossRef] [PubMed]
95. Bush, N.; Robinson, M.; Bryan, M.; Staud, R.; Boissoneault, J. Task-dependent functional connectivity of pain-related brain regions is related to magnitude of placebo analgesia. *J. Pain* **2021**, *22*, 603. [CrossRef]
96. Wanigasekera, V.; Wartolowska, K.; Huggins, J.P.; Duff, E.P.; Vennart, W.; Whitlock, M.; Massat, N.; Pauer, L.; Rogers, P.; Hoggart, B.; et al. Disambiguating pharmacological mechanisms from placebo in neuropathic pain using functional neuroimaging. *Br. J. Anaesth.* **2018**, *120*, 299–307. [CrossRef]
97. Crawford, L.S.; Mills, E.P.; Hanson, T.; Macey, P.M.; Glarin, R.; Macefield, V.G.; Keay, K.A.; Henderson, L.A. Brainstem Mechanisms of Pain Modulation: A within-Subjects 7T fMRI Study of Placebo Analgesic and Nocebo Hyperalgesic Responses. *J. Neurosci.* **2021**, *41*, 9794–9806. [CrossRef]
98. Ruscheweyh, R.; Kühnel, M.; Filippopulos, F.; Blum, B.; Eggert, T.; Straube, A. Altered experimental pain perception after cerebellar infarction. *Pain* **2014**, *155*, 1303–1312. [CrossRef]
99. Tinnermann, A.; Geuter, S.; Sprenger, C.; Finsterbusch, J.; Büchel, C. Interactions between brain and spinal cord mediate value effects in nocebo hyperalgesia. *Science* **2017**, *358*, 105–108. [CrossRef] [PubMed]

100. Bingel, U.; Wiech, K.; Ritter, C.; Wanigasekera, V.; Ní Mhuircheartaigh, R.; Lee, M.C.; Ploner, M.; Tracey, I. Hippocampus mediates nocebo impairment of opioid analgesia through changes in functional connectivity. *Eur. J. Neurosci.* **2022**, *56*, 3967–3978. [CrossRef] [PubMed]

101. Zunhammer, M.; Bingel, U.; Wager, T.D. Placebo Effects on the Neurologic Pain Signature: A Meta-analysis of Individual Participant Functional Magnetic Resonance Imaging Data. *JAMA Neurol.* **2018**, *75*, 1321–1330. [CrossRef]

102. Cai, L.; He, L. Placebo effects and the molecular biological components involved. *Gen. Psychiatry* **2019**, *32*, e100089. [CrossRef]

103. Hall, K.T.; Loscalzo, J.; Kaptchuk, T.J. Genetics and the placebo effect: The placebome. *Trends Mol. Med.* **2015**, *21*, 285–294. [CrossRef] [PubMed]

104. Hall, K.T.; Loscalzo, J.; Kaptchuk, T. Pharmacogenomics and the Placebo Response. *ACS Chem. Neurosci.* **2018**, *9*, 633–635. [CrossRef] [PubMed]

105. Colloca, L.; Wang, Y.; Martinez, P.E.; Chang, Y.C.; Ryan, K.A.; Hodgkinson, C.; Goldman, D.; Dorsey, S.G. OPRM1 rs1799971, COMT rs4680, and FAAH rs324420 genes interact with placebo procedures to induce hypoalgesia. *Pain* **2019**, *160*, 1824–1834. [CrossRef] [PubMed]

106. Peciña, M.; Love, T.; Stohler, C.S.; Goldman, D.; Zubieta, J.K. Effects of the Mu opioid receptor polymorphism (OPRM1 A118G) on pain regulation, placebo effects and associated personality trait measures. *Neuropsychopharmacology* **2015**, *40*, 957–965. [CrossRef]

107. Wang, R.S.; Hall, K.T.; Giulianini, F.; Passow, D.; Kaptchuk, T.J.; Loscalzo, J. Network analysis of the genomic basis of the placebo effect. *JCI Insight* **2017**, *2*, e93911. [CrossRef] [PubMed]

108. Weimer, K.; Hahn, E.; Mönnikes, N.; Herr, A.K.; Stengel, A.; Enck, P. Are Individual Learning Experiences More Important Than Heritable Tendencies? A Pilot Twin Study on Placebo Analgesia. *Front. Psychiatry* **2019**, *10*, 679. [CrossRef]

109. Raffaeli, W.; Tenti, M.; Corraro, A.; Malafoglia, V.; Ilari, S.; Balzani, E.; Bonci, A. Chronic Pain: What Does It Mean? A Review on the Use of the Term Chronic Pain in Clinical Practice. *J. Pain Res.* **2021**, *14*, 827–835. [CrossRef]

110. Vase, L.; Robinson, M.E.; Verne, N.G.; Price, D.D. Increased placebo analgesia over time in irritable bowel syndrome (IBS) patients is associated with desire and expectation but not endogenous opioid mechanisms. *Pain* **2005**, *115*, 338–347. [CrossRef]

111. Kaptchuk, T.J.; Kelley, J.M.; Conboy, L.A.; Davis, R.B.; Kerr, C.E.; Jacobson, E.E.; Kirsch, I.; Schyner, R.N.; Nam, B.H.; Nguyen, L.T.; et al. Components of placebo effect: Randomised controlled trial in patients with irritable bowel syndrome. *BMJ* **2008**, *336*, 999–1003. [CrossRef]

112. Klinger, R.; Kothe, R.; Schmitz, J.; Kamping, S.; Flor, H. Placebo effects of a sham opioid solution: A randomized controlled study in patients with chronic low back pain. *Pain* **2017**, *158*, 1893–1902. [CrossRef]

113. Olson, E.M.; Akintola, T.; Phillips, J.; Blasini, M.; Haycock, N.R.; Martinez, P.E.; Greenspan, J.D.; Dorsey, S.G.; Wang, Y.; Colloca, L. Effects of sex on placebo effects in chronic pain participants: A cross-sectional study. *Pain* **2021**, *162*, 531–542. [CrossRef]

114. Machado, G.C.; Maher, C.G.; Ferreira, P.H.; Pinheiro, M.B.; Lin, C.W.; Day, R.O.; McLachlan, A.J.; Ferreira, M.L. Efficacy and safety of paracetamol for spinal pain and osteoarthritis: Systematic review and meta-analysis of randomised placebo controlled trials. *BMJ* **2015**, *350*, h1225. [CrossRef]

115. Roelofs, P.D.; Deyo, R.A.; Koes, B.W.; Scholten, R.J.; van Tulder, M.W. Non-steroidal anti-inflammatory drugs for low back pain. *Cochrane Database Syst. Rev.* **2008**, CD000396. [CrossRef] [PubMed]

116. Chaparro, L.E.; Furlan, A.D.; Deshpande, A.; Mailis-Gagnon, A.; Atlas, S.; Turk, D.C. Opioids compared with placebo or other treatments for chronic low back pain: An update of the Cochrane Review. *Spine* **2014**, *39*, 556–563. [CrossRef] [PubMed]

117. Henschke, N.; Kuijpers, T.; Rubinstein, S.M.; van Middelkoop, M.; Ostelo, R.; Verhagen, A.; Koes, B.W.; van Tulder, M.W. Injection therapy and denervation procedures for chronic low-back pain: A systematic review. *Eur. Spine J.* **2010**, *19*, 1425–1449. [CrossRef]

118. Müller, M.; Kamping, S.; Benrath, J.; Skowronek, H.; Schmitz, J.; Klinger, R.; Flor, H. Treatment history and placebo responses to experimental and clinical pain in chronic pain patients. *Eur. J. Pain* **2016**, *20*, 1530–1541. [CrossRef] [PubMed]

119. Constantino, M.J.; Arnkoff, D.B.; Glass, C.R.; Ametrano, R.M.; Smith, J.Z. Expectations. *J. Clin. Psychol.* **2011**, *67*, 184–192. [CrossRef]

120. Peerdeman, K.J.; van Laarhoven, A.I.M.; Keij, S.M.; Vase, L.; Rovers, M.M.; Peters, M.L.; Evers, A.W.M. Relieving patients' pain with expectation interventions: A meta-analysis. *Pain* **2016**, *157*, 1179–1191. [CrossRef]

121. Colloca, L.; Akintola, T.; Haycock, N.R.; Blasini, M.; Thomas, S.; Phillips, J.; Corsi, N.; Schenk, L.A.; Wang, Y. Prior Therapeutic Experiences, Not Expectation Ratings, Predict Placebo Effects: An Experimental Study in Chronic Pain and Healthy Participants. *Psychother. Psychosom.* **2020**, *89*, 371–378. [CrossRef]

122. Kupers, R.; Maeyaert, J.; Boly, M.; Faymonville, M.E.; Laureys, S. Naloxone-insensitive epidural placebo analgesia in a chronic pain patient. *Anesthesiology* **2007**, *106*, 1239–1242. [CrossRef]

123. De Leon-Casasola, O.A. Opioids for chronic pain: New evidence, new strategies, safe prescribing. *Am. J. Med.* **2013**, *126*, S3–S11. [CrossRef] [PubMed]

124. Meske, D.S.; Lawal, O.D.; Elder, H.; Langberg, V.; Paillard, F.; Katz, N. Efficacy of opioids versus placebo in chronic pain: A systematic review and meta-analysis of enriched enrollment randomized withdrawal trials. *J. Pain Res.* **2018**, *11*, 923–934. [CrossRef] [PubMed]

125. Martins, D.; Veronese, M.; Turkheimer, F.E.; Howard, M.A.; Williams, S.C.R.; Dipasquale, O. A candidate neuroimaging biomarker for detection of neurotransmission-related functional alterations and prediction of pharmacological analgesic response in chronic pain. *Brain Commun.* **2022**, *4*, fcab302. [CrossRef] [PubMed]

126. Ballantyne, J.C.; Shin, N.S. Efficacy of opioids for chronic pain: A review of the evidence. *Clin. J. Pain* **2008**, *24*, 469–478. [CrossRef]

127. Thompson, S.J.; Pitcher, M.H.; Stone, L.S.; Tarum, F.; Niu, G.; Chen, X.; Kiesewetter, D.O.; Schweinhardt, P.; Bushnell, M.C. Chronic neuropathic pain reduces opioid receptor availability with associated anhedonia in rat. *Pain* **2018**, *159*, 1856–1866. [CrossRef]

128. DaSilva, A.F.; Zubieta, J.K.; DosSantos, M.F. Positron emission tomography imaging of endogenous mu-opioid mechanisms during pain and migraine. *Pain Rep.* **2019**, *4*, e769. [CrossRef]

129. Maarrawi, J.; Peyron, R.; Mertens, P.; Costes, N.; Magnin, M.; Sindou, M.; Laurent, B.; Garcia-Larrea, L. Differential brain opioid receptor availability in central and peripheral neuropathic pain. *Pain* **2007**, *127*, 183–194. [CrossRef]

130. Harris, R.E.; Clauw, D.J.; Scott, D.J.; McLean, S.A.; Gracely, R.H.; Zubieta, J.K. Decreased central mu-opioid receptor availability in fibromyalgia. *J. Neurosci.* **2007**, *27*, 10000–10006. [CrossRef]

131. Rossettini, G.; Colombi, A.; Carlino, E.; Manoni, M.; Mirandola, M.; Polli, A.; Camerone, E.M.; Testa, M. Unraveling Negative Expectations and Nocebo-Related Effects in Musculoskeletal Pain. *Front. Psychol.* **2022**, *13*, 789377. [CrossRef]

132. Crombez, G.; Van Ryckeghem, D.M.L.; Eccleston, C.; Van Damme, S. Attentional bias to pain-related information: A meta-analysis. *Pain* **2013**, *154*, 497–510. [CrossRef] [PubMed]

133. Pincus, T.; Morley, S. Cognitive-processing bias in chronic pain: A review and integration. *Psychol. Bull.* **2001**, *127*, 599–617. [CrossRef]

134. Schoth, D.E.; Liossi, C. Biased interpretation of ambiguous information in patients with chronic pain: A systematic review and meta-analysis of current studies. *Health Psychol.* **2016**, *35*, 944–956. [CrossRef]

135. Rizvi, S.J.; Gandhi, W.; Salomons, T. Reward processing as a common diathesis for chronic pain and depression. *Neurosci. Biobehav. Rev.* **2021**, *127*, 749–760. [CrossRef]

136. Apkarian, A.V.; Sosa, Y.; Krauss, B.R.; Thomas, P.S.; Fredrickson, B.E.; Levy, R.E.; Harden, R.N.; Chialvo, D.R. Chronic pain patients are impaired on an emotional decision-making task. *Pain* **2004**, *108*, 129–136. [CrossRef] [PubMed]

137. Becker, S.; Kleinböhl, D.; Baus, D.; Hölzl, R. Operant learning of perceptual sensitization and habituation is impaired in fibromyalgia patients with and without irritable bowel syndrome. *Pain* **2011**, *152*, 1408–1417. [CrossRef] [PubMed]

138. Verdejo-García, A.; López-Torrecillas, F.; Calandre, E.P.; Delgado-Rodríguez, A.; Bechara, A. Executive function and decision-making in women with fibromyalgia. *Arch. Clin. Neuropsychol.* **2009**, *24*, 113–122. [CrossRef]

139. Walteros, C.; Sánchez-Navarro, J.P.; Muñoz, M.A.; Martínez-Selva, J.M.; Chialvo, D.; Montoya, P. Altered associative learning and emotional decision making in fibromyalgia. *J. Psychosom. Res.* **2011**, *70*, 294–301. [CrossRef] [PubMed]

140. Berger, S.E.; Baria, A.T.; Baliki, M.N.; Mansour, A.; Herrmann, K.M.; Torbey, S.; Huang, L.; Parks, E.L.; Schnizter, T.J.; Apkarian, A.V. Risky monetary behavior in chronic back pain is associated with altered modular connectivity of the nucleus accumbens. *BMC Res. Notes* **2014**, *7*, 739. [CrossRef]

141. Finan, P.H.; Smith, M.T. The comorbidity of insomnia, chronic pain, and depression: Dopamine as a putative mechanism. *Sleep Med. Rev.* **2013**, *17*, 173–183. [CrossRef]

142. Taylor, A.M.W.; Becker, S.; Schweinhardt, P.; Cahill, C. Mesolimbic dopamine signaling in acute and chronic pain: Implications for motivation, analgesia, and addiction. *Pain* **2016**, *157*, 1194–1198. [CrossRef]

143. Borsook, D.; Erpelding, N.; Becerra, L. Losses and gains: Chronic pain and altered brain morphology. *Expert Rev. Neurother.* **2013**, *13*, 1221–1234. [CrossRef]

144. Vachon-Presseau, E.; Abdullah, T.B.; Berger, S.E.; Huang, L.; Griffith, J.W.; Schnitzer, T.J.; Apkarian, A.V. Validating a biosignature-predicting placebo pill response in chronic pain in the settings of a randomized controlled trial. *Pain* **2022**, *163*, 910–922. [CrossRef]

145. Carlino, E.; Vase, L. Can knowledge of Placebo and Nocebo Mechanisms Help Improve Randomized Clinical Trials? *Int. Rev. Neurobiol.* **2018**, *138*, 329–357. [CrossRef]

146. Benedetti, F.; Carlino, E.; Piedimonte, A. Increasing uncertainty in CNS clinical trials: The role of placebo, nocebo, and Hawthorne effects. *Lancet Neurol.* **2016**, *15*, 736–747. [CrossRef]

147. Vase, L.; Petersen, G.L.; Riley, J.L., 3rd; Price, D.D. Factors contributing to large analgesic effects in placebo mechanism studies conducted between 2002 and 2007. *Pain* **2009**, *145*, 36–44. [CrossRef]

148. Petersen, G.L.; Finnerup, N.B.; Colloca, L.; Amanzio, M.; Price, D.D.; Jensen, T.S.; Vase, L. The magnitude of nocebo effects in pain: A meta-analysis. *Pain* **2014**, *155*, 1426–1434. [CrossRef] [PubMed]

149. Tsutsumi, Y.; Tsujimoto, Y.; Tajika, A.; Omae, K.; Fujii, T.; Onishi, A.; Kataoka, Y.; Katsura, M.; Noma, H.; Sahker, E.; et al. Proportion attributable to contextual effects in general medicine: A meta-epidemiological study based on Cochrane reviews. *BMJ Evid. Based Med.* **2023**, *28*, 40–47. [CrossRef] [PubMed]

150. Zou, K.; Wong, J.; Abdullah, N.; Chen, X.; Smith, T.; Doherty, M.; Zhang, W. Examination of overall treatment effect and the proportion attributable to contextual effect in osteoarthritis: Meta-analysis of randomised controlled trials. *Ann. Rheum. Dis.* **2016**, *75*, 1964–1970. [CrossRef] [PubMed]

151. Jonas, W.B.; Crawford, C.; Colloca, L.; Kaptchuk, T.J.; Moseley, B.; Miller, F.G.; Kriston, L.; Linde, K.; Meissner, K. To what extent are surgery and invasive procedures effective beyond a placebo response? A systematic review with meta-analysis of randomised, sham controlled trials. *BMJ Open* **2015**, *5*, e009655. [CrossRef] [PubMed]

152. Karlsson, M.; Bergenheim, A.; Larsson, M.E.H.; Nordeman, L.; van Tulder, M.; Bernhardsson, S. Effects of exercise therapy in patients with acute low back pain: A systematic review of systematic reviews. *Syst. Rev.* **2020**, *9*, 182. [CrossRef]

53. Artus, M.; van der Windt, D.A.; Jordan, K.P.; Hay, E.M. Low back pain symptoms show a similar pattern of improvement following a wide range of primary care treatments: A systematic review of randomized clinical trials. *Rheumatology* **2010**, *49*, 2346–2356. [CrossRef] [PubMed]
54. Hayden, J.A.; Wilson, M.N.; Riley, R.D.; Iles, R.; Pincus, T.; Ogilvie, R. Individual recovery expectations and prognosis of outcomes in non-specific low back pain: Prognostic factor review. *Cochrane Database Syst. Rev.* **2019**, CD011284. [CrossRef] [PubMed]
55. Mohamed Mohamed, W.J.; Joseph, L.; Canby, G.; Paungmali, A.; Sitilertpisan, P.; Pirunsan, U. Are patient expectations associated with treatment outcomes in individuals with chronic low back pain? A systematic review of randomised controlled trials. *Int. J. Clin. Pract.* **2020**, *74*, e13680. [CrossRef] [PubMed]
56. Wassinger, C.A.; Edwards, D.C.; Bourassa, M.; Reagan, D.; Weyant, E.C.; Walden, R.R. The Role of Patient Recovery Expectations in the Outcomes of Physical Therapist Intervention: A Systematic Review. *Phys. Ther.* **2022**, *102*, pzac008. [CrossRef] [PubMed]
57. Kinney, M.; Seider, J.; Beaty, A.F.; Coughlin, K.; Dyal, M.; Clewley, D. The impact of therapeutic alliance in physical therapy for chronic musculoskeletal pain: A systematic review of the literature. *Physiother. Theory Pract.* **2020**, *36*, 886–898. [CrossRef] [PubMed]
58. Bajcar, E.A.; Bąbel, P. How Does Observational Learning Produce Placebo Effects? A Model Integrating Research Findings. *Front. Psychol.* **2018**, *9*, 2041. [CrossRef]
59. Colloca, L. Placebo, nocebo, and learning mechanisms. *Handb. Exp. Pharm.* **2014**, *225*, 17–35. [CrossRef]
60. Peerdeman, K.J.; van Laarhoven, A.I.; Peters, M.L.; Evers, A.W. An Integrative Review of the Influence of Expectancies on Pain. *Front. Psychol.* **2016**, *7*, 1270. [CrossRef]
61. Schwartz, M.; Fischer, L.M.; Bläute, C.; Stork, J.; Colloca, L.; Zöllner, C.; Klinger, R. Observing treatment outcomes in other patients can elicit augmented placebo effects on pain treatment: A double-blinded randomized clinical trial with patients with chronic low back pain. *Pain* **2022**, *163*, 1313–1323. [CrossRef]
62. Price, D.D.; Milling, L.S.; Kirsch, I.; Duff, A.; Montgomery, G.H.; Nicholls, S.S. An analysis of factors that contribute to the magnitude of placebo analgesia in an experimental paradigm. *Pain* **1999**, *83*, 147–156. [CrossRef]
63. Bordin, E.S. The generalizability of the psychoanalytic concept of the working alliance. *Psychother. Theory Res. Pract.* **1979**, *16*, 252–260. [CrossRef]
64. Fuentes, J.; Armijo-Olivo, S.; Funabashi, M.; Miciak, M.; Dick, B.; Warren, S.; Rashiq, S.; Magee, D.J.; Gross, D.P. Enhanced therapeutic alliance modulates pain intensity and muscle pain sensitivity in patients with chronic low back pain: An experimental controlled study. *Phys. Ther.* **2014**, *94*, 477–489. [CrossRef] [PubMed]
65. Kelley, J.M.; Lembo, A.J.; Ablon, J.S.; Villanueva, J.J.; Conboy, L.A.; Levy, R.; Marci, C.D.; Kerr, C.E.; Kirsch, I.; Jacobson, E.E.; et al. Patient and practitioner influences on the placebo effect in irritable bowel syndrome. *Psychosom. Med.* **2009**, *71*, 789–797. [CrossRef] [PubMed]
66. Di Blasi, Z.; Harkness, E.; Ernst, E.; Georgiou, A.; Kleijnen, J. Influence of context effects on health outcomes: A systematic review. *Lancet* **2001**, *357*, 757–762. [CrossRef] [PubMed]
67. Wartolowska, K.A.; Hohenschurz-Schmidt, D.; Vase, L.; Aronson, J.K. The importance of using placebo controls in nonpharmacological randomised trials. *Pain* **2022**, *164*, 921–925. [CrossRef]
68. Rief, W.; Glombiewski, J.A. The hidden effects of blinded, placebo-controlled randomized trials: An experimental investigation. *Pain* **2012**, *153*, 2473–2477. [CrossRef]
69. Shah, E.; Triantafyllou, K.; Hana, A.A.; Pimentel, M. Adverse events appear to unblind clinical trials in irritable bowel syndrome. *Neurogastroenterol. Motil.* **2014**, *26*, 482–488. [CrossRef]
70. Freed, B.; Williams, B.; Situ, X.; Landsman, V.; Kim, J.; Moroz, A.; Bang, H.; Park, J.J. Blinding, sham, and treatment effects in randomized controlled trials for back pain in 2000–2019: A review and meta-analytic approach. *Clin. Trials* **2021**, *18*, 361–370. [CrossRef]
71. Frisaldi, E.; Shaibani, A.; Benedetti, F. Why We should Assess Patients' Expectations in Clinical Trials. *Pain Ther.* **2017**, *6*, 107–110. [CrossRef]
72. Zeppieri, G., Jr.; George, S.Z. Patient-defined desired outcome, success criteria, and expectation in outpatient physical therapy: A longitudinal assessment. *Health Qual. Life Outcomes* **2017**, *15*, 29. [CrossRef]
73. Zeppieri, G., Jr.; Lentz, T.A.; Atchison, J.W.; Indelicato, P.A.; Moser, M.W.; Vincent, K.R.; George, S.Z. Preliminary results of patient-defined success criteria for individuals with musculoskeletal pain in outpatient physical therapy settings. *Arch. Phys. Med. Rehabil.* **2012**, *93*, 434–440. [CrossRef] [PubMed]
74. Rutherford, B.R.; Sneed, J.R.; Roose, S.P. Does study design influence outcome? The effects of placebo control and treatment duration in antidepressant trials. *Psychother. Psychosom.* **2009**, *78*, 172–181. [CrossRef] [PubMed]

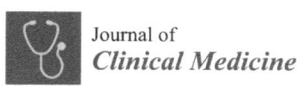

Journal of
Clinical Medicine

Review

The Biology of Chronic Pain and Its Implications for Pain Neuroscience Education: State of the Art

Kory Zimney [1,*], Wouter Van Bogaert [2,3,4,5] and Adriaan Louw [6]

[1] Department of Physical Therapy, University of South Dakota, 414 East Clark St., Vermillion, SD 57069, USA
[2] Pain in Motion Research Group (PAIN), Department of Physiotherapy, Human Physiology and Anatomy, Faculty of Physical Education and Physiotherapy, Vrije Universiteit Brussel, Laarbeeklaan 121, 1000 Brussels, Belgium
[3] Research Foundation–Flanders (FWO), Leuvenseweg 38, 1000 Brussels, Belgium
[4] Interuniversity Centre for Health Economics Research (I-CHER), Department of Public Health (GEWE), Faculty of Medicine and Pharmacy, Vrije Universiteit Brussel, Laarbeeklaan 103, 1000 Brussels, Belgium
[5] Department of Physical Medicine and Physiotherapy, University Hospital Brussels, Laarbeeklaan 101, 1000 Brussels, Belgium
[6] Evidence in Motion, 618 Broad Street, Suite B, Story City, IA 50248, USA
* Correspondence: kory.zimney@usd.edu

Abstract: Pain is an individualized experience for the person suffering from chronic pain. Significant strides have been made in the last few decades in understanding various biological changes that coincide with chronic pain. This state-of-the-art overview looks at the current evidence related to the biology of chronic pain and the implications these findings have on the delivery of pain neuroscience education (PNE). The paper summarizes the various (epi)genetic, neural, endocrine, and immune factors discovered and explored in the scientific literature concerning chronic pain. Each of these biological factors has various implications for the content and delivery of PNE. We discuss the future directions these biological factors have for the clinical implementation of PNE by linking the importance of behavior change, optimizing the learning environment, and using an individualized multimodal treatment approach with PNE. In addition, future directions for research of PNE based on these biological factors are provided with importance placed on individualized patient-centered care and how PNE can be used with traditional modes of care and growing trends with other care methods. PNE was originally and continues to be rooted in understanding chronic pain biology and how that understanding can improve patient care and outcomes.

Keywords: chronic pain; pain neuroscience education; epigenetic factors; neural factors; endocrine factors; immune factors

Citation: Zimney, K.; Van Bogaert, W.; Louw, A. The Biology of Chronic Pain and Its Implications for Pain Neuroscience Education: State of the Art. *J. Clin. Med.* **2023**, *12*, 4199. https://doi.org/10.3390/jcm12134199

Academic Editor: Guy Hans

Received: 16 May 2023
Revised: 6 June 2023
Accepted: 14 June 2023
Published: 21 June 2023

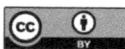
1. Introduction

Thomas Kuhn's The Structure of Scientific Revolutions [1] pointed out two primary mechanisms required for science to advance. One is the gradual accumulation of knowledge or facts; the other is the rapid shift in integrating the facts that occurs when a new theory or paradigm is proposed. In the scientific area of the biology of chronic pain, continual advancements in understanding the basic facts of the biology within patients suffering from chronic pain have occurred through the decades. One such advancement led to the initial paradigm shift in patient education by Louie Gifford and David Butler [2] with the concept of educating patients about pain, not just their injury, during clinical practice. Later, the idea of explaining pain was formally introduced into the research literature through a randomized control trial by Lorimer Moseley [3]. Following this first trial, the paradigm shift led to an explosion of research and facts around the benefits of pain neuroscience education (PNE) in the past two decades.

PNE can be described as different educational methods used with individuals to change someone's understanding of pain. It uses various change strategies, psychologically informed practices, and modern pain-related biological science to elicit conceptual change within the individual to reduce fear, anxiety, and worry about their pain condition. This shift in the conceptual understanding of pain for an individual can then lead to alterations in their attitudes, beliefs, and behaviors [4].

To date, numerous systematic reviews and meta-analyses have shown the benefits of PNE in various areas, such as self-reported pain reduction, lower disability, decreased fear-avoidance and pain catastrophizing, improved pain knowledge, increased movement, and lower healthcare costs [5–13]. While there is evidence in place showing that PNE has positive benefits, there are still other studies that show little to no effects with the use of PNE [14,15]. Future work needs to continue exploring nuances of education and therapist-patient interaction during the educational process to improve the outcomes with the use of PNE and when it may provide benefit and when it will be less useful. Research shows small to moderate effect sizes with the general use of PNE when delivered within a multimodal treatment plan, typically combined with exercise. Unfortunately, the exact dosage regarding the amount of information, length of time to deliver the education, and the best setting, whether in groups or individual, is still unknown. To improve these effect sizes, the individualization of PNE may need to be tailored to the individual patient in front of us and their specific biological, emotional, and social needs. Educational strategies, such as PNE, also need to be delivered with care as potential nocebo effects can occur [16,17]. Pain is an individual human experience; thus, the care for an individual needs to be on a personal level [18]. This is sometimes at odds with much of current healthcare practice and payment systems that want to reduce treatment delivery into simpler, linear models and methods, specifically since these can be more easily controlled for direct cause and effect research purposes, standardized for ease of delivery, and monitored more closely for payment. One thing that the study of the biology of pain has taught us is that simple does not fit into the model or method of treatment very well, but complex and nonlinear models and methods of treatment do [19,20].

This state-of-the-art paper provides an overview of the current evidence regarding the biology of chronic pain and the implications for PNE for people with chronic pain within the new paradigm shift of understanding and educating individuals on the complexity of pain. Although the biology of chronic pain literature is extensive, this paper aims to highlight a few of the significant biological discoveries in the past few decades and how they continue to shape the delivery of PNE. The primary areas covered will be genetic (more specifically epigenetic), neural (primarily neuroplasticity and processing within the brain), endocrine (related to autonomic responses to stress and sleep), and immune factors. While there are other factors potentially involved for people with chronic pain, this paper will explore specifically these four factors in terms of how they pertain to pain education content and delivery changes within this new paradigm.

2. State of the Art

Pain is an unpleasant sensory and emotional experience associated with, or resembling that associated with, actual or potential tissue damage [21]. In the revised 2020 International Association for the Study of Pain definition, key notes were added. One of those solidified the idea that pain is a complex process influenced by varying biological, psychological, and social factors. This state of the art will further explore this complicated intertwining of these regarding how psychological and social factors can change biology and how biological factors can affect psychology and social aspects (Table 1).

2.1. (Epi)genetic Factors

Genetics plays a role in pain, especially in those with chronic pain, as genetic risk factors have been found in several chronic pain conditions [22]. The various genes associated with chronic pain are long and complex, including genes from serotonergic, glutamatergic, GABAergic, cytokines, growth factors, and more [23–25]. Though genetics is an essential factor in someone's pain experience, it alone cannot explain the whole picture, as demonstrated through multiple twin studies [26,27]. Another scientific finding currently at the center of modern medicine is epigenetics [28]. Epigenetics has shown us that gene expression is not solely based on someone's genetic background. Instead, the environment and the individual's health also influence genetic expression. A common metaphor that can be used to explain the relevance of epigenetics is to consider people's genetic structure as a full set of piano keys, with epigenetics being the mechanism determining which keys are being played [29]. This understanding requires us to take a much broader look into someone's health and pain condition and look beyond the body, considering their lived environment and contextual factors [30–33]. Indeed, current evidence shows that physical activity and psychological stress (e.g., fear) can induce epigenetic changes in relation to pain [29]. Whereas physical activity was found to positively influence the (epi)genetic processes regarding nociceptive modulation, stress response, and the pathophysiology of chronic diseases, intense psychological stress seems to negatively influence such processes, which can even result in increased pain sensitivity [29,34]. Moreover, such stress-induced changes seem to be maintained long after the stressful event has ended [34]. Additionally, epigenetics is also suggested to play a role in the transition from acute to chronic pain, as well as the neuroplasticity responsible for the hyperexcitability of the central nervous system, which is often present in people with chronic pain [34–36]. The importance of such knowledge on epigenetics in PNE is to help patients understand the intricacies of genetics that might make them more sensitive to pain and how the environment can change the expression of those genes through the epigenetic process. Specifically, clinicians can emphasize the role of environmental and lifestyle factors in the complexity of pain sensitivity. Clinicians can also assist patients in understanding that some individuals might be more genetically prone to being hypersensitive and that epigenetic influences can amplify or limit this predisposition. Overall, the care for people with chronic pain needs to extend to the larger conversation regarding social determinants of health and its role in an individual's experience but also the larger societal issues of their role in the pain epidemic [30–32]. This provides a ripe ground for a powerful combination of acceptance and understanding of their biological response to the condition yet hope for change within other factors they control.

2.2. Neural Factors

Looking at neural-related changes during pain led to the introduction of Gate Theory, one of the most significant paradigm shifts in the study of pain [37]. The idea that neural processing could be altered and changed at different levels was novel then. This idea regarding neural processing changes at the spinal cord level has been a springboard into the complexity of the pain experience. This theory pointed out that the simple cause-and-effect process does not occur with pain, especially as pain persists. Once this shift occurred to recognize that pain was not a cause-and-effect mechanism, it opened study into neuroplasticity and memory at multiple levels, from the peripheral receptor at various points through the nervous system all the way up to the brain. It is well understood that the biology of pain changes the structure and function of the nervous system, which also changes the pain experience [38–41]. Hasmi, et al. [40], showed a dramatic shift in information processing as pain persists and that emotional circuits become much more activated over time during the pain experience. Other research has also shown us that pain changes the brain, and other social determinants of health can also affect brain development [42,43]. These two findings have had profound implications on PNE. As pain persists, we need to consider the emotional needs of our patients, and education should be directed in that area. In addition, the social determinants of an individual have a significant effect on their health. Thus, attention must be placed in that direction during our educational and treatment process. This emphasis also ties into the need to consider the patient's emotional state when delivering PNE and potential interactions when utilizing mindfulness stress-based reduction techniques in conjunction with or before education [44].

Another discovery area specific to neuroplasticity and chronic pain is the functional and structural changes to the spinal and cortical representation of the patient's body image and schema, along with tactile acuity abilities [45–52]. These findings highlight the importance of evaluating tactile acuity [46] and motor imagery [53] with patients suffering from chronic pain along with the value of utilizing graded motor imagery techniques and sensory discrimination training [51,54–56]. Explaining these concepts to patients is integral to the treatment process. Compliance with self-management is vital with these interventions because of the repetition needed for beneficial neuroplastic changes. Patient education and support have been linked to improved compliance with chronic conditions [57]. Helping the patient understand these conscious and unconscious representation alterations of their body can provide an essential link in their understanding of their "abnormal" feelings and awareness of the affected area of the body as "normal" consequences of neurobiological changes that can occur in the body especially as pain persists. This deeper understanding can be a motivational catalyst for carrying out self-management with the interventions.

Another component of the "dark side" of neuroplasticity as it relates to chronic pain is involved with memory and learning [58]. These neuroplastic changes involved with pain memories deepen the argument that chronic pain is a disease of the nervous system and which distinguishes itself from the phenomena of acute pain and notification of tissue injury. The idea of pain memories has increased in acceptance since the early experiments within Melzack's lab at McGill University [59]. Recent research has shown that pain threshold levels [60] and muscle strength [61] are altered in individuals after injury compared to those without a history of injury. This finding has implications within PNE as part of the educational process to help patients understand how the performance of activities will involve overcoming these painful memories and retraining the nervous system.

2.3. Endocrine Factors

The relationship between stress and pain has long been established, with stress being able to induce either hyper- or hypoalgesia as well as allodynia in patients [62,63]. The concept of increased nerve sensitivity (hyperalgesia and allodynia) is a clinical presentation that does not imply a mechanism but has been identified during studies where individuals have reduced pain pressure thresholds when encountering a stress enhanced environment or situation [64,65]. The analgesic effect of stress depends on the type of stressor, but it can also differ between patients, particularly those with chronic pain [66]. Besides pain modulation, stress can induce or worsen other complaints, such as fatigue or cognitive symptoms, in people with chronic pain [67–69]. Such induction or worsening of symptoms due to stress can be described as stress intolerance [68]. Recently, Wyns, et al. [68], have provided an excellent overview of how stress intolerance plays a significant role in chronic pain. Two of the primary hormonal outputs of the endocrine system during the Hypothalamus–Pituitary–Adrenal (HPA) activation are cortisol and adrenaline. The paradigm shift from the pain education level with this knowledge is the importance of reducing stress and improving the environment to allow learning to occur [62]. The increased threat of pain enhances increased sensitization with associative fear learning, and it can amplify pain [70]. This concept that stress and emotions play a significant role in pain experiences must be a significant component of the educational process [71]. Not only is it a relevant concept to discuss with the patients as part of their education, but it can also aid clinicians in establishing a proper context to provide the education. Creating a safe learning environment is vital for the patient to learn the ideas of pain science and understand that it is more about the nerve sensitivity than the state of the tissues [72]. Another valuable concept in PNE is creating an optimal learning environment. Alterations of endocrine function can influence the learning environment. Being in pain can impair a patient's value-based goal-directed behavior [73] through the effects of the stress response system. This response can be mediated by the latter's influence on the prefrontal cortex neural networks [74]. As such, PNE needs to be directed toward not just the accumulation of knowledge about pain by the patient but relevant knowledge that will spark goal-directed behavior to improve their functional status.

The endocrine system is also closely linked to sleep, as it is influenced heavily by circadian rhythms and sleep–wake states that alter hormonal control within individuals [75,76]. These alterations in endocrine function associated with sleep disturbances and chronic pain are connected to the Hypothalamus–Pituitary–Adrenal (HPA) axis which mediates an individual's response to both physical and psychological stress [77]. The alterations in the HPA axis have been found to affect cortisol levels leading to various pain sensitivity problems [78]. The endocrine changes in cortisol levels due to sleep disturbance and chronic pain are also tightly interrelated with the immune system and change with pro-inflammatory cytokine production. Another interesting link between chronic pain and sleep disturbance is melatonin production. Some individuals suffering from various chronic pain conditions have seen improvements in pain when taking exogenous melatonin [79,80]. This understanding of the links between chronic pain and sleep disturbance can be vital while delivering PNE to help patients make meaningful connections to various health changes related to endocrine function changes and provide reasoning behind the importance of sleep hygiene within a complete multimodal treatment plan.

Table 1. Evidence regarding biological factors involved in pain and implications for pain neuroscience education.

Biological Factor	First Author, Reference	Investigated Mechanism	Implication for Pain Neuroscience Education
(Epi)genetic	Zorina-Lichtenwalter [17]	Genetic contributions to chronic pain	Educate the patient on the role of genetic factors in the variability of stimuli responses.
	Polli [24]	Physical and psychological stressors can induce epigenetic changes in relation to chronic pain	Explain to the patient how various stressors can alter genetic expression to explain why certain stimuli can be experienced differently in other contexts.
	Nirvanie-Persaud [29]	Epigenetics play a role in the transition from acute to chronic pain	Provide understanding to the patient of how various factors, including genetic and environmental, may have led to persistent pain.
	Mauceri [30]	Epigenetic changes can facilitate peripheral and central sensitization processes	Explain to the patient how their increased sensitivity can partially be explained and maintained by changes on the genetic level.
Neural	Hasmi [35]	Shift of pain processing from nociceptive to emotional circuits with chronification of pain	Consider and discuss emotional components during the patient's education and care, especially as pain persists.
	Bosnar Puretic [36]	Neuroplasticity can lead to central sensitization process	Educate the patient on the key concept of neuroplasticity and how the nervous system changes and sensitizes over time to help focus more on the sensitivity of the nervous system and less on damage to the tissues as pain persists.
	Catley [41]	Spinal and cortical representation changes in people with chronic pain	Educate the patient on the concept of body representation changes that can occur with chronic pain and the need for various interventions (i.e., GMI and sensory discrimination) to facilitate recovery.
	Price [53]	Linking of pain and memory mechanisms with chronic pain	Provide understanding to the patient of the concept of "pain memories" and how treatment needs to work on overcoming pain memories that might be maladaptive to function.

Table 1. *Cont.*

Biological Factor	First Author, Reference	Investigated Mechanism	Implication for Pain Neuroscience Education
Endocrine	Lunde [58]	Stress response system implications within chronic pain	Educate the patient on the link between chronic pain and the stress response system to provide an understanding of the individual's pain experience.
	Wyns [61]	Stress intolerance role in chronic pain	Explain to the patient why various stress management interventions can assist in improving chronic pain limitations.
	Haack [70]	Sleep deficiency and chronic pain alterations in endocrine function	Educate the patient on the important link between poor sleep and changes in endocrine function.
Immune	Marchand [74]	Inflammatory mediators released from immune cells contribute to persistent pain states	Educate the patient on the link between the immune system and chronic pain is critical. These facts also help explain why pain may increase or decrease based on immune system response and may not be due to tissue changes.
	Totsch [76]	Diet can influence pain through the immune system	Include education on why diet changes in a multimodal treatment could be beneficial.
	Besedovsky [77]	Sleep can influence pain through the immune system	Educate the patient on improving sleep hygiene as part of the multimodal treatment.

2.4. Immune Factors

The immune system has a very prominent role in chronic pain [81,82]. Research has found a long list of inflammatory molecules involved in the experience of pain (e.g., mast cells, cytokines, macrophages, neutrophils, and T and B cells). In addition, extensive study has investigated various immune mediators and cytokines that can alter pain processing (e.g., TNFα, IL-1β, NGF, bradykinin, serotonin, and chemokines). Understanding an individual's complex immune system processes opens an extensive door as part of the educational process with the patient. Appreciating this complexity helps them understand further that their body is not damaged but is overprotective and can be retrained [71]. In addition, understanding the immune system's involvement in chronic pain has also been linked to the importance of dietary interventions to reduce the potential inflammation-mediated disorder [83]. Not only diet, but sleep [84] and stress reduction through touch [85] and meditation [86–88] also have links to immune system function and pain. These findings further support using a multimodal approach with PNE to maximize the effects of any one treatment through the combined impact of linking treatments to improve the individual's health on multiple levels. It also provides an explanation of why previous individual treatments had little to no effect but still might be beneficial. A common metaphor to explain this is that a car with four flat tires does not run well unless all four tires are inflated properly. Pumping up one tire is an important step in the process, but until the other three tires are inflated, it will appear as if the efforts made pumping up one tire were meaningless. This is true for important interventions: exercise, sleep hygiene, stress reduction, diet, etc., alone may seem pointless but when all of them are working, positive changes can be seen.

3. Future Directions for Clinical Practice

Understanding the complex biological systems interaction that interplays in chronic pain has carried over to changes in treatment, especially around PNE. Figure 1 depicts the timeline of PNE from the 1990s with a gradual refining of the use of PNE over the decades. PNE has continued to evolve from its early days as a clinical concept in the 1990s, moving into the initial research testing phase in the 2000s, and becoming more widely accepted through the depth of evidence supporting the use of PNE from 2010 to

2020. Future directions will need to look at PNE plus the other multimodal treatments in conjunction with each other within a patient-centered approach to care. During this more individualized approach, PNE plus the other interventions must tie together the biological factors (epigenetic, neural, endocrine, immune, and others) that work at different levels in each patient encountered during clinical practice. The various colors within the figure symbolize the potential different levels at which each of these factors may be involved with individual patients (Figure 1).

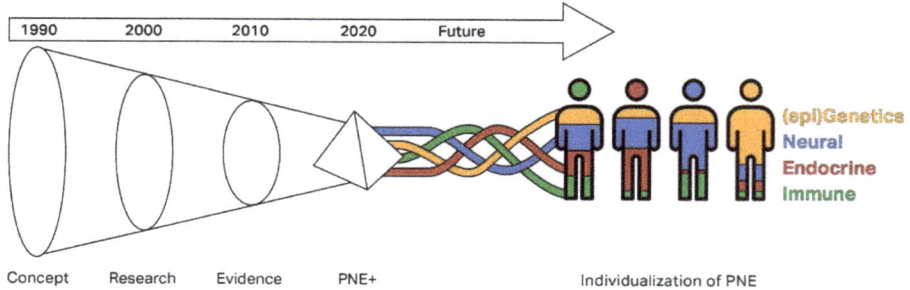

Figure 1. Timeline of PNE in clinical practice with future directions.

PNE is not about the result of making the patient more knowledgeable about pain; more importantly, it is about the process of using the knowledge gained to facilitate behavior change in a complex environment [71,89–92]. Part of the behavior change for patients is the reconceptualization process of their pain experience through a deeper understanding of the complex biology occurring within themselves [71,72,90] Some excellent qualitative studies looking into the reconceptualization process can be constructive for clinical practice. They recognized that patients would go through various degrees of reconceptualization [90]. Patients go through their journey to reconceptualize their pain experience from one bound in a biomedical viewpoint toward a broader biopsychosocial view. Within the roots of the reconceptualization process is the psycho–neuro–endocrine–immune changes occurring within the patient's biology. Since the patient needs to undergo this change process, the clinician must understand the stages of change that patients will go through because the educational needs at each step differ [93–95]. Clinicians need to consider the various processes of change and utilize skills and techniques to help patients progress in the change process (e.g., consciousness-raising, self-reevaluation, counterconditioning, helping relationships, and self-liberation) [95]. Another important factor is that patients must find personal relevance in their education [90]. Pain knowledge alone is useless to patients unless they find meaning specific to their condition. Stories and metaphors are a mainstay in PNE, but these stories must make sense to the patient in their context, not the clinicians [96,97]. Skillful patient history-taking is needed to explore the patient's prior level of beliefs about their condition and the treatments that might be beneficial [90,98]. For some patients, it will be essential to dispel previous myths (de-educate) before moving forward with new knowledge (re-educate) and helping them reconceptualize their pain experience [99].

Keeping in mind that the change in the various biological factors discussed happens concurrently as part of the behavior change process during PNE, integrating motivational interviewing is a skill clinicians should consider using to assist with this behavior change process. When motivational interviewing techniques are implemented, the needed biological changes can occur [100]. The reader should review the manuscript by Nijs, et al. [91] for a complete practical guide for clinicians along with Miller and Rollnick's book: Motivational Interviewing: Helping people change [101]. Motivational interviewing is a crucial behavioral strategy used to assist patients in the behavior change process and sets the stage for the patient to be more receptive to many of the concepts of PNE to assist in the pain reconceptualization process [102]. The general qualities of motivational interviewing are essential to carry through the pain education process [101]. Motivational interviewing and

PNE should contain a guiding style of communication that fits between good listening and giving information. PNE and motivational interviewing should also be designed to empower the patient to change by drawing out their own meaning and capacity for change. Lastly, both should be based on a respectful and curious way of being with people that facilitates the change process and honors the patient's autonomy. The motivational interviewing fundamental methods of engaging, focusing, evoking, and planning can help the clinician create the "flow" of conversation through the educational session.

For behavior change to occur, the clinician needs to assist in creating the right environment for the patient. The right environment encompasses physical, emotional, learning space, and psychologically safe aspects. Patients with chronic pain need to be open to change; they need safety, and their physical and, potentially more importantly, emotional needs must be met [92]. Research has shown that meeting the patient's emotional needs is often the most critical as the relationship between the provider and the patient progresses along with the length of time the patient has their condition [103]. The clinician needs to see the biological links and importance of the neural, endocrine, and immune systems in the concept of the right environment playing a role in the treatment process. The famous quote of Theodore Roosevelt that addresses this concept is fitting to remember: "No one cares how much you know, until they know how much you care". Meeting these emotional needs of the patient is grounded in our understanding of the basic science of the shift in brain processing as the pain becomes chronic in the more emotionally related brain areas [42]. The emotional safety of an individual is built through the reciprocal nature of trust within the healthcare relationship [104,105]. Trust is a vital component of the therapeutic alliance [106,107]. PNE that provides an evidence-based biological understanding of the patient's pain experience, that answers the patient's questions, and that helps them make sense of their pain can be a vehicle to build trust between the patient and provider [97,108].

PNE alone for a complex dynamic systems problem such as chronic pain has little effect when delivered in isolation [6]. The evidence continues to support that PNE works best when delivered as part of a larger treatment plan tying together all the treatment options (nutrition, sleep, stress reduction, meditation, breathing, exercise, manual therapies, etc.) into a coherent message providing hope. All these treatment interventions can work in a symbiotic nature when we recognize the principles of the biological processes occurring as we deliver each mode of treatment. When we embrace a complexity mindset to chronic pain resulting from complex, dynamic, and individually unique interactions between the various factors within the more extensive system [20], it allows for a way toward better health and recovery from chronic pain, i.e., when we can utilize a variety of treatments that have various interactions within an individual and their biology and overall pain experience. Although, clinically, therapists have to appreciate that there is heterogeneity in each individual's pain problem, there are also overlapping items that can help us classify pain mechanisms [109–114] and lead the clinician toward various treatment options that are the most plausible for improved outcomes (Figure 2).

---

1) Pain reconceptualization is a vital part of the behavior change process and should be guided by clinicians who understand the stages of change the patient goes through.

2) Motivational interviewing techniques should be integrated with PNE to create the right environment for patients to be open to change.

3) Clinicians need to provide an optimal and trusted learning environment by offering a biological understanding of the patient's pain experience.

4) PNE works best as part of a multimodal treatment plan tailored to the patient's individual pain experience, and and utilizing the principles of the biological processes occurring within the individual. A patient-centered and individualized approach is essential for effective PNE, and research needs to inform care specific to these items.

Figure 2. Key messages for clinical practice.

4. Future Directions for Research

The next evolution in PNE research needs to move beyond the general question of whether it works. If we fully embrace the multidimensional nature of chronic pain, we need to recognize the inherent limitation of any research directed toward a single domain and expect meaningful outcomes. A one-size-fits-all approach is most likely not going to suit any specific individual. The NIH National Pain Strategy points to the need for care to be patient-centered, compassionate, and individualized for every patient. If this is the treatment goal, PNE research needs to inform care specific to these items.

PNE must break from the idea of rote intervention employed equally to all patients. Future studies should explore the uniqueness and complexities of each patient and how this affects the communication style of the therapist, the patient-centered content to be delivered, and the individualized value-centered goals and outcomes of the education. Specific studies are needed to examine how the patient's various personal and social factors and the concordance of those factors with the therapist can alter the outcomes and the potential content that needs to be provided along with the delivery style. More patient-centered research is necessary to examine learning styles, stages of behavior change, levels of therapeutic alliance, implicit biases, and other factors that can alter the learning experience and how that will affect the outcomes for the patient receiving the interventions. Because of the various interactions with other treatments, ongoing research needs to explore the effects of diverse PNE approaches and interactions when provided with multiple treatment interventions. Given the ongoing digitalization of healthcare, studies examining the possibilities of eHealth for PNE are needed. Specifically, the cost-effectiveness of such eHealth applications to deliver an individually tailored education to (multiple) patients would be worthwhile to investigate. In addition, the study designs will require more pragmatic approaches of using multiple methods to develop these complex interactions [115,116]. These designs will require nonlinear and iterative development of interventions. Different methodologies should be considered, such as cluster randomized trials, stepped-wedge designs, or preference trials.

Because of the individualized experience of each patient, ongoing phenomenological and grounded theory qualitative study needs to be conducted to assist the clinician and the researcher in embracing and fully understanding the patient's pain experience. This enhanced understanding can lead to a greater non-judgmental and empathetic understanding of the patient, thus enhancing the therapeutic alliance [117] (Figure 3).

---

1) A patient-centered and individualized approach is essential for effective PNE, and research needs to inform care specific to these items.

2) Future studies should explore the uniqueness and complexities of each patient and how this affects the therapist's communication, the patient-centered content, and the individualized value-centered goals and outcomes of the education.

3) Ongoing research needs to explore the effects of diverse PNE approaches when provided with multiple treatment interventions, including the possibilities of eHealth for PNE and using multiple methods for intervention development.

Figure 3. Key messages for research.

5. Conclusions

This state-of-the-art paper has explored some of the more relevant advances in the biological understanding of pain related to (epi)genetic, neural, endocrine, and immune factors. The depth and breadth of our knowledge of these factors have grown substantially in the past few decades. This evidence has and should be used to help patients understand the complexity of pain, especially as it persists. The use of PNE is rooted in assisting patients in understanding these complex biological processes occurring in them by utilizing stories and metaphors to help them move through a behavior change process to improve function and potentially reduce pain as they regain quality of life.

Author Contributions: Conceptualization, K.Z., W.V.B. and A.L.; writing—original draft preparation, K.Z.; writing review and editing; W.V.B. and A.L. All authors have read and agreed to the published version of the manuscript.

Funding: W.V.B. is funded by the Research Foundation Flanders (FWO), Brussels, Belgium (nr. 1S61521N), though the funder played no role in the design, conduct, or reporting of this study.

Institutional Review Board Statement: Not applicable.

Informed Consent Statement: Not applicable.

Data Availability Statement: Not applicable.

Conflicts of Interest: The authors declare no conflict of interest.

References

1. Kuhn, T.S. *The Structure of Scientific Revolutions*, 1st ed.; University of Chicago Press: Chicago, IL, USA, 1962.
2. Gifford, L.S.; Butler, D.S. The integration of pain sciences into clinical practice. *J. Hand Ther.* **1997**, *10*, 86–95. [CrossRef] [PubMed]
3. Moseley, G. Combined physiotherapy and education is efficacious for chronic low back pain. *Aust. J. Physiol.* **2002**, *48*, 297–302. [CrossRef]
4. Moseley, G.L.; Butler, D.S. Fifteen years of explaining pain: The past, present, and future. *J. Pain* **2015**, *16*, 807–813. [CrossRef] [PubMed]
5. Clarke, C.L.; Ryan, C.G.; Martin, D.J. Pain neurophysiology education for the management of individuals with chronic low back pain: A systematic review and meta-analysis. *Man. Ther.* **2011**, *16*, 544–549. [CrossRef] [PubMed]
6. Louw, A.; Zimney, K.; Puentedura, E.J.; Diener, I. The efficacy of pain neuroscience education on musculoskeletal pain: A systematic review of the literature. *Physiother. Theory Pract.* **2016**, *32*, 332–355. [CrossRef] [PubMed]
7. Saracoglu, I.; Akin, E.; Aydin Dincer, G.B. Efficacy of adding pain neuroscience education to a multimodal treatment in fibromyalgia: A systematic review and meta-analysis. *Int. J. Rheum. Dis.* **2022**, *25*, 394–404. [CrossRef] [PubMed]
8. Silva, V.A.G.; Maujean, A.; Campbell, L.; Sterling, M. A Systematic Review and Meta-analysis of the Effectiveness of Psychological Interventions Delivered by Physiotherapists on Pain, Disability and Psychological Outcomes in Musculoskeletal Pain Conditions. *Clin. J. Pain* **2018**, *34*, 838–857. [CrossRef] [PubMed]
9. Watson, J.A.; Ryan, C.G.; Cooper, L.; Ellington, D.; Whittle, R.; Lavender, M.; Dixon, J.; Atkinson, G.; Cooper, K.; Martin, D.J. Pain neuroscience education for adults with chronic musculoskeletal pain: A mixed-methods systematic review and meta-analysis. *J. Pain* **2019**, *20*, e1140–e1141. [CrossRef]
10. Wood, L.; Hendrick, P.A. A systematic review and meta-analysis of pain neuroscience education for chronic low back pain: Short-and long-term outcomes of pain and disability. *Eur. J. Pain* **2019**, *23*, 234–249. [CrossRef]
11. Tegner, H.; Frederiksen, P.; Esbensen, B.A.; Juhl, C. Neurophysiological Pain-education for Patients with Chronic Low Back Pain-A Systematic Review and Meta-analysis. *Clin. J. Pain* **2018**, *34*, 778–786. [CrossRef] [PubMed]
12. Traeger, A.C.; Hübscher, M.; Henschke, N.; Moseley, G.L.; Lee, H.; McAuley, J.H. Effect of Primary Care–Based Education on Reassurance in Patients with Acute Low Back Pain: Systematic Review and Meta-analysis. *JAMA Intern. Med.* **2015**, *175*, 733–743. [CrossRef]
13. Watson, J.A.; Ryan, C.G.; Atkinson, G.; Williamson, P.; Ellington, D.; Whittle, R.; Dixon, J.; Martin, D.J. Inter-individual differences in the responses to pain neuroscience education in adults with chronic musculoskeletal pain: A systematic review and meta-analysis of randomized controlled trials. *J. Pain* **2021**, *22*, 9–20. [CrossRef]
14. Lane, E.; Magel, J.S.; Thackeray, A.; Greene, T.; Fino, N.F.; Puentedura, E.J.; Louw, A.; Maddox, D.; Fritz, J.M. Effectiveness of training physical therapists in pain neuroscience education for patients with chronic spine pain: A cluster-randomized trial. *Pain* **2022**, *163*, 852–860. [CrossRef]
15. Traeger, A.C.; Lee, H.; Hübscher, M.; Skinner, I.W.; Moseley, G.L.; Nicholas, M.K.; Henschke, N.; Refshauge, K.M.; Blyth, F.M.; Main, C.J.; et al. Effect of intensive patient education vs placebo patient education on outcomes in patients with acute low back pain: A randomized clinical trial. *JAMA Neurol.* **2019**, *76*, 161–169. [CrossRef]
16. Benedetti, F.; Lanotte, M.; Lopiano, L.; Colloca, L. When words are painful: Unraveling the mechanisms of the nocebo effect. Research Support, Non-U.S. Gov't Review. *Neuroscience* **2007**, *147*, 260–271. [CrossRef] [PubMed]
17. Bedell, S.E.; Graboys, T.B.; Bedell, E.; Lown, B. Words that harm, words that heal. *Arch Intern Med.* **2004**, *164*, 1365–1368. [CrossRef]
18. Gillespie, H.; Kelly, M.; Duggan, S.; Dornan, T. How do patients experience caring? Scoping review. *Patient Educ. Couns.* **2017**, *100*, 1622–1633. [CrossRef]
19. Peppin, J.F.; Cheatle, M.D.; Kirsh, K.L.; McCarberg, B.H. The complexity model: A novel approach to improve chronic pain care. *Pain Med.* **2015**, *16*, 653–666. [CrossRef] [PubMed]

20. Hush, J.M. Low back pain: It is time to embrace complexity. *Pain* **2020**, *161*, 2248–2251. [CrossRef]
21. Raja, S.N.; Carr, D.B.; Cohen, M.; Finnerup, N.B.; Flor, H.; Gibson, S.; Keefe, F.J.; Mogil, J.S.; Ringkamp, M.; Sluka, K.A.; et al. The revised International Association for the Study of Pain definition of pain: Concepts, challenges, and compromises. *Pain* **2020**, *161*, 1976–1982. [CrossRef] [PubMed]
22. Zorina-Lichtenwalter, K.; Meloto, C.B.; Khoury, S.; Diatchenko, L. Genetic predictors of human chronic pain conditions. *Neuroscience* **2016**, *338*, 36–62. [CrossRef]
23. Woolf, C.J.; Ma, Q. Nociceptors--noxious stimulus detectors. *Neuron* **2007**, *55*, 353–364. [CrossRef] [PubMed]
24. Raouf, R.; Quick, K.; Wood, J.N. Pain as a channelopathy. *J. Clin. Investig.* **2010**, *120*, 3745–3752. [CrossRef]
25. Cregg, R.; Momin, A.; Rugiero, F.; Wood, J.N.; Zhao, J. Pain channelopathies. *J. Physiol.* **2010**, *588*, 1897–1904. [CrossRef] [PubMed]
26. Battie, M.C.; Videman, T.; Kaprio, J.; Gibbons, L.E.; Gill, K.; Manninen, H.; Saarela, J.; Peltonen, L. The Twin Spine Study: Contributions to a changing view of disc degeneration. *Spine J.* **2009**, *9*, 47–59. [CrossRef]
27. MacGregor, A.J.; Andrew, T.; Sambrook, P.N.; Spector, T.D. Structural, psychological, and genetic influences on low back and neck pain: A study of adult female twins. *Arthritis Care Res.* **2004**, *51*, 160–167. [CrossRef] [PubMed]
28. Feinberg, A.P. Epigenetics at the epicenter of modern medicine. *JAMA* **2008**, *299*, 1345–1350. [CrossRef] [PubMed]
29. Polli, A.; Ickmans, K.; Godderis, L.; Nijs, J. When environment meets genetics: A clinical review of the epigenetics of pain, psychological factors, and physical activity. *Arch. Phys. Med. Rehabil.* **2019**, *100*, 1153–1161. [CrossRef] [PubMed]
30. Wilkinson, R.G.; Marmot, M. *Social Determinants of Health: The Solid Facts*; World Health Organization: Geneva, Switzerland, 2003.
31. Marmot, M. Social determinants of health inequalities. *Lancet* **2005**, *365*, 1099–1104. [CrossRef]
32. Karran, E.L.; Grant, A.R.; Moseley, G.L. Low back pain and the social determinants of health: A systematic review and narrative synthesis. *Pain* **2020**, *161*, 2476–2493. [CrossRef] [PubMed]
33. Carlino, E.; Benedetti, F. Different contexts, different pains, different experiences. *Neuroscience* **2016**, *338*, 19–26. [CrossRef] [PubMed]
34. Nirvanie-Persaud, L.; Millis, R.M.; Persaud, L.N. Epigenetics and Pain: New Insights to an Old Problem. *Cureus* **2022**, *14*, e29353. [CrossRef]
35. Mauceri, D. Role of Epigenetic Mechanisms in Chronic Pain. *Cells* **2022**, *11*, 2613. [CrossRef]
36. Lopez-Munoz, E.; Mejia-Terrazas, G.E. Epigenetics and Postsurgical Pain: A Scoping Review. *Pain Med.* **2022**, *23*, 246–262. [CrossRef] [PubMed]
37. Melzack, R.; Wall, P.D. Pain Mechanisms: A New Theory: A gate control system modulates sensory input from the skin before it evokes pain perception and response. *Science* **1965**, *150*, 971–979. [CrossRef]
38. Mansour, A.R.; Baliki, M.N.; Huang, L.; Torbey, S.; Herrmann, K.M.; Schnitzer, T.J.; Apkarian, A.V. Brain white matter structural properties predict transition to chronic pain. *Pain* **2013**, *154*, 2160–2168. [CrossRef] [PubMed]
39. Baliki, M.N.; Petre, B.; Torbey, S.; Herrmann, K.M.; Huang, L.; Schnitzer, T.J.; Fields, H.L.; Apkarian, A.V. Corticostriatal functional connectivity predicts transition to chronic back pain. *Nat. Neurosci.* **2012**, *15*, 1117–1119. [CrossRef]
40. Hashmi, J.A.; Baliki, M.N.; Huang, L.; Baria, A.T.; Torbey, S.; Hermann, K.M.; Schnitzer, T.J.; Apkarian, A.V. Shape shifting pain: Chronification of back pain shifts brain representation from nociceptive to emotional circuits. *Brain* **2013**, *136*, 2751–2768. [CrossRef] [PubMed]
41. Bosnar Puretić, M.; Demarin, V. Neuroplasticity mechanisms in the pathophysiology of chronic pain. *Acta Clin. Croat.* **2012**, *51*, 425–429.
42. Jackson, J.L.; Grant, V.; Barnett, K.S.; Ball, M.K.; Khalid, O.; Texter, K.; Laney, B.; Hoskinson, K.R. Structural racism, social determinants of health, and provider bias: Impact on brain development in critical congenital heart disease. *Can. J. Cardiol.* **2022**, *39*, 133–143. [CrossRef]
43. Hilal, S.; Brayne, C. Epidemiologic Trends, Social Determinants, and Brain Health: The Role of Life Course Inequalities. *Stroke* **2022**, *53*, 437–443. [CrossRef] [PubMed]
44. Goldsmith, E.S.; Koffel, E.; Ackland, P.; Hill, J.; Landsteiner, A.; Miller, W.; Stroebel, B.; Ullman, K.; Wilt, T.; Duan-Porter, W. *Implementation of Psychotherapies and Mindfulness-Based Stress Reduction for Chronic Pain and Chronic Mental Health Conditions: A Systematic Review*; Department of Veterans Affairs: Washington, DC, USA, 2021.
45. Bray, H.; Moseley, G.L. Disrupted working body schema of the trunk in people with back pain. *Br. J. Sports Med.* **2011**, *45*, 168–173. [CrossRef]
46. Catley, M.J.; O'Connell, N.E.; Berryman, C.; Ayhan, F.F.; Moseley, G.L. Is tactile acuity altered in people with chronic pain? A systematic review and meta-analysis. *J. Pain* **2014**, *15*, 985–1000. [CrossRef]
47. Haggard, P.; Iannetti, G.D.; Longo, M.R. Spatial sensory organization and body representation in pain perception. *Curr. Biol.* **2013**, *23*, R164–R176. [CrossRef]
48. Moseley, G.L. I can't find it! Distorted body image and tactile dysfunction in patients with chronic back pain. *Pain* **2008**, *140*, 239–243. [CrossRef] [PubMed]
49. Tsay, A.; Allen, T.J.; Proske, U.; Giummarra, M.J. Sensing the body in chronic pain: A review of psychophysical studies implicating altered body representation. *Neurosci. Biobehav. Rev.* **2015**, *52*, 221–232. [CrossRef]
50. Flor, H.; Braun, C.; Elbert, T.; Birbaumer, N. Extensive reorganization of primary somatosensory cortex in chronic back pain patients. *Neurosci. Lett.* **1997**, *224*, 5–8. [CrossRef] [PubMed]

1. Moseley, G.L.; Flor, H. Targeting Cortical Representations in the Treatment of Chronic Pain: A Review. *Neurorehabil. Neural. Repair.* **2012**, *26*, 646–652. [CrossRef] [PubMed]

2. Elbert, T.; Flor, H.; Birbaumer, N.; Knecht, S.; Hampson, S.; Larbig, W. Extensive reorganization of the somatosensory cortex in adult humans after nervous system injury. *Neuroreport* **1994**, *5*, 2593–2597. [CrossRef] [PubMed]

3. Moseley, G.L. Why do people with complex regional pain syndrome take longer to recognize their affected hand? *Neurology* **2004**, *62*, 2182–2186. [CrossRef]

4. Moseley, G.L.; Zalucki, N.M.; Wiech, K. Tactile discrimination, but not tactile stimulation alone, reduces chronic limb pain. *Pain* **2008**, *137*, 600–608. [CrossRef] [PubMed]

5. Louw, A.; Farrell, K.; Zimney, K.; Feller, K.; Jones, C.; Martin, B.; Rettenmeier, M.; Theisen, M.; Wedeking, D. Pain and Decreased Range of Motion in Knees and Shoulders: A Brief Sensory Remapping Intervention. *Pain Rehabil. J. Physiother. Pain Assoc.* **2017**, *2017*, 20–30.

6. Walz, A.D.; Usichenko, T.; Moseley, G.L.; Lotze, M. Graded Motore Imagery and the Impact of Pain Processing in a Case of CRPS. *Clin. J. Pain* **2013**, *29*, 276–279. [CrossRef]

7. Gold, D.T.; McClung, B. Approaches to patient education: Emphasizing the long-term value of compliance and persistence. *Am. J. Med.* **2006**, *119*, S32–S37. [CrossRef]

8. Price, T.J.; Inyang, K.E. Commonalities between pain and memory mechanisms and their meaning for understanding chronic pain. *Prog. Mol. Biol. Transl. Sci.* **2015**, *131*, 409–434.

9. Reichling, D.B.; Levine, J.D. Critical role of nociceptor plasticity in chronic pain. *Trends Neurosci.* **2009**, *32*, 611–618. [CrossRef]

10. Sueki, D.G.; Dunleavy, K.; Puentedura, E.J.; Heard, L.; Van Der Heide, P.; Cheng, M.-S. The Differing Effects of Nociception and Pain Memory on Pain Thresholds in Participants with and without a History of Injury: A Pretest-Posttest Quasi Experimental Study. *J. Behav. Brain Sci.* **2022**, *12*, 359–379. [CrossRef]

11. Sueki, D.G.; Dunleavy, K.; Puentedura, E.J.; Heard, L.; Van der Heide, P.; Cheng, M.-S. The differing effects of nociception and pain memory on isometric muscle strength in participants with and without a history of injury: A quasi-experimental study. *Am. J. Phys. Med. Rehabil.* **2023**, accepted online version 10-1097. [CrossRef] [PubMed]

12. Timmers, I.; Quaedflieg, C.W.; Hsu, C.; Heathcote, L.C.; Rovnaghi, C.R.; Simons, L.E. The interaction between stress and chronic pain through the lens of threat learning. *Neurosci. Biobehav. Rev.* **2019**, *107*, 641–655. [CrossRef]

13. Lunde, C.E.; Sieberg, C.B. Walking the tightrope: A proposed model of chronic pain and stress. *Front. Neurosci.* **2020**, *14*, 270. [CrossRef] [PubMed]

14. Bement, M.H.; Weyer, A.; Keller, M.; Harkins, A.L.; Hunter, S.K. Anxiety and stress can predict pain perception following a cognitive stress. *Physiol. Behav.* **2010**, *101*, 87–92. [CrossRef]

15. Crettaz, B.; Marziniak, M.; Willeke, P.; Young, P.; Hellhammer, D.; Stumpf, A.; Burgmer, M. Stress-induced allodynia–evidence of increased pain sensitivity in healthy humans and patients with chronic pain after experimentally induced psychosocial stress. *PLoS ONE* **2013**, *8*, e69460. [CrossRef] [PubMed]

16. Loffler, M.; Schneider, P.; Schuh-Hofer, S.; Kamping, S.; Usai, K.; Treede, R.D.; Nees, F.; Flor, H. Stress-induced hyperalgesia instead of analgesia in patients with chronic musculoskeletal pain. *Neurobiol. Pain* **2023**, *13*, 100110. [CrossRef] [PubMed]

17. Dennis, N.L.; Larkin, M.; Derbyshire, S.W. 'A giant mess'–making sense of complexity in the accounts of people with fibromyalgia. *Br. J. Health Psychol.* **2013**, *18*, 763–781. [CrossRef] [PubMed]

18. Wyns, A.; Hendrix, J.; Lahousse, A.; De Bruyne, E.; Nijs, J.; Godderis, L.; Polli, A. The Biology of Stress Intolerance in Patients with Chronic Pain—State of the Art and Future Directions. *J. Clin. Med.* **2023**, *12*, 2245. [CrossRef]

19. Galvez-Sanchez, C.M.; Duschek, S.; Reyes Del Paso, G.A. Psychological impact of fibromyalgia: Current perspectives. *Psychol. Res. Behav. Manag.* **2019**, *12*, 117–127. [CrossRef]

20. Madden, V.J.; Harvie, D.S.; Parker, R.; Jensen, K.B.; Vlaeyen, J.W.; Moseley, G.L.; Stanton, T.R. Can pain or hyperalgesia be a classically conditioned response in humans? A systematic review and meta-analysis. *Pain Med.* **2016**, *17*, 1094–1111. [CrossRef] [PubMed]

71. Leake, H.B.; Moseley, G.L.; Stanton, T.R.; O'Hagan, E.T.; Heathcote, L.C. What do patients value learning about pain? A mixed methods survey on the relevance of target concepts following pain science education. *Pain* **2021**, *162*, 2558–2568. [CrossRef]

72. Moseley, G.L. Reconceptualising pain according to modern pain science. *Phys. Ther. Rev.* **2007**, *12*, 169–178. [CrossRef]

73. Smeets, T.; Van Ruitenbeek, P.; Hartogsveld, B.; Quaedflieg, C.W. Stress-induced reliance on habitual behavior is moderated by cortisol reactivity. *Brain Cogn.* **2019**, *133*, 60–71. [CrossRef] [PubMed]

74. Hermans, E.J.; Henckens, M.J.; Joëls, M.; Fernández, G. Dynamic adaptation of large-scale brain networks in response to acute stressors. *Trends Neurosci.* **2014**, *37*, 304–314. [CrossRef] [PubMed]

75. Aldabal, L.; Bahammam, A.S. Metabolic, endocrine, and immune consequences of sleep deprivation. *Open Respir. Med. J.* **2011**, *5*, 31–43. [CrossRef] [PubMed]

76. Kukushkin, M.; Poluektov, M. Current views on chronic pain and its relationship to the state of sleep. *Neurosci. Behav. Physiol.* **2019**, *49*, 13–19. [CrossRef]

77. Haack, M.; Simpson, N.; Sethna, N.; Kaur, S.; Mullington, J. Sleep deficiency and chronic pain: Potential underlying mechanisms and clinical implications. *Neuropsychopharmacology* **2020**, *45*, 205–216. [CrossRef] [PubMed]

78. Balbo, M.; Leproult, R.; Van Cauter, E. Impact of sleep and its disturbances on hypothalamo-pituitary-adrenal axis activity. *Int. J. Endocrinol.* **2010**, *2010*, 759234. [CrossRef]

79. Citera, G.; Arias, M.; Maldonado-Cocco, J.; La'zaro, M.; Rosemffet, M.; Brusco, L.; Scheines, E.; Cardinalli, D. The effect of melatonin in patients with fibromyalgia: A pilot study. *Clin. Rheumatol.* **2000**, *19*, 9–13. [CrossRef] [PubMed]
80. Mozaffari, S.; Rahimi, R.; Abdollahi, M. Implications of melatonin therapy in irritable bowel syndrome: A systematic review. *Curr. Pharm. Des.* **2010**, *16*, 3646–3655. [CrossRef]
81. Marchand, F.; Perretti, M.; McMahon, S.B. Role of the immune system in chronic pain. *Nat. Rev. Neurosci.* **2005**, *6*, 521–532. [CrossRef] [PubMed]
82. Totsch, S.K.; Sorge, R.E. Immune system involvement in specific pain conditions. *Mol. Pain* **2017**, *13*, 1744806917724559. [CrossRef]
83. Totsch, S.K.; Waite, M.E.; Sorge, R.E. Dietary influence on pain via the immune system. *Prog. Mol. Biol. Transl. Sci.* **2015**, *131*, 435–469.
84. Besedovsky, L.; Lange, T.; Born, J. Sleep and immune function. *Pflügers Arch. Eur. J. Physiol.* **2012**, *463*, 121–137. [CrossRef]
85. Garrard, C.T. *The Effect of Therapeutic Touch on Stress Reduction and Immune Function in Persons with AIDS*; The University of Alabama at Birmingham: Birmingham, AL, USA, 1995.
86. Zeidan, F.; Gordon, N.S.; Merchant, J.; Goolkasian, P. The effects of brief mindfulness meditation training on experimentally induced pain. *J. Pain* **2010**, *11*, 199–209. [CrossRef] [PubMed]
87. Zeidan, F.; Martucci, K.T.; Kraft, R.A.; Gordon, N.S.; McHaffie, J.G.; Coghill, R.C. Brain mechanisms supporting the modulation of pain by mindfulness meditation. *J. Neurosci.* **2011**, *31*, 5540–5548. [CrossRef]
88. Salomons, T.V.; Kucyi, A. Does meditation reduce pain through a unique neural mechanism? *J. Neurosci.* **2011**, *31*, 12705–12707. [CrossRef]
89. Fletcher, C.; Bradnam, L.; Barr, C. The relationship between knowledge of pain neurophysiology and fear avoidance in people with chronic pain: A point in time, observational study. *Physiother. Theory Pract.* **2016**, *32*, 271–276. [CrossRef]
90. King, R.; Robinson, V.; Elliott-Button, H.L.; Watson, J.A.; Ryan, C.G.; Martin, D.J. Pain reconceptualisation after pain neurophysiology education in adults with chronic low back pain: A qualitative study. *Pain Res. Manag.* **2018**, *2018*, 3745651. [CrossRef] [PubMed]
91. Nijs, J.; Wijma, A.J.; Willaert, W.; Huysmans, E.; Mintken, P.; Smeets, R.; Goossens, M.; van Wilgen, C.P.; Van Bogaert, W.; Louw, A. Integrating motivational interviewing in pain neuroscience education for people with chronic pain: A practical guide for clinicians. *Phys. Ther.* **2020**, *100*, 846–859. [CrossRef]
92. Wijma, A.J.; Speksnijder, C.M.; Crom-Ottens, A.F.; Knulst-Verlaan, J.C.; Keizer, D.; Nijs, J.; van Wilgen, C.P. What is important in transdisciplinary pain neuroscience education? A qualitative study. *Disabil. Rehabil.* **2018**, *40*, 2181–2191. [CrossRef]
93. Prochaska, J.O.; Norcross, J.C. Stages of change. *Psychother. Theory Res. Pract. Train.* **2001**, *38*, 443. [CrossRef]
94. Hutchison, A.J.; Breckon, J.D.; Johnston, L.H. Physical activity behavior change interventions based on the transtheoretical model: A systematic review. *Health Educ. Behav.* **2009**, *36*, 829–845. [CrossRef] [PubMed]
95. Prochaska, J.O.; Velicer, W.F. The transtheoretical model of health behavior change. *Am. J. Health Promot.* **1997**, *12*, 38–48. [CrossRef] [PubMed]
96. Leventhal, H.; Ian, B. The common-sense model of self-regulation of health and illness. In *The Self-Regulation of Health and Illness Behaviour*; Routledge: Oxfordshire, UK, 2012; pp. 56–79.
97. Bunzli, S.; Smith, A.; Schütze, R.; Lin, I.; O'Sullivan, P. Making sense of low back pain and pain-related fear. *J. Orthop. Sports Phys. Ther.* **2017**, *47*, 628–636. [CrossRef]
98. Wijma, A.J.; van Wilgen, C.P.; Meeus, M.; Nijs, J. Clinical biopsychosocial physiotherapy assessment of patients with chronic pain: The first step in pain neuroscience education. *Physiother. Theory Pract.* **2016**, *32*, 368–384. [CrossRef] [PubMed]
99. Louw, A.; Zimney, K.; Johnson, E.A.; Kraemer, C.; Fesler, J.; Burcham, T. De-educate to re-educate: Aging and low back pain. *Aging Clin. Exp. Res.* **2017**, *29*, 1261–1269. [CrossRef]
100. Rubak, S.; Sandbæk, A.; Lauritzen, T.; Christensen, B. Motivational interviewing: A systematic review and meta-analysis. *Br. J. Gen. Pract.* **2005**, *55*, 305–312. [PubMed]
101. Miller, W.R.; Rollnick, S. *Motivational Interviewing: Helping People Change*; Guilford Press: New York, NY, USA, 2012.
102. Alperstein, D.; Sharpe, L. The efficacy of motivational interviewing in adults with chronic pain: A meta-analysis and systematic review. *J. Pain* **2016**, *17*, 393–403. [CrossRef] [PubMed]
103. Arora, N.K.; Gustafson, D.H. Perceived Helpfulness of Physicians' Communication Behavior and Breast Cancer Patients' Level of Trust Over Time. *J. Gen. Intern. Med.* **2009**, *24*, 252–255. [CrossRef]
104. Thorne, S.E.; Robinson, C.A. Reciprocal trust in health care relationships. *J. Adv. Nurs.* **1988**, *13*, 782–789. [CrossRef]
105. Mechanic, D.; Meyer, S. Concepts of trust among patients with serious illness. *Soc. Sci. Med.* **2000**, *51*, 657–668. [CrossRef]
106. Miciak, M. Bedside Matters: A Conceptual Framework of the Therapeutic Relationship in Physiotherapy. Ph.D. Thesis, University of Alberta, Edmonton, AB, Canada, 2015.
107. Pearson, S.; Raeke, L. Patients' Trust in Physicians: Many Theories, Few Measures, and Little Data. *J. Gen. Intern. Med.* **2000**, *15*, 509–513. [CrossRef]
108. O'Keeffe, M.; Cullinane, P.; Hurley, J.; Leahy, I.; Bunzli, S.; O'Sullivan, P.B.; O'Sullivan, K. What Influences Patient-Therapist Interactions in Musculoskeletal Physical Therapy? Qualitative Systematic Review and Meta-Synthesis. *Phys. Ther.* **2016**, *96*, 609–622. [CrossRef]
109. Smart, K.; Doody, C. Mechanisms-based clinical reasoning of pain by experienced musculoskeletal physiotherapists. *Physiotherapy* **2006**, *92*, 171–178. [CrossRef]

10. Chimenti, R.L.; Frey-Law, L.A.; Sluka, K.A. A mechanism-based approach to physical therapist management of pain. *Phys. Ther.* **2018**, *98*, 302–314. [CrossRef]
11. Smart, K.M.; Blake, C.; Staines, A.; Thacker, M.; Doody, C. Mechanisms-based classifications of musculoskeletal pain: Part 1 of 3: Symptoms and signs of central sensitisation in patients with low back (+/−leg) pain. *Man. Ther.* **2012**, *17*, 336–344. [CrossRef]
12. Smart, K.M.; Blake, C.; Staines, A.; Thacker, M.; Doody, C. Mechanisms-based classifications of musculoskeletal pain: Part 2 of 3: Symptoms and signs of peripheral neuropathic pain in patients with low back (+/−leg) pain. *Man. Ther.* **2012**, *17*, 345–351. [CrossRef] [PubMed]
13. Smart, K.M.; Blake, C.; Staines, A.; Thacker, M.; Doody, C. Mechanisms-based classifications of musculoskeletal pain: Part 3 of 3: Symptoms and signs of nociceptive pain in patients with low back (+/−leg) pain. *Man. Ther.* **2012**, *17*, 352–357. [CrossRef] [PubMed]
14. Maixner, W.; Fillingim, R.B.; Williams, D.A.; Smith, S.B.; Slade, G.D. Overlapping chronic pain conditions: Implications for diagnosis and classification. *J. Pain* **2016**, *17*, T93–T107. [CrossRef] [PubMed]
15. Campbell, M.; Fitzpatrick, R.; Haines, A.; Kinmonth, A.L.; Sandercock, P.; Spiegelhalter, D.; Tyrer, P. Framework for design and evaluation of complex interventions to improve health. *BMJ* **2000**, *321*, 694–696. [CrossRef]
16. Croot, L.; O'Cathain, A.; Sworn, K.; Yardley, L.; Turner, K.; Duncan, E.; Hoddinott, P. Developing interventions to improve health: A systematic mapping review of international practice between 2015 and 2016. *Pilot Feasibility Stud.* **2019**, *5*, 127. [CrossRef]
17. Bachelor, A. Clients' perception of the therapeutic alliance: A qualitative analysis. *J. Couns. Psychol.* **1995**, *42*, 323. [CrossRef]

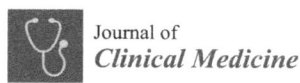

Journal of
Clinical Medicine

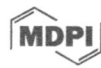

Review

Habituation to Pain in Patients with Chronic Pain: Clinical Implications and Future Directions

Maite M. van der Miesen [1,*], Catherine J. Vossen [1,2] and Elbert A. Joosten [1,2]

[1] Department of Anesthesiology and Pain Management, School for Mental Health and Neuroscience (MHeNS), Faculty of Health, Medicine and Life Sciences (FHML), Maastricht University, 6229 ER Maastricht, The Netherlands; c.vossen@mumc.nl (C.J.V.); bert.joosten@mumc.nl (E.A.J.)
[2] Department of Anesthesiology and Pain Medicine, Maastricht University Medical Centre, 6229 HX Maastricht, The Netherlands
* Correspondence: m.vandermiesen@maastrichtuniversity.nl

Abstract: In this review, the latest insights into habituation to pain in chronic pain are summarized. Using a systematic search, results of studies on the evidence of habituation to (experimental) pain in migraine, chronic low back pain, fibromyalgia, and a variety of chronic pain indications are presented. In migraine, reduced habituation based on self-report and the EEG-based N1 and N2–P2 amplitude is reported, but the presence of contradictory results demands further replication in larger, well-designed studies. Habituation to pain in chronic low back pain seems not to differ from controls, with the exception of EEG measures. In fibromyalgia patients, there is some evidence for reduced habituation of the N2–P2 amplitude. Our analysis shows that the variability between outcomes of studies on habituation to pain is high. As the mechanisms underlying habituation to pain are still not fully understood and likely involve several pathways, it is now too early to conclude that habituation to pain is related to clinical outcomes and can be used as a diagnostic marker. The review ends with a discussion on future directions for research including the use of standard outcome measures to improve comparisons of habituation to pain in patients and controls, as well as a focus on individual differences.

Keywords: chronic pain; habituation; sensitization; migraine; fibromyalgia; chronic low back pain

Citation: van der Miesen, M.M.; Vossen, C.J.; Joosten, E.A. Habituation to Pain in Patients with Chronic Pain: Clinical Implications and Future Directions. *J. Clin. Med.* **2023**, *12*, 4305. https://doi.org/10.3390/jcm12134305

Academic Editors: Jo Nijs and Andrea Polli

Received: 17 May 2023
Revised: 18 June 2023
Accepted: 20 June 2023
Published: 27 June 2023

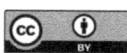
1. Introduction

Habituation is a simple non-associative form of learning that is defined as a response decrement resulting from repeated stimulation, which does not involve sensory adaptation or motor fatigue [1]. Habituation has been reported for numerous stimuli such as auditory, visual, and sensory and has been measured in humans using reflexes, ratings, and physiological measures such as skin conductance, electroencephalography (EEG), and functional magnetic resonance imaging (fMRI) [2]. In addition to habituation, sensitization to repetitive stimulation might occur, which is defined as an increase in response [1,3]. In the field of pain, habituation is usually studied using external stimuli such as heat or electrical current [4].

Reduced habituation has been suggested to occur in a number of neuropsychiatric disorders such as autism [2]. For chronic pain, however, this is not yet well established. Although deficits in habituation may occur in relation to chronic pain, most research in the field has focused on sensitization processes, especially central sensitization. Central sensitization is defined by the International Association for the Study of Pain (IASP) as an increased responsiveness of the central nervous system to normal or subthreshold input [5]. Central sensitization is thought to be implicated in several chronic pain disorders such as fibromyalgia (see, e.g., [6]) and is characterized by hyperalgesia (increase in sensitivity) and allodynia (pain due to a stimulus that would normally not cause pain). Interestingly, central sensitization is often studied based on the cellular level. Recently, researchers argued that the behavioral approach, such as measuring pain ratings as an outcome, should be more emphasized in research on sensitization to pain [7]. Notably, in this review, when discussing sensitization, we refer to an increase in pain on the behavioral level.

For both healthy individuals and chronic pain patients, the mechanism of habituation and sensitization to pain is not fully understood. Several theories have been proposed such as the dual-process theory [8]. This theory states that habituation and sensitization processes may interact to produce the behavioral outcome [8]. One recent proposed mechanism is stimulus-dependent feedback inhibition or inhibitory potentiation, which decreases incoming stimuli [9]. Prior experience, thus, affects the firing of neurons. This mechanism can be seen as a form of predictive coding [9].

Reduced habituation to pain in chronic pain patients has been mainly reported in the indications migraine, chronic low back pain (CLBP), and fibromyalgia [4]. Although numerous studies have been published, no review of the literature is, to our knowledge, available. The main aim of this review is, therefore, to summarize the literature on habituation to pain based on effects of repeated painful stimulation in chronic pain patients (with a focus on migraine, CLBP, and fibromyalgia) as well as its potential treatment targets and clinical implications. We hope that this review may serve as a knowledge basis to design new innovative studies on habituation to pain in chronic pain.

In this review, results of patients versus controls are discussed. When comparing two groups with respect to habituation, several terms are used such as altered, decreased, or impaired habituation. McDiarmid and colleagues (2017) formulated recommendations to interpret the responses of repeated stimulation, i.e., habituation curves or trajectories [2]. In the literature included in the review, however, these recommendations have not been fully implemented, and a quantifiable measure of habituation is not available. For the current review, therefore, we used the term *reduced* habituation to pain if patients showed less habituation following repeated painful stimulation as compared to controls (i.e., the decrease in VAS was less than in controls). Furthermore, reduced habituation in patients may also include and be indicative for sensitization to pain. If available, the direction of the effect, i.e., whether patients and/or controls showed habituation, no change, or sensitization to pain, is discussed and presented in tables.

2. Materials and Methods

The search was preregistered at the Open Science Framework (osf.io/nypbw). Articles were selected using a systematic search of PubMed, PsycINFO, and Web of Science databases (up until January 2023). For extensive search criteria and the selection procedure of included articles, see the Supplementary Materials (Figure S1). The articles included from our systematic search were split into those investigating healthy individuals (revised manuscript submitted) and chronic pain patients, which are the focus of this review.

3. Results

The systematic database search of PubMed, PsycINFO, and Web of Science resulted in the inclusion of $n = 40$ articles. The results of this search showed that most studies were performed in patients with headache disorders (mostly migraine, $n = 17$), CLBP ($n = 7$), and fibromyalgia ($n = 7$) (see Figure 1A). Therefore, we subdivided these sections accordingly. Sample sizes varied greatly between nine and 199 included participants (Figure 1B). Most research included self-report ratings of pain ($n = 25$), whereas EEG was the most used method ($n = 30$) followed by solely self-report ratings ($n = 8$) (Figure 1C). Heat stimuli using a thermode and heat stimuli using a laser were most frequently used for repeated painful stimulation (Figure 1D). Only two studies investigated long-term habituation to pain [10,11], whereas all other studies investigated short-term habituation to pain. For this, a wide range of stimulus repetitions were used, with a median of 30 (Figure 1E). The majority of these studies performed individual calibration to decide on the stimulus intensity, whereas 42.5% of the studies used a fixed intensity level (Figure 1F).

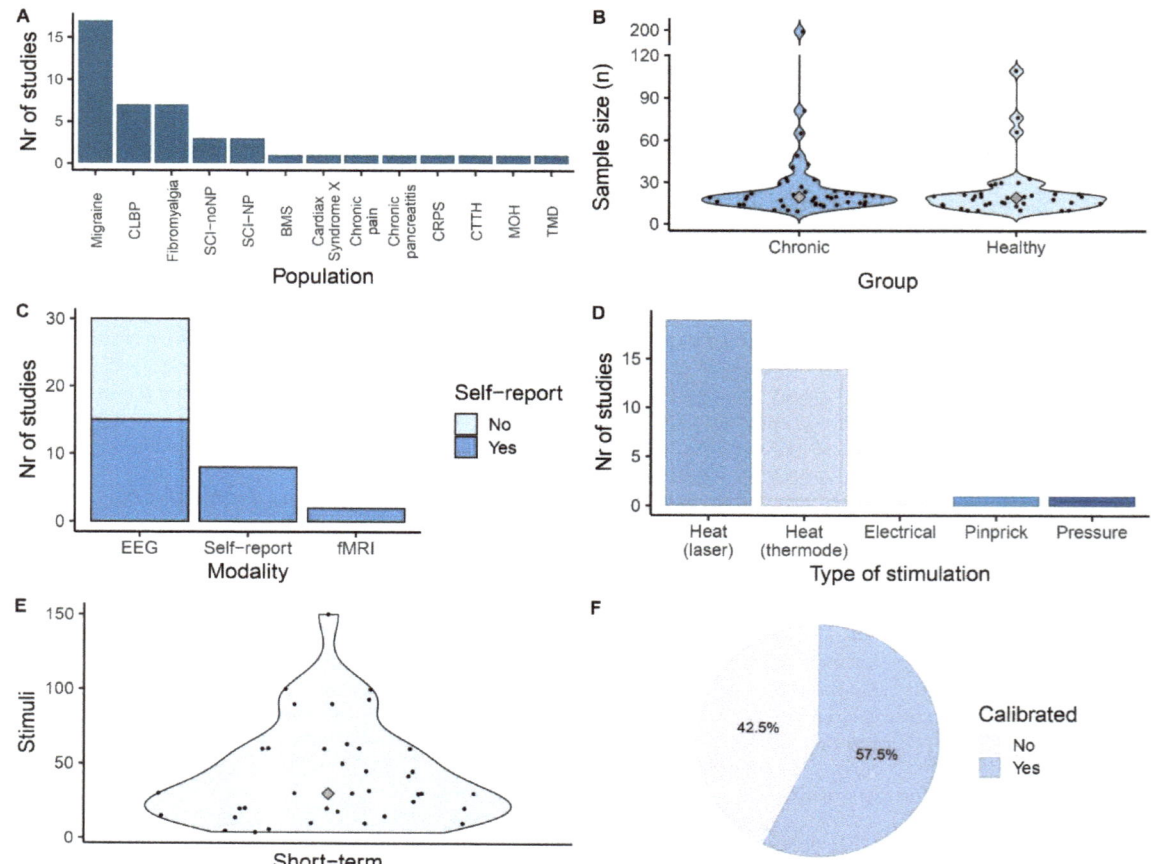

Figure 1. Overview of included studies. Gray diamonds indicate the median. (**A**) Number of studies per chronic pain indication. (**B**) Sample sizes for chronic and healthy populations. (**C**) Number of studies per modality and whether they included self-report. (**D**) Type of stimulation used. (**E**) Number of stimuli to measure habituation. (**F**) Use of individual calibration in studies. BMS, burning mouth syndrome; CLBP, chronic low back pain; CRPS, complex regional pain syndrome; CTTH, chronic tension-type headache; EEG, electroencephalography; fMRI, functional magnetic resonance imaging; MOH, medication-overuse headache; SCI-NP, spinal cord injury with neuropathic pain; SCI-noNP, spinal cord injury without neuropathic pain; TMD, temporomandibular disorder.

3.1. Headache Disorders

Headache disorders are among the most common chronic central nervous system disorders, with migraine being the indication most studied [12]. In migraine research, several research lines have focused on habituation to sensory stimuli (e.g., visual, auditory, and painful responses) [13]. It has been hypothesized that reduced habituation to pain in migraine patients may be caused by increased cortical excitability, decreased inhibition, or decreased pre-activation levels [14]. Data on habituation to pain using self-report and EEG, with a focus on migraine patients are presented in Figure 2 and Table 1.

For self-report using electrical stimuli, reduced habituation was reported at the trigeminal area but not at the tibial region [15]. Other studies that included different stimulation sites showed similar habituation for self-report at different stimulation sites [16,17]. Studies using heat stimuli showed mixed effects: habituation in both patients and in controls [16], reduced habituation in patients with migraine with aura for predicted pain [18], or reduced habituation in patients without aura [19]. Interestingly, a large study using laser stimuli showed no self-reported habituation differences between migraine patients and controls [20], which contrasts with earlier findings [17,21].

Results from evoked potentials with heat stimuli showed similar habituation [16] or reduced habituation in patients versus controls [18,19]. Several studies focused on laser-evoked potentials (LEPs) and reported a reduced N2–P2 amplitude habituation in migraine patients [17,21–24]. Another study reporting evidence for reduced habituation of the N2–P2 amplitude showed that this effect over time was accompanied by increased connectivity between the thalamus and somatosensory areas in migraine patients, but not in controls [14]. Contradictorily, an observer-blinded longitudinal study with large sample sizes ($n = 30$–49) using advanced statistical models did not report any group differences and noted similar habituation of the N2–P2 amplitude for migraine patients and controls [20]. The authors of the latter study provided a detailed comparison of studies using LEP's in migraine patients and argued that the evidence for reduced habituation in migraine patients is low [20]. Results for N1 amplitude habituation are less frequently reported and also mixed, with two studies reporting differences [23,25], although the latter did not compare groups directly, and one study reported no group differences [20].

Furthermore, it was shown that LEP amplitudes did not differ between chronic tension-type headache (CTTH) patients and healthy controls, although migraine patients showed reduced habituation compared to CTTH patients [23]. Additionally, the LEP amplitudes were not influenced by migraine phase [17,20], visually induced analgesia [26], or the presence or absence of aura [20]. Menstrual phase affected the amount of habituation in both migraine patients and healthy controls [24].

In summary, taking into account the large variability in study design, parameters, and outcome measures, it is tentatively concluded that there is only limited evidence that migraine patients show reduced habituation for both self-report and the N1 and N2–P2 amplitude. This conclusion takes into consideration that several studies reported contradictory effects (see Figure 2), and one blinded study with a large sample size did not report differences [20]. More conclusive evidence is needed, and this should be based on large-scale randomized study designs.

Table 1. Overview of habituation to pain in chronic headache disorders. ↘: decrease over time (habituation). →: no significant change. ↗: increase over time (sensitization). <: reduced habituation in the chronic pain patient compared to the control group. =: no significant difference in habituation between the groups. C, control; CHEP, contact heat-evoked potential; CTTH, chronic tension-type headache; EEG, electroencephalography; ISI, inter-stimulus interval; M, migraine; MOA, migraine without aura; MOH, medication-overuse headache; MWA, migraine with aura; NRS, numeric rating scale; PREP, pain-related evoked potential; sLORETA, standardized low-resolution brain electromagnetic tomography; VAS, visual analogue scale.

	Sample Size	Timescale	Type of Stimuli	Site	Nr of Stimuli for Habituation Analysis	Duration	ISI	Habituation Measurement	Habituation Analysis	Main Habituation Result
Bassez et al., 2020 [14]	M = 23 C = 20	Short-term	Heat (CO$_2$ laser)	Right forehead	15	Intensity (and, thus, duration) varied per participant, 15–45 ms	Self-paced, ± 10 s	EEG: N2–P2 amplitude Dynamic causal modelling	% change between first and third block Connectivity changes over blocks	M < C Increased thalamo-somatosensory connectivity in migraine patients
Beese et al., 2015 [16]	M = 22 (12 with aura) C = 22	Short-term	Heat (thermode)	Volar forearm, left and right cheek	20	-	15–18 s	NRS: single trial CHEP: N2–P2 amplitude	Average of first 5 trials vs. last 5 trials Average of first 5 trials vs. last 5 trials	NRS for each site and block: M ↘ C ↘ N2–P2 for each site and block: M ↘ C ↘
de Tommaso et al., 2005 [17]	M = 14 (without aura) C = 10	Short-term	Heat (CO$_2$ laser)	Right and left hand and supraorbital zone	60	20 ms	10 s	NRS: single trial EEG: N2–P2 amplitude	Trend over block Trend over block	NRS both hand and face: M ↗ < C ↘ N2–P2 both hand and face: M → < C ↘ No differences between migraine phase
de Tommaso et al., 2005 [21]	M = 14 (without aura) C = 10	Short-term	Heat (CO$_2$ laser)	Right supraorbital zone	63	20 ms	10 s	VAS: single trial EEG: N2–P2 amplitude	Trend over block Trend over block	VAS: M → C ↘ N2–P2: M → C ↘
de Tommaso et al., 2009 [24]	M = 9 (without aura) C = 10	Short-term	Heat (CO$_2$ laser)	Right dorsum of the hand and supraorbital zone	60	25 ms	10–15 s	EEG: N2–P2 amplitude	Ratio of amplitude between block 1 and 3	Both hand and face: M < C Menstrual cycle affects habituation of N2–P2
de Tommaso et al., 2015 [22]	M = 31 (without aura) C = 19	Short-term	Heat (CO$_2$ laser)	Dorsum of the right hand	30	30 ms	10 s	EEG: N2–P2 amplitude	Stimuli were divided in three blocks, % change relative to first block	M < C

Table 1. *Cont.*

	Sample Size	Timescale	Type of Stimuli	Site	Nr of Stimuli for Habituation Analysis	Duration	ISI	Habituation Measurement	Habituation Analysis	Main Habituation Result
De Tommaso et al., 2016 [27]	M = 20 C = 20	Short-term	Heat (CO_2 laser)	Dorsum of the right hand, right supraorbital zone and the skin over the right trapezius	30	30 ms	7 s	EEG: N2–P2 amplitude	Stimuli were divided in three blocks, % change relative to first block	Baseline N2–P2 hand and face: M < C Shoulder: M = C After onabotulintoxin A treatment, N2–P2 habituation at face increased, no effect on hand and shoulder habituation
De Tommaso et al., 2021 [28]	M = 17	Short-term	Heat (CO_2 laser)	Dorsum of the right hand and left and right supraorbital zone	30	30 ms	10 s	EEG: N1, N2, P2 amplitude	Ratio between average of last and first 10 stimuli	No effect of erenumab on N1 and P2 at both sides, increased habituation after erenumab at N2 of left forehead
Di Clemente et al., 2013 [25]	M = 13 (without aura) C = 15	Short-term	Heat (YAP laser)	Dorsum of the right hand and right supraorbital zone	45	-	10 s	EEG: N1 and N2-P2 amplitude	% change between first and third block	N1 hand and face: M < C N2–P2 hand and face: M = C Topiramate reduces N1 habituation deficit/affects habituation
Di Lorenzo et al., 2019 [29]	M = 18 (without aura) C = 18	Short-term	Electrical	Right supraorbital notch	10	Train of 3 0.1 ms pulses with 5 ms interal (total 10.3 ms)	30–35 s	PREP: N–P amplitude	Slope between first and second block	Before treatment: M < C After treatment: no group comparison Ketogenic diet increased habituation in migraine

Table 1. *Cont.*

	Sample Size	Timescale	Type of Stimuli	Site	Nr of Stimuli for Habituation Analysis	Duration	ISI	Habituation Measurement	Habituation Analysis	Main Habituation Result
Ferraro et al., 2012 [30]	MOH = 14 (group I treatment effective = 8; group II treatment not effective = 6) C = 14	Short-term	Heat (CO$_2$ laser)	Dorsum of the right hand and perioral region	90	10 ms	8–12 s	VAS: after each block EEG: N1 and N2-P2 amplitude	Percentage of the first block Percentage of the first block	VAS: Before treatment for hand and face: MOH group I and II < C After treatment hand: MOH group II < C and MOH group I After treatment face: MOH group I and II = C EEG: N1 hand before treatment: MOH group I and II < C N1 hand after treatment: MOH group I and II = C N1 face before treatment: MOH group II < C N1 face after treatment: MOH group I and II < C N2-P2 hand and face before treatment: MOH group I and II < C N2-P2 hand and face after treatment: MOH group II < C and MOH group I Treatment affected habituation in clinically improved patients
Gierse-Plogmeier et al., 2009 [15]	M = 20 (10 with aura) C = 20	Short-term	Electrical	Trigeminal (masseter region), peripheral (tibial region)	20	1 ms	2 s	VAS: last stimulus of train	Group comparison of difference score between trains	Trigeminal: M < C Peripheral: M = C

Table 1. *Cont.*

	Sample Size	Timescale	Type of Stimuli	Site	Nr of Stimuli for Habituation Analysis	Duration	ISI	Habituation Measurement	Habituation Analysis	Main Habituation Result
Lev et al., 2010 [19]	M = 21 (with aura) C = 22	Short-term	Heat (thermode)	Left volar forearm	60	-	–	NRS: single trial CHEP: N2-P2 amplitude and sLORETA	Group comparison of inter-train change Group comparison of inter-train change	NRS: M ↗ < C → N2-P2: M ↗ < C ↘ > M < C activity in contralateral orbitofrontal cortex M > C in contralateral primary somatosensory cortex, insula, parahippocampal cortex, and bilateral posterior cingulate cortex
Lev et al., 2013 [18]	MWA = 20 MOA = 19 C = 22	Short-term	Heat (thermode)	Left volar forearm	50	-	10 s	NRS: single trial CHEP: N2-P2 amplitude and sLORETA	Group comparison of inter-train change Group comparison of inter-train change	NRS: Predicted pain: MWA ↗ < C → and MOA → Unpredicted pain: MOA ↗ = MWA ↗ = C → N2-P2: Predicted pain: MOA → and MWA ↗ < C ↘ Unpredicted pain: MOA ↗ and MWA ↗ < C → Predicted pain: MWA < C activity in right inferior frontal gyrus and supplementary motor area MWA > C activity in primary and secondary somatosensory cortex, motor cortex, and bilateral posterior cingulate cortex MOA > C activity in right insula Unpredicted pain: MWA > C activity in bilateral medial frontal cortex, right anterior cingulate cortexMOA > C activity in right motor cortex, primary and secondary somatosensory cortex, left orbitofrontal cortex, parahippocampal cortex, and insula

Table 1. *Cont.*

	Sample Size	Timescale	Type of Stimuli	Site	Nr of Stimuli for Habituation Analysis	Duration	ISI	Habituation Measurement	Habituation Analysis	Main Habituation Result
Sava et al., 2018 [26]	M = 14 (without aura) C = 11	Short-term	Heat (thermode)	Right volar wrist or forehead	20	707 ms	10–22 s	CHEP: P1-P2 slope	Slope over average of 5 blocks	Mirror did not influence habituation in controls or migraine patients
Sebastianelli et al., 2023 [31]	M = 15	Short-term	Electrical	Supraorbital nerve at the forehead	18	Three 0.1 ms pulses with 5 ms interval	40 s	EEG: N-P amplitude	Slope of the amplitude between the first and third block	No effect of onabotulintoxin A on habituation
Uglem et al., 2017 [20]	M = 49 (27 without aura, 4 with, 18 both) C = 30	Short-term	Heat (YAP laser)	Dorsum of the right hand	42	6 ms	6–10 s	NRS: single trial EEG: N1 and N2-P2 amplitude	Multilevel models	NRS: M →= C →; N1: M →= C →; N2-P2: M ↘ = C ↘; Habituation was mainly similar between migraine phases
Valeriani et al., 2003 [23]	M = 24 (without aura) CTTH = 19 C = 28	Short-term	Heat (CO$_2$ laser)	Left and right dorsum of the hand and face	45 for face, 90 for hand	10 ms	8–12 s	EEG: N1-P1 and N2-P2 amplitude	% decrease over blocks	N1-P1 hand: M → C ↘; N1-P1 face: M → C →; N2-P2 hand: M ↘ < C; CTTH ↘ = C →↘; M ↘ < CTTH ↘; N2-P2 face: M →< C ↘; CTTH ↘ = C ↘

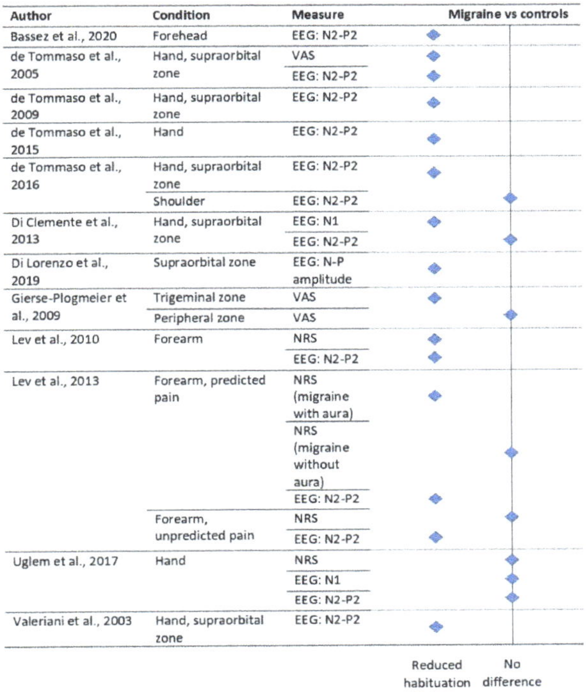

Author	Condition	Measure	Migraine vs controls
Bassez et al., 2020	Forehead	EEG: N2-P2	
de Tommaso et al., 2005	Hand, supraorbital zone	VAS	
		EEG: N2-P2	
de Tommaso et al., 2009	Hand, supraorbital zone	EEG: N2-P2	
de Tommaso et al., 2015	Hand	EEG: N2-P2	
de Tommaso et al., 2016	Hand, supraorbital zone	EEG: N2-P2	
	Shoulder	EEG: N2-P2	
Di Clemente et al., 2013	Hand, supraorbital zone	EEG: N1	
		EEG: N2-P2	
Di Lorenzo et al., 2019	Supraorbital zone	EEG: N-P amplitude	
Gierse-Plogmeier et al., 2009	Trigeminal zone	VAS	
	Peripheral zone	VAS	
Lev et al., 2010	Forearm	NRS	
		EEG: N2-P2	
Lev et al., 2013	Forearm, predicted pain	NRS (migraine with aura)	
		NRS (migraine without aura)	
		EEG: N2-P2	
	Forearm, unpredicted pain	NRS	
		EEG: N2-P2	
Uglem et al., 2017	Hand	NRS	
		EEG: N1	
		EEG: N2-P2	
Valeriani et al., 2003	Hand, supraorbital zone	EEG: N2-P2	

Reduced habituation   No difference

Figure 2. Effect of habituation to pain in migraine patients versus controls. Note: Only those studies using direct group comparisons are included. EEG, electroencephalography; NRS, numeric rating scale; VAS, visual analogue scale [14,15,17–20,22–25,29].

3.2. Chronic Low Back Pain

Chronic low back pain (CLBP) is known for its high prevalence and large global impact on health and society [32]. The majority of CLBP patients have pain without a specific patho-anatomical cause, and this pain is, therefore, described as "nonspecific" [33].

The available literature for habituation to pain in CLBP patients is relatively limited, yet still diverse (see Figure 3 and Table 2). Early short-term studies using pressure or electrical stimuli did not demonstrate any self-report differences between CLBP patients and controls, independent of the presence [34] or absence [35] of habituation to pain. CLBP patients (diverse pain population and short disease duration) and controls reported similar (long-term) habituation to pain over time, as well as within-session sensitization to pain with use of an 8 day heat paradigm [10,11]. No changes in brain activity related to differences in habituation were shown between CLBP patients and controls, both over days or within sessions [11]. In patients with painful radiculopathy, LEP habituation was reduced, although this effect was not apparent for pain ratings [36]. Two studies adopted newer analysis methods for the study of habituation. Vossen et al. (2015) explored the EEG-amplitude signal at a very detailed scale, partitioning the post-stimulus epoch in 20 ms areas under the curve (event-related fixed-interval areas; ERFIAs) in combination with multilevel modeling [37]. Reduced habituation to pain was reported in CLBP patients at 340 to 460 ms post stimulus after painful stimuli [37]. The applicability of high temporal resolution analysis of LEP signals and habituation in radiculopathy patients was shown to be limited as a result of the data quality [38].

Both short- and long-term habituation to pain in CLBP patients did not seem to differ from that noted in controls according to self-report and long-term fMRI studies (Figure 3). Temporarily restricted effects, as measured with EEG, however, were shown to effect habituation to pain in CLBP patients. The latter needs further replication to investigate the robustness and reproducibility of this effect.

Table 2. Overview of habituation to pain in CLBP. ↘: decrease over time (habituation). →: no significant change. ↗: increase over time (sensitization). <: reduced habituation in the chronic pain patient compared to the control group. =: no significant difference in habituation between the groups. BOLD, blood-oxygen-level-dependent; C, control; CLBP, chronic low back pain; EEG, electroencephalography; fMRI, functional magnetic resonance imaging; ISI, inter-stimulus interval; NRS, numeric rating scale; P, painful radiculopathy; VAS, visual analogue scale.

	Sample Size	Timescale	Type of Stimuli	Site	Nr of Stimuli for Habituation Analysis	Duration	ISI	Habituation Measurement	Habituation Analysis	Main Habituation Result
Arntz et al., 1991 [34]	CLBP = 22 C = 21	Short-term	Electrical	Thumb of left hand	20	1 s	15–45 s	VAS: pretest, last trial of blocks, post-test	Trend over time	CLBP ↘ = C ↘
Hüllemann et al., 2017 [36]	Painful radiculopathy = 27 C = 20	Short-term	Heat (YAP laser)	Middle ventral thigh	100	5 ms	8–12 s	NRS: single trail EEG: N2-P2 amplitude	Trend over blocks	P ↘ = C ↘ P ↘ < C ↘
Kersebaum et al., 2021 [38]	Painful radiculopathy n = 14 for twelve blocks and n = 18 for six blocks, controls n = 10 for twelve blocks and n = 14 for six blocks	Short-term	Heat (YAP laser)	Middle ventral thigh	100	5 ms	8–12 s	NRS: single trial EEG: N2-P2 amplitude	High-temporal-resolution analysis	NRS: over 12 blocks P ↘ C NA, over six blocks P → C → N2-P2: over 12 blocks P ↘ C NA, over six blocks P ↘ C →
May et al., 2012 [10]	CLBP = 21 C = 66	Long-term (8 days)	Heat (thermode)	Left volar forearm	480	6 s	–	VAS: average rating of last 6 stimuli	Trend over time	Within-session: CLBP ↗ = C ↗ Between-session: CLBP ↘ = C ↘
Peters et al., 1989 [35]	CLBP = 20 C = 20	Short-term	Pressure	Index finger of non-dominant hand	6	70% of pain tolerance time	4 min	VAS: single trials	Trend over time	CLBP → = C →
Rodriguez-Raecke et al., 2014 [11]	CLBP = 19 C = 21	Long-term (8 days)	Heat (thermode)	Left volar forearm	480	6 s	–	VAS: average rating of last 6 stimuli fMRI: BOLD	Trend over time Whole-brain contrast	Within-session: CLBP ↗ = C ↗ Between-session: CLBP ↘ = C ↘ CLBP = C
Vossen et al., 2015 [37]	CLBP = 65 C = 76	Short-term	Electrical	Left middle finger	150	10 ms	9–11 s	EEG: amplitude	Multilevel model with event-related fixed-interval areas	CLBP ↘ < C ↘

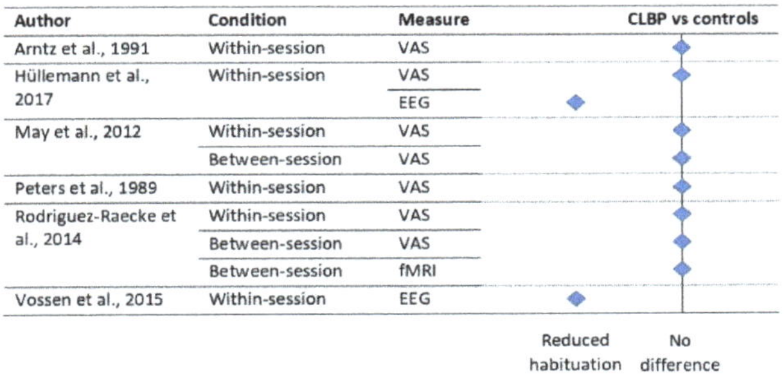

Author	Condition	Measure	CLBP vs controls
Arntz et al., 1991	Within-session	VAS	
Hüllemann et al., 2017	Within-session	VAS	
		EEG	
May et al., 2012	Within-session	VAS	
	Between-session	VAS	
Peters et al., 1989	Within-session	VAS	
Rodriguez-Raecke et al., 2014	Within-session	VAS	
	Between-session	VAS	
	Between-session	fMRI	
Vossen et al., 2015	Within-session	EEG	

Reduced habituation   No difference

Figure 3. Effect of habituation to pain in CLBP patients versus controls. Note: Only those studies using direct group comparisons are included. EEG, electroencephalography; fMRI, functional magnetic resonance imaging; VAS, visual analogue scale [10,11,34–37].

3.3. Fibromyalgia

Fibromyalgia is characterized by chronic widespread pain and potential comorbidities such as disturbed sleep and psychological problems [39].

Hollins et al. (2011) investigated habituation to pain as a function of the time course of pain ratings in patients with fibromyalgia and controls using heat pain stimuli [40]. Both fibromyalgia patients and controls displayed first an adaptation phase followed by a sensitization phase within each run. In addition, they showed habituation to pain over the runs. The magnitude of the initial adaptation phase increased over the runs. For both the habituation (within and over runs) and the sensitization to pain, no group effects were found [40]. Conversely, de Tommaso et al. (2011) did report differences in fibromyalgia patients compared tocontrols with respect to habituation of pain ratings [41] (see Figure 4). It should be taken into account that differences in sample size, stimulus type, and the way of measuring habituation make it difficult to compare the results from de Tommaso et al. (2011) with those reported by Hollins and colleagues (2011) (see Table 3). Analyses using EEG showed reduced habituation for the N2, P2, and N2–P2 amplitude in fibromyalgia patients, but not for the N1 amplitude [41]. Follow-up EEG studies from the same laboratory reported again reduced habituation to pain of the N2–P2 amplitude in fibromyalgia patients as compared to controls [42,43]. Interestingly, in a comparative study, a more pronounced reduction in habituation to pain was shown in patients with comorbid migraine or sensory deficits as compared with fibromyalgia patients without comorbidities [42]. Habituation to pain on the thigh (for the N2 component) and foot (for the P2 component) did not result in differences between fibromyalgia patients and controls [44].

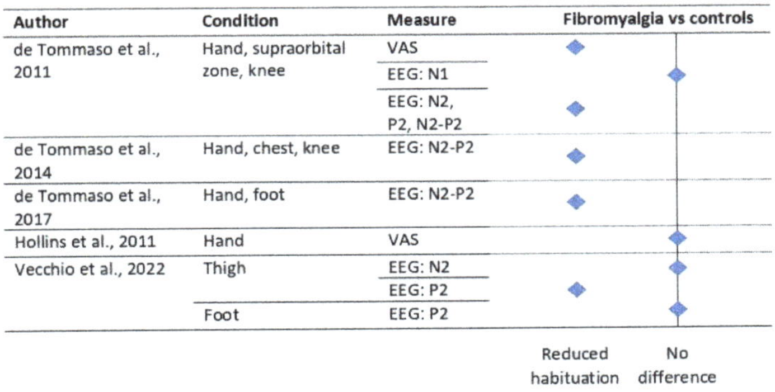

Author	Condition	Measure	Fibromyalgia vs controls
de Tommaso et al., 2011	Hand, supraorbital zone, knee	VAS	
		EEG: N1	
		EEG: N2, P2, N2-P2	
de Tommaso et al., 2014	Hand, chest, knee	EEG: N2-P2	
de Tommaso et al., 2017	Hand, foot	EEG: N2-P2	
Hollins et al., 2011	Hand	VAS	
Vecchio et al., 2022	Thigh	EEG: N2	
		EEG: P2	
	Foot	EEG: P2	

Reduced habituation   No difference

Figure 4. Effect of habituation to pain in fibromyalgia patients versus controls. Note: Only those studies using direct group comparisons are included. EEG, electroencephalography; VAS, visual analogue scale [40–44].

Table 3. Overview of habituation to pain in fibromyalgia patients. <: reduced habituation in the chronic pain patient compared to the control group. =: no significant difference in habituation between the groups. C, control; EEG, electroencephalography; F = fibromyalgia; FMD; fibromyalgia with proximal and distal denervation; FMN, fibromyalgia with normal skin biopsy; FMP, fibromyalgia with proximal denervation; ISI, inter-stimulus interval; M = migraine; TMD, temporomandibular disorder; VAS, visual analogue scale.

	Sample Size	Timescale	Type of Stimuli	Site	Nr of Stimuli for Habituation Analysis	Duration	ISI	Habituation Measurement	HabituationAnalysis	Main Habituation Result
de Tommaso et al., 2011 [41]	F = 14 C = 13	Short-term	Heat (CO_2 laser)	Dorsum of the right hand, right supraorbital zone and knee	20	25 ms	10 s	VAS: average per block EEG: N1, N2, P2, and N2-P2 amplitude	Quotient between third and first block	VAS: F < C N1: F = C N2, P2, and N2-P2: F < C No differences between sites Self-reported depressive symptoms correlate with N2 habituation
de Tommaso et al., 2014 [42]	F combined = 199 F = 94 F with M = 70F with sensory deficits = 35 C = 109	Short-term	Heat (CO_2 laser)	Dorsum of the right hand, chest and knee	10	30 ms	10 s	EEG: N2-P2 amplitude	Quotient between third and first block	All sites: F combined < C F < C F with M < C F with sensory deficits < C F with M < F with sensory deficits No correlation between habituation and self-reported depressive symptoms
de Tommaso et al., 2017 [43]	F = 50 C = 30	Short-term	Heat (CO_2 laser)	Dorsum of the right hand and foot	30	30 ms	10 s	EEG: N2-P2 amplitude	Percent amplitude change between third and first group of responses	Hand and foot: F < C
Hollins et al., 2011 [40]	F = 17 TMD = 29 C = 29	Short-term	Heat (thermode)	Base of the thumb	33	3 s	12 s	VAS: single trial	Decrease over blocks	F = TMD = C
McLoughlin et al., 2011 [45]	F = 16 C = 18	Short-term	Heat (thermode)	Left hand palm	5	20 s	20 s	VAS: single trial	Difference score	Self-reported activity correlated negatively with pain and unpleasantness difference scores in patients
Vecchio et al., 2020 [46]	F = 81	Short-term	Heat (CO_2 laser)	Dorsum of the right hand, in subgroups also thorax and dorsum of the foot	30	30 ms	10 s	EEG: N2-P2 amplitude	Ratio between third and first block	Thigh: habituation index of N2-P2 predicted intra-epidermal nerve fiber density

Table 3. *Cont.*

	Sample Size	Timescale	Type of Stimuli	Site	Nr of Stimuli for Habituation Analysis	Duration	ISI	Habituation Measurement	Habituation Analysis	Main Habituation Result
Vecchio et al., 2022 [44]	F = 41 (F with normal skin biopsy FMN = 18, F with proximal denervation FMP = 22, F with proximal and distal denervation FMD = 7) C = 15	Short-term	Heat (CO_2 laser)	Thigh and dorsum of the foot	30	30 ms	10 s	EEG: N2 and P2 amplitude	Change over time between third and first block	Thigh N2: F = C Thigh P2: F < C (all groups, FMN > FMP, FMD) Foot P2: F = C Patients with reduced intra-epidermal nerve fiber density showed less habituation of the P2 component

On the basis of the EEG studies in fibromyalgia patients, there is some evidence for reduced habituation to pain of the N2–P2 amplitude (see Figure 4). These effects demand further replication in order to infer clinical significance. Only two studies investigated self-report with contradictory findings, which needs further investigation.

3.4. Other Chronic Pain Indications

In this subsection, the studies on habituation to pain related to a variety of chronic pain indications (burning mouth syndrome, temporomandibular disorder, cardia syndrome X, chronic pancreatitis, spinal cord injury-related neuropathic pain, and complex regional pain syndrome) are summarized. Temporomandibular disorder is characterized by chronic pain located in the jaw and temporomandibular joint and is a subgroup of primary orofacial pain [47,48]. The same applies to burning mouth syndrome, which may cause a chronic burning sensation in and around the mouth [49].

Using fMRI, patients with burning mouth syndrome (BMS) showed reduced brain activity in the dorsal anterior cingulate cortex (dACC), bilateral ventral midcingulate cortex (MCC), left posterior cingulate cortex (PCC), and cerebellum over the course of four thermal stimuli [50] (see Table 4). This habituation effect of brain activity was not noted in controls, who only showed increased brain activity in the PCC over time [50]. Patients with temporomandibular disorder (TMD) did not show different habituation from both controls and fibromyalgia patients [40].

In patients with cardiac syndrome X, reduced habituation was shown after laser stimulation, which was more apparent at the chest than at the hand for self-report ratings and the N2–P2 amplitude [51]. Olesen et al. (2013) investigated contact-heat evoked potentials (CHEPs) in chronic pancreatitis patients [52]. Reduced habituation for both pain ratings and the N2–P2 amplitude over time was shown and this was more pronounced for stimulation at the chest (pancreatic area) as compared to the forearm [52]. Studies based on analysis of patients with and without spinal cord injury (SCI)-related central neuropathic pain reported mixed results (see Table 4). One study demonstrated reduced habituation to pain in patients with neuropathic pain for pain ratings and CHEPs as compared to both healthy controls and to SCI patients without central neuropathic pain [53]. Conversely, absence of any difference in habituation of CHEPs or habituation of pain ratings between SCI with and without neuropathic pain were also reported [54,55]. It should be noted that SCI is characterized by its heterogeneity based on lesion size, location, and type of injury, and that this may significantly affect the development of chronic neuropathic pain in these patients. Moreover, although all three studies tested above the level of injury, Kumru et al. (2012) stimulated at the shoulder, while Albu et al. (2015) and Lütolf et al. (2022) stimulated at the hand and forearm, respectively. This variability on top of the heterogeneity of patients described above may underlie the differences in the literature on effect of habituation to pain in patients with this indication.

In patients with complex regional pain syndrome (CRPS) both heat pain ratings and pinprick ratings did not result in (reduced) habituation or differences between patients and healthy individuals [56]. A study using EEG including chronic pain patients based on a variety of indications reported no differences in pain ratings over a series of electrical stimuli [57]. Nevertheless, both the presence of chronic pain and the hypervigilance independently affected habituation of the EEG signal at several time latencies [57].

In summary, a trend can be noted toward reduced habituation to pain in a variety of chronic pain indications. Nonetheless, the available evidence is often based on one study for a specific pain indication and with small sample sizes. These constraints do not allow making conclusive statements about differences in habituation effects specifically related to the individual indications or to chronic pain in general.

Table 4. Overview of habituation to pain in other indications. ↘: decrease over time (habituation). →: no significant change. ↗: increase over time (sensitization). <: reduced habituation in the chronic pain patient compared to the control group. =: no significant difference in habituation between the groups. BOLD, blood-oxygen-level-dependent; BMS, burning mouth syndrome; C, control; CAD, coronary artery disease; CSX, cardiac syndrome X; CHEP, contact heat evoked potential; CP, chronic pancreatitis; CRPS, complex regional pain syndrome; EEG, electroencephalography; F, fibromyalgia; ISI, inter-stimulus interval; NRS, numeric rating scale; SCI-NP, spinal cord injury with neuropathic pain; SCI-noNP, spinal cord injury without neuropathic pain; TMD, temporomandibular disorder; VAS, visual analogue scale; VRS, verbal rating scale.

	Sample Size	Timescale	Type of Stimuli	Site	Nr of Stimuli for Habituation Analysis	Duration	ISI	Habituation Measurement	Habituation Analysis	Main Habituation Result
Albu et al., 2015 [54]	SCI-noNP = 10 SCI-NP = 10 C = 10	Short-term	Heat (ther-mode)	Thenar eminence of dominant hand	10	-	20 s	NRS: single trial CHEP: N2–P2 amplitude	Percentage last stimulus with respect to first stimulus	NRS and CHEP: SCI-noNP = SCI-NP = C
Hollins et al., 2011 [40]	F = 17 TMD = 29 C = 29	Short-term	Heat (ther-mode)	Base of the thumb	33	3 s	12 s	VAS: single trial	Decrease over blocks	F = TMD = C
Kumru et al., 2012 [53]	SCI-noNP = 22 SCI-NP = 32 C = 16	Short-term	Heat (ther-mode)	Shoulder	14	-	30 s	NRS: single trial CHEP: N2–P2 amplitude	% change of last compared to first stimulus	NRS and CHEP: SCI-NP < SCI-noNP SCI-NP < C
Lütolf et al., 2022 [55]	SCI-noNP = 13, SCI-NP = 17, C = 14	Short-term	Heat (ther-mode)	Right volar forearm	10	-	15–19 s	NRS: single trial	Percentage decrease	SCI-noNP = SCI-NP = C
Olesen et al., 2013 [52]	Chronic pancreatitis = 15 C = 15	Short-term	Heat (ther-mode)	Right forearm and upper abdominal area	93	-	8–12 s	VAS: first and last stimulus of block CHEP: N1 and N2–P2 amplitude	Change over blocks	Abdominal: CP → < C ↘ Forearm: CP → < C ↘ Abdominal: N1: CP = C N2–P2: CP → < C ↘ Forearm: N1: CP = C N2–P2: CP → = C ↘
Scheuren et al., 2023 [56]	CRPS = 20, C = 16	Short-term	Heat (ther-mode), pinprick	Affected and control area	15	-	13–17s	NRS: single trial	% change in third compared to first block and trend over blocks	Heat: CRPS → = C → Pinprick: CRPS → = C →

Table 4. Cont.

Sample Size	Timescale	Type of Stimuli	Site	Nr of Stimuli for Habituation Analysis	Duration	ISI	Habituation Measurement	Habituation Analysis	Main Habituation Result
Shinozaki et al., 2016 [50] BMS = 16 C = 15	Short-term	Heat (thermode)	Right palm and right lower lip	4	32 s	104 s	NRS: single trial fMRI: BOLD	Stimulus 1 compared to 4	NRS: Lip: BMS → C ↘ Palm: BMS → C → fMRI: Lip: Reduced activity in BMS patients over time in the right dorsal anterior cingulate cortex, bilateral ventral midcingulate cortex, left posterior cingulate cortex, right angular gyrus, and left cerebellum. Increased activity in controls over time in the left posterior cingulate cortex.
Valeriani et al., 2005 [51] Cardiac syndrome X = 16 Coronary artery disease = 10 C = 13	Short-term	Heat (CO_2 laser)	Dorsum of the right hand and chest	90	10 ms	8–12 s	VAS: per block EEG: N1–P1 and N2–P2 amplitude	Trend over blocks	Chest: VAS and N2-P2: Cardiac SX ↘ Cardiac SX = CAD = C and CAD ↘ N1–P1: Cardiac SX = CAD = C Hand: VAS: Cardiac SX ↗ < C ↘ and CAD ↘ N1–P1: Cardiac SX = CAD = C N2–P2: Cardiac SX = CAD = C
Vossen et al., 2018 [57] Chronic pain (various) = 33 C = 33	Short-term	Electrical	Left middle finger	25	10 ms	9–11 s	VRS: single trial EEG: amplitude	Multilevel model with event-related fixed-interval areas	VRS: Chronic pain ↘ = C ↘ No influence of hypervigilance on pain ratings Chronic pain status and hypervigilance independently influenced the EEG-amplitude

4. Treatments and Clinical Implications

In this section, the clinical implications for habituation (or sensitization) to pain in chronic pain patients and potential treatments targeting (reduced) habituation are discussed.

4.1. Habituation to Pain and Clinical Outcomes

Our search revealed that most studies on habituation to pain and clinical outcomes were related to fibromyalgia or migraine patients (see Tables 1 and 3).

In fibromyalgia, habituation was shown to be correlated with pain at tender points [42], and patients with reduced habituation showed greater widespread pain [43]. De Tommaso et al. (2011) furthermore reported a correlation between reduced habituation of the (EEG-based) N2 amplitude and self-reported depressive symptoms in fibromyalgia patients [41], although this was not replicated in a larger scale study [42]. Furthermore, an association of habituation to pain with self-reported daily activity was reported [45]. Two studies investigated the relation between EEG signal intensity and intra-epidermal nerve fiber density (IENFD) in fibromyalgia patients. Reduced habituation of the N2–P2 component [46] or P2 component [44] was reported to be related to reduced IENFD. Subgroup analysis of those fibromyalgia patients with a reduced distal IENFD revealed that the P2 component increased over time [44].

In migraine patients, reduced habituation at the trigeminal area was correlated with migraine attack frequency [15]. Changes in brain activity in the somatosensory cortex and parietal cortex were shown to be correlated with attacks per month, whereas orbitofrontal activity correlated with disease duration [18]. Disease duration was further correlated with reduced habituation between migraine phases based on the EEG-signal (i.e., N2–P2 amplitude) [20]. Habituation to pain did not correlate with number of days until the next attack in the migraine patients [20].

In conclusion, some evidence exists that cortical habituation might be linked to the severity and frequency of pain complaints in fibromyalgia or migraine patients, as well as to IENFD in fibromyalgia patients.

4.2. Treatments Targeting Habituation to Pain

Currently, the literature on the treatments and effects on habituation to pain is limited to headache patients only. In medication-overuse headache patients, habituation of the N2–P2 amplitude was partially restored after 6 weeks in those that had clinically improved after an acute medication withdrawal treatment [30]. These findings suggest that medication overuse aggravates symptoms by central sensitization. In another study, preventive application of topiramate, an antiepileptic drug targeting among others GABA (more inhibition) and glutamate (less excitation), normalized the habituation pattern to nociceptive stimulation in migraine patients for the N1 amplitude, but at the same time did not result in effects on habituation of the N2–P2 amplitude [25]. The authors reasoned that topiramate has an effect on the sensory-discriminative component involved in habituation to pain, i.e., the secondary somatosensory cortex. Moreover, treatment with a ketogenic diet improved habituation of electrical evoked potentials, although a comparison to controls without the diet was not available [29]. A ketogenic diet has several mechanisms of action, including enhancing GABA transmission, and increasing BDNF expression and attenuation of inflammation [58]. With respect to the N2–P2 amplitude, one study reported that onabotulintoxin A (affecting neurotransmitter release) was effective for reduced habituation to pain, but only in the trigeminal area [27,59]. Furthermore, this treatment was shown to be more effective in migraine patients with severe reduced habituation [27]. This effect was, however, not shown in a similar study using electrical stimuli [31]. Furthermore, a recent pilot study reported that Erenumab (an antibody against receptors of the nociceptive neurotransmitter calcitonin gene-related peptide (CGRP)) affected the initially reduced habituation of the N2 amplitude in migraineurs [28]. On the basis of the findings of this pilot study, further confirmation is needed based on large-scale (randomized) studies.

Numerous other pharmacological options are available for chronic pain treatment, such as nonsteroidal anti-inflammatory drugs (NSAIDs), opioids, pregabalin, and selective serotonin and noradrenalin reuptake inhibitors (SNRIs) [60]. It would be interesting to investigate the effects of these treatments on habituation to pain.

4.3. Discussion and Future Directions

Possible treatments for habituation to pain may target different mechanisms as described above. These underlying mechanisms are complex and include various extra- and intracellular pathways. For example, topiramate has been reported to act via multiple mechanisms of action, such as the blockage of voltage-gated sodium channels, the enhancement of GABA-A receptors, the inhibition of L-type voltage-gated calcium channels, and/or the blockage of AMPA receptors [61]. These mechanisms are known to be involved in the development and maintenance of chronic pain and can be used as targets. GABA-neurotransmission is often linked to habituation of cellular processes in the CNS as its release was shown to be increased as a result of short-term habituation to an olfactory stimulus in *Drosophila* [9]. The mechanism of action of a ketogenic diet appears to include an anti-inflammatory and glycolytic metabolism pathway and with that appears to be an anticonvulsant. Similar to seizures, chronic pain is postulated to be related to increased excitability of neurons [62]; therefore, it is reasonable to study effects of this ketogenic diet on habituation to pain. An fMRI study in healthy participants reported evidence for a role of dopamine in habituation to pain, based on use of the dopamine D2 receptor antagonist haloperidol [63].

A recent review focusing on the genetic and molecular changes involved in habituation in general illustrated the complexity of the mechanism of action and molecules involved in habituation. In this review, various cellular pathways were highlighted, and the identification of 258 genes were reported as possible targets for drugs [64]. From this perspective, future research could investigate the effects of many more candidate drugs and their effect on habituation (and sensitization) to pain.

In conclusion, the mechanisms underlying habituation to pain are poorly understood and likely to be related to a complex set of pathways including those related to inflammation, immune responses, neurotrophins, and/or neurotransmission. Research should focus on which pathways and molecules are most dominant in order to target them specifically, and this then may result in major impact on habituation to pain. In addition, further research may include other chronic pain indications and pharmacological options targeting habituation to pain.

For now, no diagnostic markers are available for the prediction of habituation to pain. In addition, it is unclear when reduced habituation is of clinical relevance. For example, is a decrease of 0.5 point versus a 1.0 point decrease on the VAS after repeated stimulation an indication of reduced habituation to pain? Overall, it is too early to state that habituation trajectories (the response pattern resulting from repeated painful stimulation) are linked to clinical outcomes and could be used as a diagnostic marker for the prediction of chronic pain. Specifically for migraine patients, Brighina and colleagues stated that lack of habituation to pain probably represents a more general marker of neural dysfunction, with overlap of migraine with other pathologies such as chronic pain and Parkinson's disease [65].

5. Challenges in the Field

There are several challenges in the field of habituation to pain in chronic pain conditions. Importantly, chronic pain indications are very heterogeneous. In addition, even within each individual chronic pain condition, there might be age and sex differences and differences in medication use (e.g., [11,38,43]). Furthermore, the experimental pain paradigms used are very diverse, including different modalities (e.g., heat and electric), stimulation sites, and the measure of habituation. Moreover, the link to clinical outcomes and experience of (chronic) pain in the studies is limited. The baseline pain levels of patients could potentially affect habituation, but this has not yet been investigated, with the exception of one study reporting reduced habituation in patients with greater widespread pain [43]. Furthermore, the experimental pain paradigms used in the studies included in this systematic review are not necessarily clinical pain-provoking. The latter would be of interest for the field. However, in addition to these differences, it is still of interest to investigate whether the antinociceptive system(s) differ in patients with chronic pain as compared to pain-free subjects. It is hypothesized that several neuroplasticity changes have already occurred (e.g., central sensitization) in chronic pain patients, and these changes may contribute to reduced habituation to pain [6,66,67]. In conclusion, although it is a challenge to standardize experimental pain paradigms in relation to specific pain indications it should be given much more attention in future studies. This is needed to better understand general effects on habituation to pain in chronic pain.

6. Future Directions for Research

Future research in chronic pain patients may inform us on the robustness of differences in habituation to pain in chronic pain patients as compared to (for instance) healthy controls and its underlying mechanisms. Neural measures such as EEG and fMRI could be analyzed in more detail using, for example, multilevel models for increased understanding of habituation to pain in chronic pain patients. Currently, evidence linking the self-report (behavioral) and EEG or fMRI (neural) measures is limited.

A second point which can be concluded from our review is that most studies were based on small sample sizes (median = 19.5) and did not always include a control group. Hence, there is a need for larger, blinded studies (i.e., the assessor is blinded for the group), including control groups and randomized controlled trials for potential treatment effects. In addition, direct group comparisons are necessary to obtain more conclusive results. Our review showed that one group sometimes showed significant habituation, while the other group did not; hence, it was concluded that there was no difference between patients and controls. However, without directly comparing groups, this conclusion cannot be made [68].

In general, chronic pain indications are very heterogeneous, and this makes generalization of conclusions often very difficult. An alternative might be to focus on individual differences in habituation to pain. Studying individual characteristics and differences may result into a better understanding of the heterogeneity in both patients and controls, and these effects may then be linked to clinical outcomes. Current studies in chronic pain patients did not focus on individual differences or age- and sex-related differences. This, however, would be an interesting topic for further research as studies in healthy individuals pointed out large individual differences (e.g., [69]), but conflicting evidence for age and sex (e.g., [38,70–72]. Ideally, individual differences in habituation to pain could also be used in prediction models for chronic pain or treatment effects. Longitudinal designs might then help to unravel the role of habituation in (the transition to) chronic pain. Investigation of a surgical population as they may develop postoperative (chronic) pain is recommended [73].

An important issue in the correct analysis of studies on habituation to pain is the use and selection of statistical tests. In order to test and improve comparison of effects in studies on habituation to pain, we are in need of clear standardized measures to compare across studies and between patients and controls. Currently, there are several outcome measures for habituation to pain such as direct comparison of trials, linear effects (e.g., tested with a repeated-measures ANOVA), percentage change over averaged trials, habituation quotient (i.e., ratio between the average response in the first and last block), or fitting a (linear or quadratic) slope. With this variability in outcome measures, a standardized systematic comparison (such as in a meta-analysis) is not possible. Recently, recommendations for interpreting different habituation (to pain) patterns have been proposed [2]. With this, effects on habituation to pain might possibly be linked to phenotypes. On some occasions, it could be that patients show similar reduced habituation, but that the control group shows a different effect (see Figure 5), which is not captured in statistical tests.

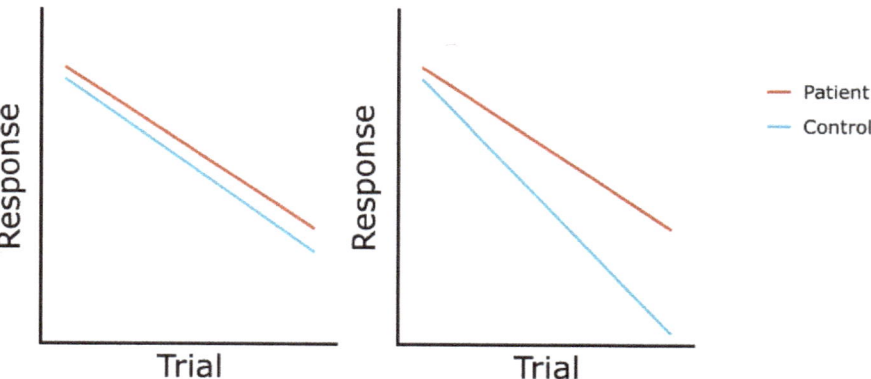

Figure 5. Example of patient groups that show similar habituation, whereas control groups differ in their response. With conventional analyses, panel one will result in no group differences whereas panel two will result in group differences, complicating the conclusion of patient vs. control effects.

Therefore, we propose the fitting of a slope as indicator of the trajectory of the habituation (linear, quadratic, etc.). The use of these slopes and trajectory of habituation to pain has several advantages over current measures; it does not require any calculation of the dependent variable (such as averaging), it is easy interpretable and indicates the direction of effects, i.e., habituation or sensitization, and, when tested against zero, it can also indicate the significance of changes compared to zero (see Figure 6). However, it would require a fixed number of trials to be comparable across studies, and it can be influenced by other factors such as interstimulus interval and type of stimulation. This is in general of influence for habituation to pain, which is why the field will greatly benefit from standard setups and measures. If the field progresses to standard protocols and outcome measures as they are currently used in quantitative sensory testing (QST), it will be possible to increase the understanding of habituation to pain and its potential role and link to chronic pain [74,75]. In addition, recently developed statistical analysis methods, such as the high-temporal-resolution EEG analysis method and the event-related fixed-interval area method, are promising improvements in the detailed investigation of habituation of pain [38,76].

Furthermore, recommendations such as the use of standard terminology, comparison of similar outcome measures (i.e., not comparing EEG effects with rating effects), taking into account the use of different timescales when analyzing and interpreting the data, and taking into account individual differences will improve future study design and analyses.

Limitations

In this review, the effects of habituation to non-painful stimuli, the pain threshold, physiological measures such as skin conductance, and stimulation paradigms where the intensity was adjusted were not included (e.g., [77,78]). Thus, reduced habituation to pain in chronic pain patients may exist according to the use of different measures, and future research is needed to explore these measures. Furthermore, this review focused mainly on habituation to pain but not on sensitization to pain in chronic pain patients. These closely related processes should preferably be described and studied together, but most studies only deal with either habituation or sensitization to pain.

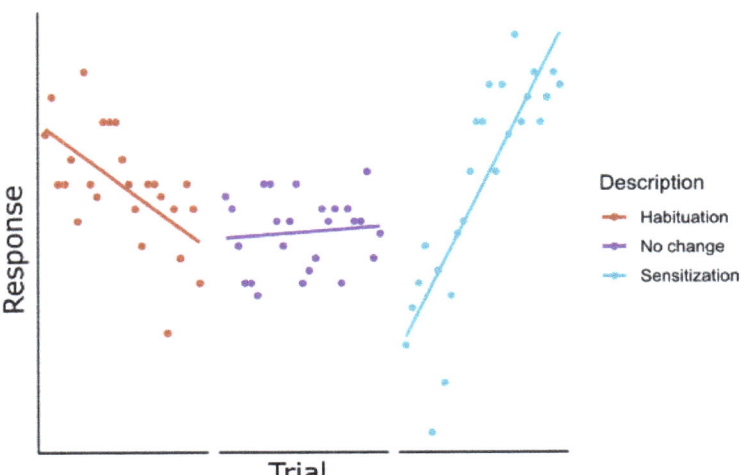

Figure 6. Example of data with a fitted (linear) slope that indicates the direction of the effect (after tested against zero), i.e., habituation, no change, or sensitization.

7. Conclusions

This review systematically summarized the available evidence on habituation to pain in different chronic pain indications. Although several studies reported reduced habituation to pain in migraine for self-report and the EEG-based N1 and N2–P2 amplitude, further evidence and confirmation based on larger, well-designed studies is needed. In CLBP patients, the evidence argues against any general differences, except for EEG measures. In fibromyalgia, there is evidence for reduced habituation to pain of the N2–P2 amplitude. Currently, the evidence of a diagnostic marker or linking habituation to pain to clinical outcomes is limited. Future studies should include standard outcome measures to improve the comparison of habituation to pain in chronic pain patients and controls. The mechanisms underlying habituation to pain are poorly understood and likely to be related to a complex set of pathways. Recent use of genetic and molecular analysis techniques allows for better understanding and selection of new pharmacological treatment options which then may help to reduce pain in chronic pain patients.

Supplementary Materials: The following supporting information can be downloaded at https://www.mdpi.com/article/10.3390/jcm12134305/s1: Material and Methods; Figure S1. Flow diagram of selection and inclusion; Table S1: Inclusion and exclusion criteria.

Funding: This research received no external funding.

Data Availability Statement: No new data were created or analyzed in this study. Data sharing is not applicable to this article.

Acknowledgments: The authors would like to thank Iris Coppieters for helpful comments on the manuscript. Our dear colleague Amanda Kaas significantly contributed to the topic and preregistration of the review but sadly passed away before the manuscript was finished.

Conflicts of Interest: The authors declare no conflict of interest.

References

1. Rankin, C.H.; Abrams, T.; Barry, R.J.; Bhatnagar, S.; Clayton, D.F.; Colombo, J.; Coppola, G.; Geyer, M.A.; Glanzman, D.L.; Marsland, S. Habituation revisited: An updated and revised description of the behavioral characteristics of habituation. *Neurobiol. Learn. Mem.* **2009**, *92*, 135–138. [CrossRef]
2. McDiarmid, T.A.; Bernardos, A.C.; Rankin, C.H. Habituation is altered in neuropsychiatric disorders-A comprehensive review with recommendations for experimental design and analysis. *Neurosci. Biobehav. Rev.* **2017**, *80*, 286–305. [CrossRef]

3. Thompson, R.F.; Spencer, W.A. Habituation: A model phenomenon for the study of neuronal substrates of behavior. *Psychol. Rev.* **1966**, *73*, 16. [CrossRef]
4. De Paepe, A.L.; Williams, A.C.C.; Crombez, G. Habituation to pain: A motivational-ethological perspective. *Pain* **2019**, *160*, 1693–1697. [CrossRef]
5. IASP. International Association for the Study of Pain (IASP). Available online: https://www.iasp-pain.org/resources/terminology/. (accessed on 11 April 2023).
6. Harte, S.E.; Harris, R.E.; Clauw, D.J. The neurobiology of central sensitization. *J. Appl. Biobehav. Res.* **2018**, *23*, e12137. [CrossRef]
7. van den Broeke, E.; Crombez, G.; Vlaeyen, J.W. Re-conceptualizing sensitization in pain: A case for a behavioural approach. *PsychArchives* **2023**. [CrossRef]
8. Groves, P.M.; Thompson, R.F. Habituation: A dual-process theory. *Psychol. Rev.* **1970**, *77*, 419. [CrossRef]
9. Ramaswami, M. Network plasticity in adaptive filtering and behavioral habituation. *Neuron* **2014**, *82*, 1216–1229. [CrossRef] [PubMed]
10. May, A.; Rodriguez-Raecke, R.; Schulte, A.; Ihle, K.; Breimhorst, M.; Birklein, F.; Jürgens, T.P. Within-session sensitization and between-session habituation: A robust physiological response to repetitive painful heat stimulation. *Eur. J. Pain* **2012**, *16*, 401–409. [CrossRef]
11. Rodriguez-Raecke, R.; Ihle, K.; Ritter, C.; Muhtz, C.; Otte, C.; May, A. Neuronal differences between chronic low back pain and depression regarding long-term habituation to pain. *Eur. J. Pain* **2014**, *18*, 701–711. [CrossRef]
12. Leonardi, M.; Steiner, T.J.; Scher, A.T.; Lipton, R.B. The global burden of migraine: Measuring disability in headache disorders with WHO's Classification of Functioning, Disability and Health (ICF). *J. Headache Pain* **2005**, *6*, 429–440. [CrossRef]
13. Casillo, F.; Sebastianelli, G.; Di Renzo, A.; Cioffi, E.; Parisi, V.; Di Lorenzo, C.; Serrao, M.; Coppola, G. The monoclonal CGRP-receptor blocking antibody erenumab has different effects on brainstem and cortical sensory-evoked responses. *Cephalalgia* **2022**, *42*, 1236–1245. [CrossRef]
14. Bassez, I.; Van de Steen, F.; Ricci, K.; Vecchio, E.; Gentile, E.; Marinazzo, D.; de Tommaso, M. Dynamic Causal Modelling of the Reduced Habituation to Painful Stimuli in Migraine: An EEG Study. *Brain Sci.* **2020**, *10*, 712. [CrossRef] [PubMed]
15. Gierse-Plogmeier, B.; Colak-Ekici, R.; Wolowski, A.; Gralow, I.; Marziniak, M.; Evers, S. Differences in trigeminal and peripheral electrical pain perception in women with and without migraine. *J. Headache Pain* **2009**, *10*, 249–254. [CrossRef]
16. Beese, L.C.; Putzer, D.; Osada, N.; Evers, S.; Marziniak, M. Contact heat evoked potentials and habituation measured interictally in migraineurs. *J. Headache Pain* **2015**, *16*, 1. [CrossRef]
17. de Tommaso, M.; Lo Sito, L.; Di Fruscolo, O.; Sardaro, M.; Pia Prudenzano, M.; Lamberti, P.; Livrea, P. Lack of habituation of nociceptive evoked responses and pain sensitivity during migraine attack. *Clin. Neurophysiol.* **2005**, *116*, 1254–1264. [CrossRef] [PubMed]
18. Lev, R.; Granovsky, Y.; Yarnitsky, D. Enhanced pain expectation in migraine: EEG-based evidence for impaired prefrontal function. *Headache* **2013**, *53*, 1054–1070. [CrossRef] [PubMed]
19. Lev, R.; Granovsky, Y.; Yarnitsky, D. Orbitofrontal disinhibition of pain in migraine with aura: An interictal EEG-mapping study. *Cephalalgia* **2010**, *30*, 910–918. [CrossRef] [PubMed]
20. Uglem, M.; Omland, P.M.; Stjern, M.; Gravdahl, G.B.; Sand, T. Habituation of laser-evoked potentials by migraine phase: A blinded longitudinal study. *J. Headache Pain* **2017**, *18*, 100. [CrossRef]
21. de Tommaso, M.; Libro, G.; Guido, M.; Losito, L.; Lamberti, P.; Livrea, P. Habituation of single CO_2 laser-evoked responses during interictal phase of migraine. *J. Headache Pain* **2005**, *6*, 195–198. [CrossRef]
22. de Tommaso, M.; Trotta, G.; Vecchio, E.; Ricci, K.; Van de Steen, F.; Montemurno, A.; Lorenzo, M.; Marinazzo, D.; Bellotti, R.; Stramaglia, S. Functional Connectivity of EEG Signals Under Laser Stimulation in Migraine. *Front. Hum. Neurosci.* **2015**, *9*, 640. [CrossRef]
23. Valeriani, M.; de Tommaso, M.; Restuccia, D.; Le Pera, D.; Guido, M.; Iannetti, G.D.; Libro, G.; Truini, A.; Di Trapani, G.; Puca, F.; et al. Reduced habituation to experimental pain in migraine patients: A CO_2 laser evoked potential study. *Pain* **2003**, *105*, 57–64. [CrossRef]
24. de Tommaso, M.; Valeriani, M.; Sardaro, M.; Serpino, C.; Fruscolo, O.D.; Vecchio, E.; Cerbo, R.; Livrea, P. Pain perception and laser evoked potentials during menstrual cycle in migraine. *J. Headache Pain* **2009**, *10*, 423–429. [CrossRef]
25. Di Clemente, L.; Puledda, F.; Biasiotta, A.; Viganò, A.; Vicenzini, E.; Truini, A.; Cruccu, G.; Di Piero, V. Topiramate modulates habituation in migraine: Evidences from nociceptive responses elicited by laser evoked potentials. *J. Headache Pain* **2013**, *14*, 25. [CrossRef]
26. Sava, S.L.; de Pasqua, V.; de Noordhout, A.M.; Schoenen, J. Visually induced analgesia during face or limb stimulation in healthy and migraine subjects. *J. Pain Res.* **2018**, *11*, 1821–1828. [CrossRef] [PubMed]
27. De Tommaso, M.; Delussi, M.; Ricci, K.; Montemurno, A.; Carbone, I.; Vecchio, E. Effects of onabotulintoxinA on habituation of laser evoked responses in chronic migraine. *Toxins* **2016**, *8*, 163. [CrossRef]
28. de Tommaso, M.; Delussi, M.; Gentile, E.; Ricci, K.; Quitadamo, S.G.; Libro, G. Effect of single dose Erenumab on cortical responses evoked by cutaneous a-delta fibers: A pilot study in migraine patients. *Cephalalgia* **2021**, *41*, 1004–1014. [CrossRef]
29. Di Lorenzo, C.; Coppola, G.; Bracaglia, M.; Di Lenola, D.; Sirianni, G.; Rossi, P.; Di Lorenzo, G.; Parisi, V.; Serrao, M.; Cervenka, M.C.; et al. A ketogenic diet normalizes interictal cortical but not subcortical responsivity in migraineurs. *BMC Neurol* **2019**, *19*, 136. [CrossRef] [PubMed]

0. Ferraro, D.; Vollono, C.; Miliucci, R.; Virdis, D.; De Armas, L.; Pazzaglia, C.; Le Pera, D.; Tarantino, S.; Balestri, M.; Di Trapani, G.; et al. Habituation to pain in "medication overuse headache": A CO_2 laser-evoked potential study. *Headache* **2012**, *52*, 792–807. [CrossRef] [PubMed]

1. Sebastianelli, G.; Casillo, F.; Di Renzo, A.; Abagnale, C.; Cioffi, E.; Parisi, V.; Di Lorenzo, C.; Serrao, M.; Pierelli, F.; Schoenen, J.; et al. Effects of Botulinum Toxin Type A on the Nociceptive and Lemniscal Somatosensory Systems in Chronic Migraine: An Electrophysiological Study. *Toxins* **2023**, *15*, 76. [CrossRef]

2. Hoy, D.; Bain, C.; Williams, G.; March, L.; Brooks, P.; Blyth, F.; Woolf, A.; Vos, T.; Buchbinder, R. A systematic review of the global prevalence of low back pain. *Arthritis Rheum.* **2012**, *64*, 2028–2037. [CrossRef] [PubMed]

3. Maher, C.; Underwood, M.; Buchbinder, R. Non-specific low back pain. *Lancet* **2017**, *389*, 736–747. [CrossRef]

4. Arntz, A.; Merckelbach, H.; Peters, M.; Schmidt, A.J. Chronic low back pain, response specificity and habituation to painful stimuli. *J. Psychophysiol.* **1991**, *5*, 177–188.

5. Peters, M.L.; Schmidt, A.J.; Van den Hout, M.A. Chronic low back pain and the reaction to repeated acute pain stimulation. *Pain* **1989**, *39*, 69–76. [CrossRef] [PubMed]

6. Hüllemann, P.; von der Brelie, C.; Manthey, G.; Düsterhöft, J.; Helmers, A.K.; Synowitz, M.; Baron, R. Reduced laser-evoked potential habituation detects abnormal central pain processing in painful radiculopathy patients. *Eur. J. Pain* **2017**, *21*, 918–926. [CrossRef]

7. Vossen, C.J.; Vossen, H.G.; Joosten, E.A.; van Os, J.; Lousberg, R. Does habituation differ in chronic low back pain subjects compared to pain-free controls? A cross-sectional pain rating ERP study reanalyzed with the ERFIA multilevel method. *Medicine* **2015**, *94*, e865. [CrossRef] [PubMed]

8. Kersebaum, D.; Fabig, S.C.; Sendel, M.; Muntean, A.C.; Baron, R.; Hullemann, P. Revealing the time course of laser-evoked potential habituation by high temporal resolution analysis. *Eur. J. Pain* **2021**, *25*, 2112–2128. [CrossRef]

9. Häuser, W.; Ablin, J.; Fitzcharles, M.-A.; Littlejohn, G.; Luciano, J.V.; Usui, C.; Walitt, B. Fibromyalgia. *Nat. Rev. Dis. Prim.* **2015**, *1*, 15022. [CrossRef]

10. Hollins, M.; Harper, D.; Maixner, W. Changes in pain from a repetitive thermal stimulus: The roles of adaptation and sensitization. *Pain* **2011**, *152*, 1583–1590. [CrossRef]

11. de Tommaso, M.; Federici, A.; Santostasi, R.; Calabrese, R.; Vecchio, E.; Lapadula, G.; Iannone, F.; Lamberti, P.; Livrea, P. Laser-evoked potentials habituation in fibromyalgia. *J. Pain* **2011**, *12*, 116–124. [CrossRef]

12. de Tommaso, M.; Nolano, M.; Iannone, F.; Vecchio, E.; Ricci, K.; Lorenzo, R.; Delussi, M.; Girolamo, F.; Lavolpe, V.; Provitera, V.; et al. Update on laser-evoked potential findings in fibromyalgia patients in light of clinical and skin biopsy features. *J. Neurol.* **2014**, *261*, 461–472. [CrossRef] [PubMed]

13. de Tommaso, M.; Ricci, K.; Libro, G.; Vecchio, E.; Delussi, M.; Montemurno, A.; Lopalco, G.; Iannone, F. Pain Processing and Vegetative Dysfunction in Fibromyalgia: A Study by Sympathetic Skin Response and Laser Evoked Potentials. *Pain Res. Treat.* **2017**, *2017*, 9747148. [CrossRef]

14. Vecchio, E.; Quitadamo, S.G.; Ricci, K.; Libro, G.; Delussi, M.; Lombardi, R.; Lauria, G.; de Tommaso, M. Laser evoked potentials in fibromyalgia with peripheral small fiber involvement. *Clin. Neurophysiol.* **2022**, *135*, 96–106. [CrossRef]

15. McLoughlin, M.J.; Stegner, A.J.; Cook, D.B. The relationship between physical activity and brain responses to pain in fibromyalgia. *J. Pain* **2011**, *12*, 640–651. [CrossRef]

16. Vecchio, E.; Lombardi, R.; Paolini, M.; Libro, G.; Delussi, M.; Ricci, K.; Quitadamo, S.G.; Gentile, E.; Girolamo, F.; Iannone, F.; et al. Peripheral and central nervous system correlates in fibromyalgia. *Eur. J. Pain* **2020**, *24*, 1537–1547. [CrossRef]

17. Gauer, R.; Semidey, M.J. Diagnosis and treatment of temporomandibular disorders. *Am. Fam. Physician* **2015**, *91*, 378–386.

18. Nicholas, M.; Vlaeyen, J.W.S.; Rief, W.; Barke, A.; Aziz, Q.; Benoliel, R.; Cohen, M.; Evers, S.; Giamberardino, M.A.; Goebel, A.; et al. The IASP classification of chronic pain for ICD-11: Chronic primary pain. *Pain* **2019**, *160*, 28–37. [CrossRef] [PubMed]

19. Jääskeläinen, S.K.; Woda, A. Burning mouth syndrome. *Cephalalgia* **2017**, *37*, 627–647. [CrossRef]

50. Shinozaki, T.; Imamura, Y.; Kohashi, R.; Dezawa, K.; Nakaya, Y.; Sato, Y.; Watanabe, K.; Morimoto, Y.; Shizukuishi, T.; Abe, O.; et al. Spatial and Temporal Brain Responses to Noxious Heat Thermal Stimuli in Burning Mouth Syndrome. *J. Dent. Res.* **2016**, *95*, 1138–1146. [CrossRef]

51. Valeriani, M.; Sestito, A.; Le Pera, D.; De Armas, L.; Infusino, F.; Maiese, T.; Sgueglia, G.A.; Tonali, P.A.; Crea, F.; Restuccia, D.; et al. Abnormal cortical pain processing in patients with cardiac syndrome X. *Eur. Heart J.* **2005**, *26*, 975–982. [CrossRef] [PubMed]

52. Olesen, S.S.; Hansen, T.M.; Graversen, C.; Valeriani, M.; Drewes, A.M. Cerebral excitability is abnormal in patients with painful chronic pancreatitis. *Eur. J. Pain* **2013**, *17*, 46–54. [CrossRef]

53. Kumru, H.; Soler, D.; Vidal, J.; Tormos, J.M.; Pascual-Leone, A.; Valls-Sole, J. Evoked potentials and quantitative thermal testing in spinal cord injury patients with chronic neuropathic pain. *Clin. Neurophysiol.* **2012**, *123*, 598–604. [CrossRef] [PubMed]

54. Albu, S.; Gómez-Soriano, J.; Avila-Martin, G.; Taylor, J. Deficient conditioned pain modulation after spinal cord injury correlates with clinical spontaneous pain measures. *Pain* **2015**, *156*, 260–272. [CrossRef]

55. Lütolf, R.; Rosner, J.; Curt, A.; Hubli, M. Indicators of central sensitization in chronic neuropathic pain after spinal cord injury. *Eur. J. Pain* **2022**, *26*, 2162–2175. [CrossRef]

56. Scheuren, P.S.; De Schoenmacker, I.; Rosner, J.; Brunner, F.; Curt, A.; Hubli, M. Pain-autonomic measures reveal nociceptive sensitization in complex regional pain syndrome. *Eur. J. Pain* **2023**, *27*, 72–85. [CrossRef] [PubMed]

57. Vossen, C.J.; Luijcks, R.; van Os, J.; Joosten, E.A.; Lousberg, R. Does pain hypervigilance further impact the lack of habituation to pain in individuals with chronic pain? A cross-sectional pain ERP study. *J. Pain Res.* **2018**, *11*, 395–405. [CrossRef]

58. Masino, S.A.; Rho, J.M. Mechanisms of Ketogenic Diet Action. In *Jasper's Basic Mechanisms of the Epilepsies*; Noebels, J.L., Avoli, M.; Rogawski, M.A., Olsen, R.W., Delgado-Escueta, A.V., Eds.; National Center for Biotechnology Information (US): Bethesda, MD, USA, 2012.

59. Burstein, R.; Blumenfeld, A.M.; Silberstein, S.D.; Manack Adams, A.; Brin, M.F. Mechanism of Action of OnabotulinumtoxinA in Chronic Migraine: A Narrative Review. *Headache J. Head Face Pain* **2020**, *60*, 1259–1272. [CrossRef]

60. Marcianò, G.; Vocca, C.; Evangelista, M.; Palleria, C.; Muraca, L.; Galati, C.; Monea, F.; Sportiello, L.; De Sarro, G.; Capuano, A. The Pharmacological Treatment of Chronic Pain: From Guidelines to Daily Clinical Practice. *Pharmaceutics* **2023**, *15*, 1165. [CrossRef] [PubMed]

61. Chong, M.; Libretto, S.E. The rationale and use of topiramate for treating neuropathic pain. *Clin. J. Pain* **2003**, *19*, 59–68. [CrossRef]

62. Masino, S.A.; Ruskin, D.N. Ketogenic diets and pain. *J. Child Neurol.* **2013**, *28*, 993–1001. [CrossRef]

63. Bauch, E.M.; Andreou, C.; Rausch, V.H.; Bunzeck, N. Neural Habituation to Painful Stimuli Is Modulated by Dopamine: Evidence from a Pharmacological fMRI Study. *Front. Hum. Neurosci.* **2017**, *11*, 630. [CrossRef]

64. Blok, L.E.R.; Boon, M.; van Reijmersdal, B.; Höffler, K.D.; Fenckova, M.; Schenck, A. Genetics, molecular control and clinical relevance of habituation learning. *Neurosci. Biobehav. Rev.* **2022**, *143*, 104883. [CrossRef]

65. Brighina, F.; Cosentino, G.; Fierro, B. Is lack of habituation a biomarker of migraine? A critical perspective. *J. Headache Pain* **2015**, *16*, A13. [CrossRef] [PubMed]

66. Rennefeld, C.; Wiech, K.; Schoell, E.D.; Lorenz, J.; Bingel, U. Habituation to pain: Further support for a central component. *Pain* **2010**, *148*, 503–508. [CrossRef]

67. Ji, R.R.; Kohno, T.; Moore, K.A.; Woolf, C.J. Central sensitization and LTP: Do pain and memory share similar mechanisms? *Trends Neurosci.* **2003**, *26*, 696–705. [CrossRef]

68. Nieuwenhuis, S.; Forstmann, B.U.; Wagenmakers, E.-J. Erroneous analyses of interactions in neuroscience: A problem of significance. *Nat. Neurosci.* **2011**, *14*, 1105–1107. [CrossRef] [PubMed]

69. Slepian, P.M.; France, C.R.; Rhudy, J.L.; Himawan, L.K.; Güereca, Y.M.; Kuhn, B.L.; Palit, S. Behavioral Inhibition and Behavioral Activation are Related to Habituation of Nociceptive Flexion Reflex, but Not Pain Ratings. *J. Pain* **2017**, *18*, 349–358. [CrossRef] [PubMed]

70. Edwards, R.R.; Fillingim, R.B. Effects of age on temporal summation and habituation of thermal pain: Clinical relevance in healthy older and younger adults. *J. Pain* **2001**, *2*, 307–317. [CrossRef]

71. Greffrath, W.; Baumgärtner, U.; Treede, R.D. Peripheral and central components of habituation of heat pain perception and evoked potentials in humans. *Pain* **2007**, *132*, 301–311. [CrossRef]

72. Jepma, M.; Jones, M.; Wager, T.D. The dynamics of pain: Evidence for simultaneous site-specific habituation and site-nonspecific sensitization in thermal pain. *J. Pain* **2014**, *15*, 734–746. [CrossRef]

73. Hoofwijk, D.; Fiddelers, A.A.; Peters, M.L.; Stessel, B.; Kessels, A.G.; Joosten, E.A.; Gramke, H.-F.; Marcus, M.A. Prevalence and predictive factors of chronic postsurgical pain and poor global recovery 1 year after outpatient surgery. *Clin. J. Pain* **2015**, *31*, 1017–1025. [CrossRef]

74. Rolke, R.; Baron, R.; Maier, C.A.; Tölle, T.; Treede, R.-D.; Beyer, A.; Binder, A.; Birbaumer, N.; Birklein, F.; Bötefür, I. Quantitative sensory testing in the German Research Network on Neuropathic Pain (DFNS): Standardized protocol and reference values. *Pain* **2006**, *123*, 231–243. [CrossRef] [PubMed]

75. Rolke, R.; Magerl, W.; Campbell, K.A.; Schalber, C.; Caspari, S.; Birklein, F.; Treede, R.D. Quantitative sensory testing: A comprehensive protocol for clinical trials. *Eur. J. Pain* **2006**, *10*, 77–88. [CrossRef] [PubMed]

76. Vossen, C.J.; Vossen, H.G.; Marcus, M.A.; van Os, J.; Lousberg, R. Introducing the event related fixed interval area (ERFIA) multilevel technique: A method to analyze the complete epoch of event-related potentials at single trial level. *PLoS ONE* **2013**, *8*, e79905. [CrossRef]

77. Coppola, G.; Pierelli, F.; Schoenen, J. Habituation and migraine. *Neurobiol. Learn. Mem.* **2009**, *92*, 249–259. [CrossRef]

78. Flor, H.; Diers, M.; Birbaumer, N. Peripheral and electrocortical responses to painful and non-painful stimulation in chronic pain patients, tension headache patients and healthy controls. *Neurosci. Lett.* **2004**, *361*, 147–150. [CrossRef] [PubMed]

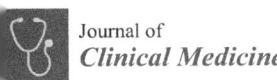

Journal of
Clinical Medicine

Review

Central Sensitization in Cancer Survivors and Its Clinical Implications: State of the Art

Tomohiko Nishigami [1,*], Masahiro Manfuku [2,3] and Astrid Lahousse [4,5,6,7]

1 Department of Physical Therapy, Faculty of Health and Welfare, Prefectural University of Hiroshima, Hiroshima 723-0053, Japan
2 Graduate School of Comprehensive Scientific Research, Prefectural University of Hiroshima, Hiroshima 723-0053, Japan; sunday_attinente@yahoo.co.jp
3 Department of Rehabilitation, Breast Care Sensyu Clinic, Osaka 596-0076, Japan
4 Pain in Motion Research Group (PAIN), Department of Physiotherapy, Human Physiology and Anatomy, Faculty of Physical Education & Physiotherapy (KIMA), Vrije Universiteit Brussel, 1090 Brussels, Belgium; astrid.lucie.lahousse@vub.be
5 Chronic Pain Rehabilitation, Department of Physical Medicine and Physiotherapy, University Hospital Brussels, 1090 Brussels, Belgium
6 Research Foundation Flanders (FWO), 1000 Brussels, Belgium
7 Rehabilitation Research (RERE) Research Group, Department of Physiotherapy, Human Physiology and Anatomy, Faculty of Physical Education & Physiotherapy (KIMA), Vrije Universiteit Brussel, 1090 Brussels, Belgium
* Correspondence: tomon@pu-hiroshima.ac.jp; Tel.: +81-848-60-1120

Abstract: Although the prevalence of cancer pain is 47% after treatment, cancer pain is often underestimated, and many patients are undertreated. The complexity of cancer pain contributes to the lack of its management. Recently, as the mechanism of cancer pain, it has become clear that central sensitization (CS) influences chronic pain conditions and the transition from acute to chronic pain. In this state-of-the-art review, we summarized the association of CS or central sensitivity syndrome with pain and the treatment for pain targeting CS in cancer survivors. The management of patients with CS should not only focus on tissue damage in either the affected body regions or within the central nervous system; rather, it should aim to target the underlying factors that sustain the CS process. Pain neuroscience education (PNE) is gaining popularity for managing chronic musculoskeletal pain and could be effective for pain and CS in breast cancer survivors. However, there is a study that did not demonstrate significant improvements after PNE, so further research is needed. Precision medicine involves the classification of patients into subgroups based on a multifaceted evaluation of disease and the implementation of treatment tailored to the characteristics of each patient, which may play a central role in the treatment of CS.

Keywords: cancer survivors; central sensitization; central sensitivity syndrome; insomnia; stress; pain neuroscience education; precision medicine

Citation: Nishigami, T.; Manfuku, M.; Lahousse, A. Central Sensitization in Cancer Survivors and Its Clinical Implications: State of the Art. *J. Clin. Med.* **2023**, *12*, 4606. https://doi.org/10.3390/jcm12144606

Academic Editor: Hubertus Axer

Received: 12 June 2023
Revised: 4 July 2023
Accepted: 6 July 2023
Published: 11 July 2023

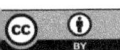
1. Introduction

In high-income nations, cancer now ranks above vascular illnesses as the main cause of mortality [1]. Additionally, it is anticipated that by 2040, the worldwide cancer burden will increase by 47% [2]. Oncology has made significant progress, and advanced cancer is no longer synonymous with terminal illness. However, providing pain treatment during the survivorship phase is gaining more importance due to the expanding population of cancer survivors [2]. The prevalence of cancer pain is 47% (95%CI 39–55) after treatment [3]. Despite this high prevalence, cancer pain is often underestimated, and many patients are undertreated [4–7]. The complexity of factors affecting cancer pain is contributed to the lack of management of cancer pain [8–10]. Pain in cancer survivors can be difficult to manage because they underwent many types of treatment, including surgery, radiation therapy, and chemotherapy, and clinicians should be cautious because the pain might be due to cancer metastasis/recurrence or other non-cancer-related causes. Therefore, to improve the lack of management of cancer pain, the International Association for the Study of Pain (IASP) defined a new classification of cancer survivor pain in ICD-11 [11]. The new classification of cancer-related pain in cancer survivors is divided into two major categories: "chronic cancer pain", such as visceral pain and bone metastasis pain due to cancer progression or metastasis, and "chronic pain after cancer treatment" related to surgery or drug treatment [11]. More recently, patients with chronic musculoskeletal pain have been classified into three pain mechanisms: "Nociceptive pain", "Neuropathic pain", and "Nociplastic pain" as a classification of pain properties [12,13] and cancer pain is classified in the same way [14]. Clinicians should consider the seven-step diagnostic approach to differentiate between predominant pain and provide appropriate pain treatment in cancer survivors [14].

Recently, as the mechanism of cancer pain, it has become clear that central sensitization (CS) influences chronic pain conditions and the transition from acute to chronic pain [15–18]. IASP defines CS as the "Increased responsiveness of nociceptive neurons in the central nervous system to their normal or subthreshold afferent input". Systematic reviews and meta-analyses of CS for musculoskeletal diseases have reported that CS influences symptom severity and pain in musculoskeletal diseases such as knee osteoarthritis and low back pain [18–22]. CS has also received attention as a mechanism for cancer pain because CS could affect pain in about 40% of breast cancer survivors [23,24]. Moreover, CS-related symptoms have the capability to predict the intensity and interference of persistent post-surgical pain 1 year after surgery [25,26]. These findings suggest that the assessment and treatment of CS are important for the appropriate treatment and management of cancer pain.

2. Objectives

This state-of-the-art review aims to investigate the relationship between CS or central sensitivity syndrome and pain in cancer survivors, as well as explore the treatment approaches targeting CS for pain management. While CS is initially observed in animal models, this review focuses on its assumed presence in humans. Additionally, the review will elaborate on the potential associations with other comorbidities that may contribute to the perpetuation of CS in cancer survivors. Furthermore, it will provide insights and directions for future research, along with discussing the clinical implications of CS in the context of pain management for cancer survivors.

3. Methodology

A comprehensive search was conducted on PubMed and Web of Science until April 2023, using keywords such as Cancer Survivors, Central Sensitization, Central sensitivity syndrome, Central Sensitization-related symptoms, Insomnia, Sleep Disturbances, Stress, Pain Neuroscience Education, and Precision Medicine in order to identify the most relevant and up-to-date evidence. Eligible articles must meet the following requirements: (1) be written in English, Dutch, French or Japanese, (2) be published in full text, and (3) be consistent with the goal of this review. The following study designs were not included in the studies: case reports, conference proceedings, abstracts, letters to the editor, statements of personal opinion, and editorials. T.N. and M.M. conducted the initial literature review, and all co-authors subsequently contributed to revisions and additions. The original draft of the text was written by T.N. and M.M., and all authors engaged in electronic communication to discuss and revise the final draft. With reference to the classification of cancer survivor pain in ICD-11 [11], cancer pain is caused by damage of primary cancer, metastasis (e.g., bone pain or visceral metastasis pain), or cancer treatments, and these treatments can induce chronic secondary pain syndromes that persist after cancer treatment such as postmastectomy pain or post-thoracotomy pain after surgery, chemotherapy-induced peripheral neuropathy (CIPN), aromatase inhibitor-induced musculoskeletal symptoms, radiation-induced neuropathy or radiation-induced fibrosis. This paper distinguishes (1) pain related to cancer or during its treatment and (2) persistent pain after treatment completion (except for maintenance therapy).

4. Pain Related to Central Sensitization in Cancer Survivors

Assessing CS in individuals remains a challenge, and an optimal clinical approach for this purpose is quantitative sensory testing (QST). QST utilizes standardized mechanical and thermal stimuli, such as von Frey filament pinprick stimuli, light touch, pressure algometers, and quantitative thermosetting, to explore the nociceptive and non-nociceptive afferent pathways in the peripheral and central nervous systems. There are two main modalities of QST: static QST and dynamic QST. Static QST is the most basic method of evaluating response to standardized stimuli. Pressure value at the moment when the pressure stimulus changes to pain is called the pressure pain threshold (PPT) and is one of the most frequently used static QST. Dynamic QST is an evaluation that reflects functional changes in the central pain regulatory system and requires a slightly more complicated method than static QST. Temporal summation of pain (TS) examines the phenomenon of pain exacerbated over time by continuous pain stimulation. Conditioned pain modulation (CPM) is the suppression of pain sensitivity at the site of evaluation by a pain stimulus applied to a remote site. TS evaluates the hyperresponsiveness of the ascending pain control system, while CPM evaluates the dysfunction of the descending inhibitory controls. The utility of QST for analyzing the various etiologies and pathologies in musculoskeletal pain disorders is evident [27]. For clinicians, there is growing interest in bedside QSTs, which do not necessitate specialized, expensive, or time-consuming equipment [28,29]. Additionally, the validity and reliability of bedside QSTs are promising [30–32]. However, future research needs to assess its added value and feasibility in clinical practice for assessing CS [33].

There is also an increasing number of reports related to hyperalgesia and CS measured using QST [25,26,34–41]. Most reports on cancer pain and QST have been mainly evaluated by PPT. Postoperative breast, head and neck, and colorectal cancer survivors have more hypersensitivity in the surgical neck, shoulder joint, and lumbar back compared to healthy controls [37–39]. Several studies have revealed that hypersensitivity has been observed in distant areas from the painful site, such as the nonoperative neck and shoulder joint [37,38] and the tibialis anterior muscle as well as the operative side and in painful areas [37,40,41]. Survivors with chronic postoperative pain after breast cancer surgery have decreased CPM and enhanced TS compared to survivors without chronic pain [42,43]. Edwards RR et al. reported that pain catastrophizing might mediate central nervous system pain-modulatory processes [43]. Scott et al. reported that radiotherapy for bone metastatic pain improves hypersensitivity at the pain site [44]. However, there are no reports on hypersensitivity at distant areas from the pain site, and the relationship between cancer pain (e.g., bone metastatic pain and visceral metastatic pain) and CS is not clear. Thus, further research is needed to determine whether the relationship between post-cancer treatment pain and CS in cancer survivors is similar for cancer pain.

5. Pain Related to Central Sensitivity Syndrome in Cancer Survivors

Yunus et al. proposed the central sensitivity syndrome as a comprehensive disease concept in which CS is involved in pathogenesis [45]. Unexplained organic symptoms related to CS common to various chronic diseases consider symptoms a single syndrome rather than in isolation. This terminology is a breakthrough that corrects the idea that different diagnoses have different mechanisms. Recently, the Central Sensitization Inventory (CSI) was proposed as an alternative method and a comprehensive screening tool for evaluating CS-related symptoms. CSI consists of symptoms associated with worsening CS, such as sleep disturbances, muscle stiffness, fatigue, sensitivity to light and smell, and stress (CS-related symptoms), and has been translated in many countries [46]. The CSI has shown excellent psychometric properties in chronic pain patients with CS-related symptoms [46] and excellent validity and internal consistency in breast cancer patients [47]. Higher CSI scores indicate a higher degree of self-reported CS-related symptoms, which can be classified into three clusters of severity: low level, medium level, and high level [48].

CS-related symptoms contribute to the prevalence of chronic pain after breast cancer surgery, pain intensity, and capacity impairment [23,35,49–51]. It has also been found that breast cancer survivors with medium and high levels of CS severity have more pain intensity and pain location than breast cancer survivors with low levels of CS severity [47]. In a longitudinal study, CS-related symptoms before and after surgery were independent predictors for pain intensity and disability of chronic pain after breast cancer surgery, in addition to treatment-related factors such as axillary lymph node dissection [25,26]. CS-related symptoms are not only associated with pain intensity and disability but also with anxiety, depression, pain catastrophizing [52,53], and fear of exercise [54]. The association between pain after cancer treatment and CS-related symptoms in cancer survivors is clear, but the association with cancer pain (e.g., bone and visceral metastases) is still unclear. However, cancer survivors with advanced cancer pain and those receiving palliative care or opioid treatment generally have more CS-related symptoms, such as insomnia and fatigue [55–58]. Thus, assessment and intervention for CS-related symptoms will be important for cancer survivors with cancer pain (e.g., bone and visceral metastases) in the future as part of cancer pain management.

6. Inflammation and Central Sensitization in Cancer Survivors

Inflammation has been shown to play a role in both the initiation and persistence of central sensitization [38,59]. Under normal conditions, astrocytes and microglia are primarily responsible for maintaining cell retention and immune responses in the spinal cord. However, when inflammation occurs, these cells become activated. For instance, activated astrocytes release inflammatory cytokines like Interleukin-1 beta (Il-1β) and Tumor Necrosis Factor-alpha (TNF-α), which contribute to the development of central sensitization [60]. Similarly, the activation of microglia leads to the release of inflammatory cytokines, Prostaglandin E2 (PGE2), Nitric Oxide (NO), and Brain-Derived Neurotrophic Factor (BDNF). Notably, BDNF can suppress the function of inhibitory Gamma-Aminobutyric Acid (GABA)-ergic neurons that densely reside in layer II of the dorsal horn of the spinal cord [61]. These mechanisms collectively contribute to the heightened excitability of spinal dorsal horn neurons and the occurrence of central sensitization. Moreover, microglia play a significant role in maintaining advanced-stage cancer pain in female rats by generating the inflammatory cytokine IL-1β and increasing the synaptic transmission of spinal nociceptive neurons [62]. Despite the likelihood of inflammation's involvement in CS among cancer survivors, there is currently only the support of preclinical experiments, and there is a lack of studies evaluating inflammatory markers in this population and investigating their association with CS. This remains an important area for future research, which will enhance our understanding of how to tackle inflammation for cancer pain and post-treatment pain in this cancer survivor population.

7. Sleep/Insomnia and Stress Related to Central Sensitization in Cancer Survivors

Sleep disturbances [63,64] and stress [65] are common comorbidities in cancer survivors, and both are associated with a worsening of pain symptoms in chronic pain patients [66,67]. Furthermore, CS-related symptoms measured using the CSI are strongly associated with sleep disturbances and stress [68,69].

For sleep, the evidence demonstrated that taking medications/opioids disrupts individuals' sleep quality since it might amplify their daytime fatigue and sleepiness, leading to napping during the day and disturbing the night rest [70]. Systematic review and meta-analysis suggested that sleep deprivation exacerbated peripheral and central pain sensitization measured using the QST in healthy individuals. However, similar results in cancer survivors with persistent pain remain unknown [71]. Furthermore, Pacho-Hernández

JC et al. reported that sleep quality mediated CS-related symptoms and quality of life in individuals with post-COVID-19 pain [72].

Stress in patients with chronic pain can modulate pain and exacerbate symptoms (such as fatigue and cognitive impairments) in response to stress [73,74]. Stress and pain demonstrate a high degree of comorbidity, indicating a considerable overlap in both conceptual and biological mechanisms [67].

However, the relationship between CS and sleep quality and stress, and whether sleep quality and stress mediate for CS, is currently unclear in cancer survivors. Thus, evidence is still scarce, but it is a potential target for treating CS.

8. Nociplastic Pain Related to Central Sensitization in Cancer Survivor

CS is one of the key mechanisms of nociplastic pain. Nociplastic pain was proposed as a third mechanistic pain descriptor in addition to nociceptive and neuropathic pain by IASP in 2017 [12]. The IASP defines nociplastic pain as "pain that arises from altered nociception despite no clear evidence of actual or threatened tissue damage causing the activation of peripheral nociceptors or evidence for disease or lesion of the somatosensory system causing the pain" [13]. The Cancer Pain Phenotyping (CANPPHE) Network reports that the grading system guideline consists of seven steps, all of which are recommended to be implemented for cancer survivors [14]. The evaluation used in CS and CS-related symptoms is also used in the guideline (e.g., evoked pain hypersensitivity phenomena, history of pain hypersensitivity, comorbidities associated with hyperalgesia). In the future, it may become more common to use these guidelines to classify and identify phenotypes rather than to evaluate only CS or CS-related symptoms. However, at present, the reliability and validity of the guideline in cancer survivors are not clear, and further research is crucial.

9. Challenges of Treating Pain in Cancer Survivors—Targeting Central Sensitization

Pharmacological treatment (NSAIDs, antidepressants, anticonvulsants, opioids, etc.) and non-pharmacological treatment (rehabilitation, cognitive behavioral interventions, etc.) are generally recommended in guidelines [8–10] for cancer pain. Pharmacological treatment is only a part of cancer pain management due to its numerous side effects. The effectiveness of the pharmacological treatment is also generally limited in patients with chronic non-cancer pain and CS. The use of opioids is not recommended for nociplastic pain involving CS [75,76]. According to the literature, opioids can lead to opiate-induced hyperalgesia, which will generate more pain in the long term and might decrease the survival rate [77,78].

What treatment is needed for CS? The management of patients with CS should not only focus on tissue damage (scar formation, muscle shortening, nerve damage, metastatic bone tumors, etc.) in either the affected body regions or within the central nervous system; rather, it should aim to target the underlying factors, including illness beliefs, stress, poor sleep, physical (in)activity, and even potentially unhealthy dietary habits, that sustain the CS process [79]. A systematic review revealed that physical therapy such as manual therapy, exercise, electrotherapy, education, and acupuncture improved CS-related variables in patients with chronic musculoskeletal pain [80]. A systematic review revealed that physical therapy results in a modest improvement in CS variables such as TS and CPM in patients with chronic musculoskeletal pain. It is not clear whether physical therapy improves CS variables in patients with cancer pain and pain after cancer treatment because the systematic review did not include them.

In the field of oncology, there have been attempts to see if these rehabilitations are effective [81–85]. International multidisciplinary roundtable reported consensus exercise guidelines [82]. The data were deemed sufficient to suggest exercise for several cancer-related health outcomes (such as fatigue, sadness, anxiety, and lymphedema). However, due to the lack of evidence, exercise for cancer pain management was not included [86]. As with other management methods, pain education is getting a lot of attention. Pain neuroscience education (PNE), an educational intervention, is gaining popularity for managing chronic musculoskeletal pain. The goal is to change the perception of pain from being caused by biological processes such as tissue damage or disease to being a necessary response to protect the body's tissues. There are some differences between PNE for musculoskeletal pain and cancer pain PNE (Table 1). In particular, the description of the anxiety and threat of cancer recurrence is characteristic [87–91]. PNE alone is not effective enough, and its benefits can increase when combined with exercise. Several systematic reviews and meta-analyses have reported that interventions combining PNE and exercise therapy for persons with chronic musculoskeletal pain have resulted in at least short-term improvements in pain and disability [91]. We reported that pain intensity and disability significantly improved, and CS-related symptoms decreased in the group that received PNE combined with physiotherapy rather than the group that received biomedical education (BME) combined with physiotherapy in a retrospective case–control study of postoperative breast cancer survivors [88]. A single-arm study in breast cancer survivors suggests that the combination of exercise therapy and educational programs improves CS-related symptoms [54], and personalized eHealth interventions, including pain science education and self-management strategies, are effective in improving pain-related function, CS-related symptoms and quality of life [89]. However, in a large randomized controlled trial (RCT) of breast cancer survivors, there were no significant differences in pain-related disability, pain intensity, or psychological symptoms between the BME plus physical therapy and PNE plus physical therapy groups [90]. The results may have been influenced by the diversity of patients, including postoperative pain, CIPN, and hormone-induced arthralgia. A systematic review including more than 4000 participants found that compared to the target group, pain education programs for cancer survivors with cancer pain showed significant improvements in pain intensity and disability, self-efficacy, pain knowledge and barriers, and medication adherence, but in less than 20% of all eligible patients [92]. Combining physical therapy with a pain education program as a non-pharmacological treatment for cancer pain with cancer survivors may effectively improve pain intensity, capacity impairment, and CS-related symptoms. However, since most intervention studies have been conducted in breast cancer survivors, it is unclear whether similar results can be obtained in other cancer survivors. Further research is also needed to determine whether the pain education program is effective for all types of cancer pain, including chronic pain after cancer treatment (postoperative pain, CIPN, etc.) and chronic cancer pain (bone metastasis pain, visceral metastasis pain, etc.).

Next to pain education, clinicians should focus on tackling insomnia and stress, which might improve CS [79]. There is evidence of treatment for insomnia and stress in cancer survivors. Cognitive behavior therapy (CBT) for insomnia (CBT-I) is the gold standard and treatment for insomnia [93]. Systematic review and meta-analysis have shown that CBT-I is strongly recommended for treating insomnia [94]. Cognitive behavioral stress management, which allows patients to better deal with the impact of the environment, had a positive effect on stress in patients with breast cancer [95]. Mindfulness-based stress reduction (MBSR) and yoga are also effective for stress in cancer survivors [96–98]. However, evidence is lacking concerning the impact of those interventions on cancer survivors' pain (cancer pain and pain after cancer treatment) and CS symptoms. The indirect effect of those interventions on CS symptoms should be further investigated in the future.

Table 1. Difference between pain neuroscience education for musculoskeletal pain and cancer pain.

Sessions	Musculoskeletal Pain	Cancer Pain
Pathoanatomic models	No reference to pathoanatomic models	Explanation of general side effects of treatment modalities (surgery, radiotherapy, chemotherapy and hormone therapy)
Acute pain vs. chronic pain	Transition from acute to chronic pain	
Nerve function	The neuron (receptor, axon, terminal) and the synapse (action potential, neurotransmitters, postsynaptic membrane potential, chemically driven ion channel)	
Peripheral and central sensitization	Peripheral sensitization (e.g., peripheral nerve injury, inflammation) Central sensitization (e.g., brain and spinal cord function, the pain matrix in the brain)	
Descending nociceptive inhibition and facilitation	Emotions, stress, sleep, physical activity, pain cognitions, and pain behavior	
Reconceptualization of pain as a normal brain response to perceived threat	Vicious cycle due to kinesiophobia and fear–avoidance models. Information about sensations that are a threat to the body is recognized as 'pain' as a normal response of the brain.	Vicious cycle due to kinesiophobia and fear–avoidance models. Threatening perception of pain as cancer recurrence or metastasis, leading to heightened anxiety and avoidance behavior.
Transfer knowledge about pain to an adaptive behavioral change	Advice on managing factors that contribute to persistent pain, such as correcting misperceptions and activity management (pacing strategies), taking into account biopsychosocial factors	

10. Future Directions for Research and Clinical Practice

Previous clinical studies have examined the efficacy of certain treatments for certain diseases and have not individually designed treatments for problems at the individual patient level. Precision medicine, which has been the focus of much attention in recent years, involves the classification of patients into subgroups based on a multifaceted evaluation of disease and the implementation of treatment tailored to the characteristics of each patient. Precision medicine is mainly used in oncology to identify the histology and genotype of cancer and optimize treatment in individual patients [99]. Precision rehabilitation has not been fully explored at this time. For precision rehabilitation, physical, cognitive, and psychosocial factors need to be measured, and the patients could be classified into subgroups based on results. Some studies classified patients based on CSI scores (low-CSI/high-CSI). High-intensity training improves symptoms of CS in patients with chronic low back pain, and this effect is greatest in those with high CSI scores at baseline. PNE is more effective in pain catastrophizing in patients with high CSI scores [100]. These studies indicate the possibility of developing precision rehabilitation, while there is still a lack of suggestions on how to deal specifically with CSS. Interventions targeting the following sub-categories (1. Emotional distress, 2. Urological and general symptoms, 3. Headache/Jaw symptoms, 4. Sleep disturbance, and 5. Muscle symptoms of CSS) may be needed (Figure 1). Furthermore, it is necessary to determine whether precision cancer pain medicine, customized according to the underlying pain mechanisms, is more effective than conventional medical care. Precision pain medicine should shift from local therapies like stretching, resistance training, and physical therapy to systemic therapies like pain education and activity level pacing (Figure 2). However, the effectiveness of precision pain medicine or precision rehabilitation is not clear for both musculoskeletal patients and cancer survivors, and further research is needed.

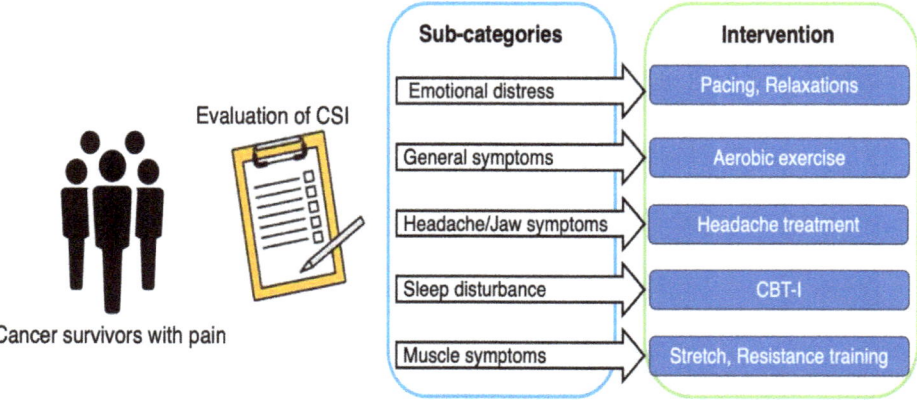

Figure 1. Central sensitivity syndrome targeted education.

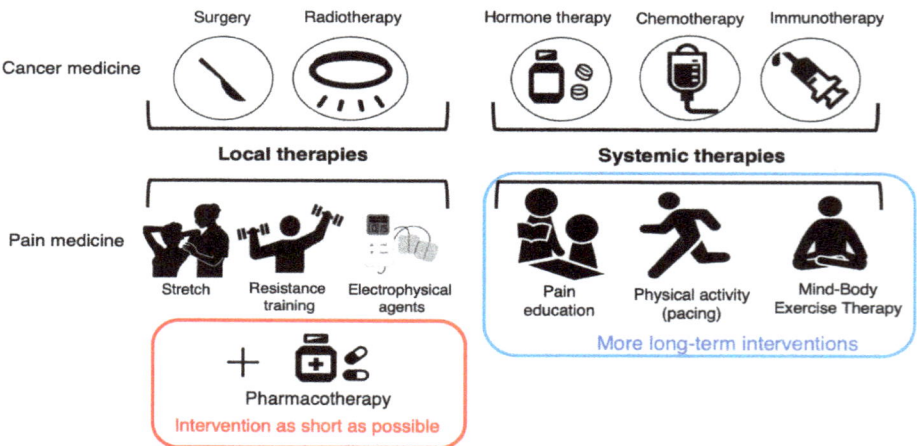

Figure 2. Multimodal therapy for cancer pain.

11. Conclusions

Evidence that CS affects cancer pain is accumulating. Recently, a seven-step diagnostic approach for differentiating the predominant pains has been developed for cancer survivors. Besides, bedside QSTs and CSI-tool could also help clinicians identify CSS. In the future, it is necessary to investigate multimodal lifestyle interventions in the long term for cancer survivors with predominant CS.

Author Contributions: Conceptualization, T.N.; Methodology, T.N.; Investigation, T.N., M.M. and A.L.; Writing—original draft preparation, T.N. and M.M.; Writing, review and editing, T.N., M.M. and A.L.; Visualization, T.N. and M.M.; Supervision, T.N. All authors have read and agreed to the published version of the manuscript.

Funding: This research did not receive any specific grant from funding agencies in the public, commercial, or not-for-profit sectors. A.L. is a research fellow funded by the Research Foundation Flanders (FWO—Fonds Wetenschappelijk Onderzoek), Belgium (grant number 11B1920N).

Institutional Review Board Statement: Not applicable.

Informed Consent Statement: Not applicable.

Data Availability Statement: Not applicable.

Conflicts of Interest: The authors declare no conflict of interest.

References

1. Mahase, E. Cancer ovet alertakes CVD to become leading cause of death in high income countries. *BMJ* **2019**, *366*, l5368. [CrossRef] [PubMed]
2. Sung, H.; Ferlay, J.; Siegel, R.L.; Laversanne, M.; Soerjomataram, I.; Jemal, A.; Bray, F. Global Cancer Statistics 2020: GLOBOCAN Estimates of Incidence and Mortality Worldwide for 36 Cancers in 185 Countries. *CA Cancer J. Clin.* **2021**, *71*, 209–249. [CrossRef] [PubMed]
3. Haenen, V.; Evenepoel, M.; De Baerdemaecker, T.; Meeus, M.; Devoogdt, N.; Morlion, B.; Dams, L.; Van Dijck, S.; Van der Gucht, E.; De Vrieze, T.; et al. Pain prevalence and characteristics in survivors of solid cancers: A systematic review and meta-analysis. *Support Care Cancer* **2022**, *31*, 85. [CrossRef]
4. Roberto, A.; Greco, M.T.; Uggeri, S.; Cavuto, S.; Deandrea, S.; Corli, O.; Apolone, G. Living systematic review to assess the analgesic undertreatment in cancer patients. *Pain Pract.* **2022**, *22*, 487–496. [CrossRef] [PubMed]
5. Greco, M.T.; Roberto, A.; Corli, O.; Deandrea, S.; Bandieri, E.; Cavuto, S.; Apolone, G. Quality of cancer pain management: An update of a systematic review of undertreatment of patients with cancer. *J. Clin. Oncol.* **2014**, *32*, 4149–4154. [CrossRef] [PubMed]
6. Breivik, H.; Cherny, N.; Collett, B.; De Conno, F.; Filbet, M.; Foubert, A.J.; Cohen, R.; Dow, L. Cancerrelated pain: A pan-European survey of prevalence, treatment, and patient attitudes. *Ann. Oncol.* **2009**, *20*, 1420–1433. [CrossRef]
7. Deandrea, S.; Montanari, M.; Moja, L.; Apolone, G. Prevalence of undertreatment in cancer pain. A review of published literature. *Ann. Oncol.* **2008**, *19*, 1985–1991. [CrossRef]
8. WHO. WHO Guidelines for the Pharmacological and Radiotherapeutic Management of Cancer Pain in Adults and Adolescents. 2018. Available online: https://apps.who.int/iris/bitstream/handle/10665/279700/9789241550390-eng.pdf (accessed on 15 April 2023).
9. Fallon, M.; Giusti, R.; Aielli, F.; Hoskin, P.; Rolke, R.; Sharma, M.; Ripamonti, C.I.; ESMO Guidelines Committee. Management of cancer pain in adult patients: ESMO Clinical Practice Guidelines. *Ann. Oncol.* **2018**, *29*, iv166–iv191. [CrossRef]
10. Swarm, R.A.; Paice, J.A.; Anghelescu, D.L.; Are, M.; Bruce, J.Y.; Buga, S.; Chwistek, M.; Cleeland, C.; Craig, D.; Gafford, E.; et al. Adult Cancer Pain, Version 3.2019, NCCN Clinical Practice Guidelines in Oncology. *J. Natl. Compr. Cancer Netw.* **2019**, *17*, 977–1007. [CrossRef]
11. Bennett, M.I.; Kaasa, S.; Barke, A.; Korwisi, B.; Rief, W.; Treede, R.D.; IASP Taskforce for the Classification of Chronic Pain. The IASP classification of chronic pain for ICD-11: Chronic cancer-related pain. *Pain* **2019**, *160*, 38–44. [CrossRef]
12. Kosek, E.; Cohen, M.; Baron, R.; Gebhart, G.F.; Mico, J.A.; Rice, A.S.C.; Rief, W.; Sluka, A.K. Do we need a third mechanistic descriptor for chronic pain states? *Pain* **2016**, *157*, 1382–1386. [CrossRef] [PubMed]
13. International Association for the Study of Pain (IASP). IASP Terminology 2022. Available online: https://www.iasp-pain.org/resources/terminology/?navItemNumber=576#Centralsensitization (accessed on 15 April 2023).
14. Nijs, J.; Lahousse, A.; Fernández-de-Las-Peñas, C.; Madeleine, P.; Fontaine, C.; Nishigami, T.; Desmedt, C.; Vanhoeij, M.; Mostaqim, K.; Cuesta-Vargas, A.I.; et al. Towards precision pain medicine for pain after cancer: The Cancer Pain Phenotyping Network multidisciplinary international guidelines for pain phenotyping using nociplastic pain criteria. *Br. J. Anaesth.* **2023**, *130*, 611–621. [CrossRef] [PubMed]
15. Nijs, J.; George, S.Z.; Clauw, D.J.; Fernández-de-las-Peñas, C.; Kosek, E.; Ickmans, K.; Fernández-Carnero, J.; Polli, A.; Kapreli, E.; Huysmans, E.; et al. Central sensitisation in chronic pain conditions: Latest discoveries and their potential for precision medicine. *Lancet Rheumatol.* **2021**, *3*, e383–e392. [CrossRef]
16. Chimenti, R.L.; Frey-Law, L.A.; Sluka, K.A. A Mechanism-Based Approach to Physical Therapist Management of Pain. *Phys. Ther.* **2018**, *98*, 302–314. [CrossRef] [PubMed]
17. Glare, P.; Aubrey, K.R.; Myles, P.S. Transition from acute to chronic pain after surgery. *Lancet* **2019**, *393*, 1537–1546. [CrossRef]
18. Den Boer, C.; Dries, L.; Terluin, B.; Van der Wouden, J.C.; Blankenstein, A.H.; Van Wilgen, C.P.; Lucassen, P.; Van der Horst, H.E. Central sensitization in chronic pain and medically unexplained symptom research: A systematic review of definitions, operationalizations and measurement instruments. *J. Psychosom. Res.* **2019**, *117*, 32–40. [CrossRef]
19. Den Bandt, H.L.; Paulis, W.D.; Beckwée, D.; Ickmans, K.; Nijs, J.; Voogt, L. Pain Mechanisms in Low Back Pain: A Systematic Review With Meta-analysis of Mechanical Quantitative Sensory Testing Outcomes in People With Nonspecific Low Back Pain. *J. Orthop. Sports Phys. Ther.* **2019**, *49*, 698–715. [CrossRef]
20. Fingleton, C.; Smart, K.; Moloney, N.; Fullen, B.M.; Doody, C. Pain sensitization in people with knee osteoarthritis: A systematic review and meta-analysis. *Osteoarthr. Cartil.* **2015**, *23*, 1043–1056. [CrossRef]
21. Touche, R.L.; Paris-Alemany, A.; Hidalgo-Pérez, A.; López-de-Uralde-Villanueva, I.; Angulo-Diaz-Parreño, S.; Muñoz-García, D. Evidence for Central Sensitization in Patients with Temporomandibular Disorders: A Systematic Review and Meta-analysis of Observational Studies. *Pain Pract.* **2018**, *18*, 388–409. [CrossRef]
22. Bartholomew, C.; Lack, S.; Neal, B. Altered pain processing and sensitisation is evident in adults with patellofemoral pain: A systematic review including meta-analysis and meta-regression. *Scand. J. Pain* **2019**, *20*, 11–27. [CrossRef]

23. De Groef, A.; Meeus, M.; De Vrieze, T.; Vos, L.; Van Kampen, M.; Geraerts, I.; Devoogdt, N. Unraveling Self-Reported Signs of Central Sensitization in Breast Cancer Survivors with Upper Limb Pain: Prevalence Rate and Contributing Factors. *Pain Physician* **2018**, *21*, E247–E256. [CrossRef] [PubMed]

24. Leysen, L.; Adriaenssens, N.; Nijs, J.; Pas, R.; Bilterys, T.; Vermeir, S.; Lahousse, A.; Beckwée, D. Chronic pain in breast cancer survivors: Nociceptive, neuropathic, or central sensitization pain? *Pain Pract.* **2019**, *19*, 183–195. [CrossRef] [PubMed]

25. Manfuku, M.; Nishigami, T.; Mibu, A.; Yamashita, H.; Imai, R.; Kanamori, H.; Sumiyoshi, K. Predictors of persistent post-surgical pain intensity and interference at 1 year after breast cancer surgery: Assessing central sensitization, central sensitivity symptoms, and psychological factors. *Breast Cancer* **2023**, *30*, 271–281. [CrossRef] [PubMed]

26. Dams, L.; Van der Gucht, E.; Haenen, V.; Lauwers, M.; De Pauw, S.; Steurs, T.; Devoogdt, N.; Smeets, A.; Bernar, K.; De Vrieze, T.; et al. Biopsychosocial risk factors for pain and painrelated disability 1 year after surgery for breast cancer. *Support Care Cancer* **2022**, *30*, 4465–4475. [CrossRef]

27. Uddin, Z.; MacDermid, J.C. Quantitative Sensory Testing in Chronic Musculoskeletal Pain. *Pain Med.* **2016**, *17*, 1694–1703. [CrossRef]

28. Edwards, R.R.; Dworkin, R.H.; Turk, D.C.; Angst, M.S.; Dionne, R.; Freeman, R.; Hansson, P.; Haroutounian, S.; Lars Arendt-Nielsen, L.; Attal, N.; et al. Patient phenotyping in clinical trials of chronic pain treatments: IMMPACT recommendations. *Pain* **2016**, *157*, 1851–1871. [CrossRef]

29. Edwards, R.R.; Schreiber, K.L.; Dworkin, R.H.; Turk, D.C.; Baron, R.; Freeman, R.; Jensen, T.S.; Latremoliere, A.; Markman, J.D.; Rice, A.S.C.; et al. Optimizing and Accelerating the Development of Precision Pain Treatments for Chronic Pain: IMMPACT Review and Recommendations. *J. Pain* **2023**, *24*, 204–225. [CrossRef]

30. Izumi, M.; Hayashi, Y.; Saito, R.; Oda, S.; Petersen, K.K.; Arendt-Nielsen, L.; Ikeuchi, M. Detection of altered pain facilitatory and inhibitory mechanisms in patients with knee osteoarthritis by using a simple bedside tool kit (QuantiPain). *Pain Rep.* **2022**, *7*, e998. [CrossRef]

31. Reimer, M.; Forstenpointner, J.; Hartmann, A.; Otto, J.C.; Vollert, J.; Gierthmühlen, J.; Klein, T.; Hüllemann, P.; Baron, R. Sensory bedside testing: A simple stratification approach for sensory phenotyping. *Pain Rep.* **2020**, *5*, e820. [CrossRef]

32. Sachau, J.; Otto, J.C.; Kirchhofer, V.; Larsen, J.B.; Kennes, L.N.; Hüllemann, P.; Arendt-Nielsen, L.; Baron, R. Development of a bedside tool-kit for assessing sensitization in patients with chronic osteoarthritis knee pain or chronic knee pain after total knee replacement. *Pain* **2022**, *163*, 308–318. [CrossRef]

33. Fillingim, R.B.; Loeser, J.D.; Baron, R.; Edwards, R.R. Assessment of Chronic Pain: Domains, Methods, and Mechanisms. *J. Pain* **2016**, *17*, T10–T20. [CrossRef]

34. Mustonen, L.; Aho, T.; Harno, H.; Sipilä, R.; Meretoja, T.; Kalso, E. What makes surgical nerve injury painful? A 4-year to 9-year follow-up of patients with intercostobrachial nerve resection in women treated for breast cancer. *Pain* **2019**, *160*, 246–256. [CrossRef] [PubMed]

35. Manfuku, M.; Nishigami, T.; Mibu, A.; Tanaka, K.; Kitagaki, K.; Sumiyoshi, K. Comparison of central sensitization-related symptoms and health-related quality of life between breast cancer survivors with and without chronic pain and healthy controls. *Breast Cancer* **2019**, *26*, 758–765. [CrossRef] [PubMed]

36. Zhu, Y.; Loggia, M.L.; Edwards, R.R.; Flowers, K.M.; Muñoz-Vergara, D.W.; Partridge, A.H.; Schreiber, K.L. Increased Clinical Pain Locations and Pain Sensitivity in Women After Breast Cancer Surgery: Influence of Aromatase Inhibitor Therapy. *Clin. J. Pain* **2022**, *38*, 721–729. [CrossRef] [PubMed]

37. Caro-Morán, E.; Fernández-Lao, C.; Díaz-Rodríguez, L.; Cantarero-Villanueva, I.; Madeleine, P.; Arroyo-Morales, M. Pressure Pain Sensitivity Maps of the Neck-Shoulder Region in Breast Cancer Survivors. *Pain Med.* **2016**, *17*, 1942–1952. [CrossRef]

38. Ortiz-Comino, L.; Fernández-Lao, C.; Castro-Martín, E.; Cantarero-Villanueva, I.; Madeleine, P.; Arroyo-Morales, M. Myofascial pain, widespread pressure hypersensitivity, and hyperalgesia in the face, neck, and shoulder regions, in survivors of head and neck cancer. *Support Care Cancer* **2020**, *28*, 2891–2898. [CrossRef]

39. Sánchez-Jiménez, A.; Cantarero-Villanueva, I.; Molina-Barea, R.; Fernández-Lao, C.; Galiano-Castillo, N.; Arroyo-Morales, M. Widespread pressure pain hypersensitivity and ultrasound imaging evaluation of abdominal area after colon cancer treatment. *Pain Med.* **2014**, *15*, 233–240. [CrossRef]

40. Fernández-Lao, C.; Cantarero-Villanueva, I.; Fernández-delasPeñas, C.; Del-Moral-Ávila, R.; Menjón-Beltrán, S.; Arroyo-Morales, M. Widespread mechanical pain hypersensitivity as a sign of central sensitization after breast cancer surgery: Comparison between mastectomy and lumpectomy. *Pain Med.* **2011**, *12*, 72–78. [CrossRef]

41. Fernández-Lao, C.; Cantarero-Villanueva, I.; Fernández-de-LasPeñas, C.; Del-Moral-Ávila, R.; Arendt-Nielsen, L.; Arroyo-Morales, M. Myofascial trigger points in neck and shoulder muscles and widespread pressure pain hypersensitivity in patients with postmastectomy pain: Evidence of peripheral and central sensitization. *Clin. J. Pain* **2010**, *26*, 798–806. [CrossRef]

42. Schreiber, K.L.; Martel, M.O.; Shnol, H.; Shaffer, J.R.; Greco, C.; Viray, N.; Taylor, L.N.; McLaughlin, M.; Brufsky, A.; Ahrendt, G.; et al. Persistent pain in postmastectomy patients: Comparison of psychophysical, medical, surgical, and psychosocial characteristics between patients with and without pain. *Pain* **2013**, *154*, 660–668. [CrossRef]

43. Edwards, R.R.; Mensing, G.; Cahalan, C.; Greenbaum, S.; Narang, S.; Belfer, I.; Schreiber, K.L.; Campbell, C.; Wasan, A.D.; Jamison, R.N. Alteration in pain modulation in women with persistent pain after lumpectomy: Influence of catastrophizing. *J. Pain Symptom Manag.* **2013**, *46*, 30–42. [CrossRef] [PubMed]

44. Scott, A.C.; McConnell, S.; Laird, B.; Colvin, L.; Fallon, M. Quantitative Sensory Testing to assess the sensory characteristics of cancer-induced bone pain after radiotherapy and potential clinical biomarkers of response. *Eur. J. Pain* **2012**, *16*, 123–133. [CrossRef] [PubMed]

45. Yunus, M.B. Central sensitivity syndromes: A unified concept for fibromyalgia and other similar maladies. *J. Indian Rheum. Assoc.* **2000**, *8*, 27–33.

46. Scerbo, T.; Colasurdo, J.; Dunn, S.; Unger, J.; Nijs, J.; Cook, C. Measurement Properties of the Central Sensitization Inventory: A Systematic Review. *Pain Pract.* **2018**, *18*, 544–554. [CrossRef] [PubMed]

47. Hurth, A.; Steege, J.N.; Scheepbouwer, P.; Roose, E.; Lahousse, A.; Leysen, L.; Stas, L.; Kregel, J.; Salvat, E.; Nijs, J. Assessment of Central Sensitization in Breast Cancer Survivors: Convergent Validity and Use of the Central Sensitization Inventory (CSI) and Its Short-Form as a Clustering Tool. *Clin. Pract.* **2021**, *11*, 607–618. [CrossRef]

48. Cuesta-Vargas, A.I.; Neblett, R.; Nijs, J.; Chiarotto, A.; Kregel, J.; Van Wilgen, C.P.; Pitance, L.; Knezevic, A.; Gatchel, R.J.; Mayer, T.G.; et al. Establishing central sensitization-related symptom severity subgroups: A multicountry study using the central sensitization inventory. *Pain Med.* **2020**, *21*, 2430–2440. [CrossRef]

49. De Groef, A.; Meeus, M.; De Vrieze, T.; Vos, L.; Van Kampen, M.; Christiaens, M.R.; Neven, P.; Geraerts, I.; Devoogdt, N. Pain characteristics as important contributing factors to upper limb dysfunctions in breast cancer survivors at long term. *Musculoskelet. Sci. Pract.* **2017**, *29*, 52–59. [CrossRef]

50. Roldán-Jiménez, C.; Martín-Martín, J.; Pajares, B.; Ribelles, N.; Alba, E.; Cuesta-Vargas, A.I. Factors associated with upper limb function in breast cancer survivors. *Phys. Med. Rehabil.* **2023**, *15*, 151–156. [CrossRef]

51. De la Rosa-Díaz, I.; Barrero-Santiago, L.; Acosta-Ramírez, P.; Martín-Peces-Barba, M.; Iglesias-Hernández, E.; Plisset, B.; Lutinier, N.; Belzanne, M.; Touche, R.L.; Grande-Alonso, M. Cross-Sectional Comparative Study on Central Sensitization-Psychosocial Associated Comorbidities and Psychological Characteristics in Breast Cancer Survivors with Nociceptive Pain and Pain with Neuropathic Features and without Pain. *Life* **2022**, *12*, 1328. [CrossRef]

52. Leysen, L.; Cools, W.; Nijs, J.; Adriaenssens, N.; Pas, R.; Van Wilgen, C.P.; Bults, R.; Roose, E.; Lahousse, A.; Beckwée, D. The mediating effect of pain catastrophizing and perceived injustice in the relationship of pain on health-related quality of life in breast cancer survivors. *Support Care Cancer* **2021**, *29*, 5653–5661. [CrossRef]

53. Lahousse, A.; Ivakhnov, S.; Nijs, J.; Beckwée, D.; De Las Peñas, C.F.; Roose, E.; Leysen, L. The mediating effect of perceived injustice and pain catastrophizing in the relationship of pain on fatigue and sleep in breast cancer survivors: A cross-sectional study. *Pain Med.* **2022**, *23*, 1299–1310. [CrossRef] [PubMed]

54. Gutiérrez-Sánchez, D.; Pajares-Hachero, B.I.; Trinidad-Fernández, M.; Escriche-Escuder, A.; Iglesias-Campos, M.; Bermejo-Pérez, M.J.; Alba-Conejo, E.; Roldán-Jiménez, C.; Cuesta-Vargas, A. The Benefits of a Therapeutic Exercise and Educational Intervention Program on Central Sensitization Symptoms and Pain-Related Fear Avoidance in Breast Cancer Survivors. *Pain Manag. Nurs.* **2022**, *23*, 467–472. [CrossRef] [PubMed]

55. Henson, L.A.; Maddocks, M.; Evans, C.; Davidson, M.; Hicks, S.; Higginson, I.J. Palliative Care and the Management of Common Distressing Symptoms in Advanced Cancer: Pain, Breathlessness, Nausea and Vomiting, and Fatigue. *J. Clin. Oncol.* **2020**, *38*, 905–914. [CrossRef] [PubMed]

56. Nzwalo, I.; Aboim, M.A.; Joaquim, N.; Marreiros, A.; Nzwalo, H. Systematic Review of the Prevalence, Predictors, and Treatment of Insomnia in Palliative Care. *Am. J. Hosp. Palliat. Care* **2020**, *37*, 957–969. [CrossRef] [PubMed]

57. Fabi, A.; Bhargava, R.; Fatigoni, S.; Guglielmo, M.; Horneber, M.; Roila, F.; Weis, J.; Jordan, K.; Ripamonti, C.I. Cancer-related fatigue: ESMO Clinical Practice Guidelines for diagnosis and treatment. *Ann. Oncol.* **2020**, *31*, 713–723. [CrossRef]

58. Wang, X.S.; Zhao, F.; Fisch, M.J.; O'Mara, A.M.; Cella, D.; Mendoza, T.R.; Cleeland, C.S. Prevalence and characteristics of moderate to severe fatigue: A multicenter study in cancer patients and survivors. *Cancer* **2014**, *120*, 425–432. [CrossRef]

59. Ji, R.R.; Nackley, A.; Huh, Y.; Terrando, N.; Maixner, W. Neuroinflammation and Central Sensitization in Chronic and Widespread Pain. *Anesthesiology* **2018**, *129*, 343–366. [CrossRef]

60. Milligan, E.D.; Watkins, L.R. Pathological and protective roles of glia in chronic pain. *Nat. Rev. Neurosci.* **2009**, *10*, 23–36. [CrossRef]

61. Coull, J.A.M.; Beggs, S.; Boudreau, D.; Boivin, D.; Tsuda, M.; Inoue, K.; Gravel, C.; Salter, M.W.; Koninck, Y.D. BDNF from microglia causes the shift in neuronal anion gradient underlying neuropathic pain. *Nature* **2005**, *438*, 1017–1021. [CrossRef]

62. Yang, Y.; Li, H.; Li, T.T.; Luo, H.; Gu, X.Y.; Lü, N.; Ji, R.R.; Zhang, Y.O. Delayed activation of spinal microglia contributes to the maintenance of bone cancer pain in female Wistar rats via P2X7 receptor and IL-18. *J. Neurosci.* **2015**, *35*, 7950–7963. [CrossRef]

63. Savard, J.; Simard, S.; Blanchet, J.; Ivers, H.; Morin, C.M. Prevalence, clinical characteristics, and risk factors for insomnia in the context of breast cancer. *Sleep* **2001**, *24*, 583–590. [CrossRef] [PubMed]

64. Leysen, L.; Lahousse, A.; Nijs, J.; Adriaenssens, N.; Mairesse, O.; Ivakhnov, S.; Bilterys, T.; Van Looveren, E.; Pas, R.; Beckwée, D. Prevalence and risk factors of sleep disturbances in breast cancer survivors: Systematic review and meta-analyses. *Support Care Cancer* **2019**, *27*, 4401–4433. [CrossRef] [PubMed]

65. Syrowatka, A.; Motulsky, A.; Kurteva, S.; Hanley, J.A.; Dixon, W.G.; Meguerditchian, A.N.; Tamblyn, R. Predictors of distress in female breast cancer survivors: A systematic review. *Breast Cancer Res. Treat.* **2017**, *165*, 229–245. [CrossRef]

66. Looveren, E.V.; Bilterys, T.; Munneke, W.; Cagnie, B.; Ickmans, K.; Mairesse, O.; Malfliet, A.; De Baets, L.; Nijs, J.; Goubert, D.; et al. The Association between Sleep and Chronic Spinal Pain: A Systematic Review from the Last Decade. *J. Clin. Med.* **2021**, *10*, 3836. [CrossRef] [PubMed]

67. Abdallah, C.G.; Geha, P. Chronic Pain and Chronic Stress: Two Sides of the Same Coin? *Chronic Stress* **2017**, *1*, 2470547017704763. [CrossRef]
68. Adams, G.R.; Gandhi, W.; Harrison, R.; Van Reekum, C.M.; Wood-Anderson, D.; Gilron, I.; Salomons, T.V. Do "central sensitization" questionnaires reflect measures of nociceptive sensitization or psychological constructs? A systematic review and meta-analyses. *Pain* **2023**, *164*, 1222–1239. [CrossRef]
69. Haruyama, Y.; Sairenchi, T.; Uchiyama, K.; Suzuki, K.; Hirata, K.; Kobashi, G. A large-scale population-based epidemiological study on the prevalence of central sensitization syndromes in Japan. *Sci. Rep.* **2021**, *11*, 23299. [CrossRef] [PubMed]
70. Rosen, I.M.; Aurora, R.N.; Kirsch, D.B.; Carden, K.A.; Malhotra, R.K.; Ramar, K.; Abbasi-Feinberg, F.; Kristo, D.A.; Martin, J.L.; Olson, E.J.; et al. Chronic Opioid Therapy and Sleep: An American Academy of Sleep Medicine Position Statement. *J. Clin. Sleep Med.* **2019**, *15*, 1671–1673. [CrossRef]
71. Chang, J.R.; Fu, S.N.; Li, X.; Li, S.X.; Wang, X.; Zhou, Z.; Pinto, S.M.; Samartzis, D.; Karppinen, J.; Wong, A.Y. The differential effects of sleep deprivation on pain perception in individuals with or without chronic pain: A systematic review and meta-analysis. *Sleep Med. Rev.* **2022**, *66*, 101695. [CrossRef]
72. Pacho-Hernández, J.C.; Fernández-de-Las-Peñas, C.; Fuensalida-Novo, S.; Jiménez-Antona, C.; Ortega-Santiago, R.; Cigarán-Mendez, M. Sleep Quality Mediates the Effect of Sensitization-Associated Symptoms, Anxiety, and Depression on Quality of Life in Individuals with Post-COVID-19 Pain. *Brain Sci.* **2022**, *12*, 1363. [CrossRef]
73. Dennis, N.L.; Larkin, M.; Derbyshire, S.W.G. 'A giant mess'—Making sense of complexity in the accounts of people with fibromyalgia. *Br. J. Health Psychol.* **2013**, *18*, 763–781. [CrossRef] [PubMed]
74. Alok, R.; Das, S.K.; Agarwal, G.G.; Salwahan, L.; Srivastava, R. Relationship of severity of depression, anxiety and stress with severity of fibromyalgia. *Clin. Exp. Rheumatol.* **2011**, *29*, 70–72.
75. Nijs, J.; Roose, E.; Lahousse, A.; Mostaqim, K.; Reynebeau, I.; De Couck, M.; Beckwee, D.; Huysmans, E.; Bults, R.; Van Wilgen, P.; et al. Pain and Opioid Use in Cancer Survivors: A Practical Guide to Account for Perceived Injustice. *Pain Physician* **2021**, *24*, 309–317.
76. Fitzcharles, M.A.; Cohen, S.P.; Clauw, D.J.; Littlejohn, G.; Usui, C.; Häuser, W. Nociplastic pain: Towards an understanding of prevalent pain conditions. *Lancet* **2021**, *397*, 2098–2110. [CrossRef]
77. Tompkin, D.A.; Campbell, C.M. Opioid-induced hyperalgesia: Clinically relevant or extraneous research phenomenon? *Curr. Pain Headache Rep.* **2011**, *15*, 129–136. [CrossRef] [PubMed]
78. Rudd, R.A.; Seth, P.; David, F.; Scholl, L. Increases in Drug and Opioid-Involved Overdose Deaths United States, 2010–2015. *Morb. Mortal. Wkly. Rep.* **2016**, *65*, 1445–1452. [CrossRef]
79. Nijs, J.; Leysen, L.; Vanlauwe, J.; Logghe, T.; Ickmans, K.; Polli, A.; Malfliet, A.; Coppieters, I.; Huysmans, E. Treatment of central sensitization in patients with chronic pain: Time for change? *Expert Opin. Pharmacother.* **2019**, *20*, 1961–1970. [CrossRef] [PubMed]
80. Arribas-Romano, A.; Fernández-Carnero, J.; Molina-Rueda, F.; Angulo-Diaz-Parreño, S.; Navarro-Santana, M.J. Efficacy of Physical Therapy on Nociceptive Pain Processing Alterations in Patients with Chronic Musculoskeletal Pain: A Systematic Review and Meta-analysis. *Pain Med.* **2020**, *21*, 2502–2517. [CrossRef]
81. Stout, N.L.; Mina, D.S.; Lyons, K.D.; Robb, K.; Silver, J.K. A systematic review of rehabilitation and exercise recommendations in oncology guidelines. *CA Cancer J. Clin.* **2021**, *71*, 149–175. [CrossRef]
82. Campbell, K.L.; Winters-Stone, K.M.; Wiskemann, J.; May, A.M.; Schwartz, A.L.; Courneya, K.S.; Zucker, D.S.; Matthews, C.E.; Ligibel, J.A.; Gerber, L.H.; et al. Exercise Guidelines for Cancer Survivors: Consensus Statement from International Multidisciplinary Roundtable. *Med. Sci. Sports Exerc.* **2019**, *51*, 2375–2390. [CrossRef]
83. Tanriverdi, A.; Kahraman, B.O.; Ergin, G.; Karadibak, D.; Savci, S. Effect of exercise interventions in adults with cancer receiving palliative care: A systematic review and meta-analysis. *Support Care Cancer* **2023**, *31*, 205. [CrossRef]
84. Guo, S.; Han, W.; Wang, P.; Wang, X.; Fang, X. Effects of exercise on chemotherapy-induced peripheral neuropathy in cancer patients: A systematic review and meta-analysis. *J. Cancer Surviv.* **2023**, *17*, 318–331. [CrossRef] [PubMed]
85. Roberts, R.E.; Rickett, K.; Feng, S.; Vagenas, D.; Woodward, N.E. Exercise therapies for preventing or treating aromatase inhibitor-induced musculoskeletal symptoms in early breast cancer. *Cochrane Database Syst. Rev.* **2020**, *1*, CD012988. [CrossRef] [PubMed]
86. Cuthbert, C.; Twomey, R.; Bansal, M.; Rana, B.; Dhruva, T.; Livingston, V.; Daun, J.T.; Culos-Reed, S.N. The role of exercise for pain management in adults living with and beyond cancer: A systematic review and meta-analysis. *Support Care Cancer* **2023**, *31*, 254. [CrossRef] [PubMed]
87. Nijs, J.; Wijma, A.J.; Leysen, L.; Pas, R.; Willaert, W.; Hoelen, W.; Ickmans, K.; Van Wilgen, C.P. Explaining pain following cancer: A practical guide for clinicians. *Braz. J. Phys. Ther.* **2019**, *23*, 367–377. [CrossRef]
88. Manfuku, M.; Nishigami, T.; Mibu, A.; Yamashita, H.; Imai, R.; Tanaka, K.; Kitagaki, K.; Hiroe, K.; Sumiyoshi, K. Effect of perioperative pain neuroscience education in patients with post-mastectomy persistent pain: A retrospective, propensity score-matched study. *Support Care Cancer* **2021**, *29*, 5351–5359. [CrossRef] [PubMed]
89. De Groef, A.; Evenepoel, M.; Van Dijck, S.; Dams, L.; Haenen, V.; Wiles, L.; Catley, M.; Vogelzang, A.; Olver, I.; Hibbert, P.; et al. Feasibility and pilot testing of a personalized eHealth intervention for pain science education and self-management for breast cancer survivors with persistent pain: A mixed-method study. *Support Care Cancer* **2023**, *31*, 119. [CrossRef]

0. Dams, L.; Van der Gucht, E.; Devoogdt, N.; Smeets, A.; Bernar, K.; Morlion, B.; Godderis, L.; Haenen, V.; De Vrieze, T.; Fieuws, S.; et al. Effect of pain neuroscience education after breast cancer surgery on pain-, physical-, and emotional functioning: A double-blinded randomized controlled trial (EduCan trial). *Pain* **2022**, *164*, 1489–1501. [CrossRef]

1. Siddall, B.; Ram, A.; Jones, M.D.; Booth, J.; Perriman, D.; Summers, S.J. Short-term impact of combining pain neuroscience education with exercise for chronic musculoskeletal pain: A systematic review and meta-analysis. *Pain* **2022**, *163*, e20–e30. [CrossRef]

2. Oldenmenger, W.H.; Geerling, J.I.; Mostovaya, I.; Vissers, K.C.P.; De Graeff, A.; Reyners, A.K.L.; Van der Linden, Y.M. A systematic review of the effectiveness of patient-based educational interventions to improve cancer-related pain. *Cancer Treat. Rev.* **2018**, *63*, 96–103. [CrossRef]

3. Qaseem, A.; Kansagara, D.; Forciea, M.A.; Cooke, M.; Denberg, T.D. Management of Chronic Insomnia Disorder in Adults: A Clinical Practice Guideline From the American College of Physicians. *Ann. Intern. Med.* **2016**, *165*, 125–133. [CrossRef] [PubMed]

4. Johnson, J.A.; Rash, J.A.; Campbell, T.S.; Savard, J.; Gehrman, P.R.; Perlis, M.; Carlson, L.E.; Garland, S.N. A systematic review and meta-analysis of randomized controlled trials of cognitive behavior therapy for insomnia (CBT-I) in cancer survivors. *Sleep Med. Rev.* **2016**, *27*, 20–28. [CrossRef] [PubMed]

5. Tang, M.; Liu, X.; Wu, Q.; Shi, Y. The Effects of Cognitive-Behavioral Stress Management for Breast Cancer Patients: A Systematic Review and Meta-analysis of Randomized Controlled Trials. *Cancer Nurs.* **2020**, *43*, 222–237. [CrossRef] [PubMed]

6. Danhauer, S.C.; Addington, E.L.; Cohen, L.; Sohl, S.J.; Van Puymbroeck, M.; Albinati, N.K.; Culos-Reed, S.N. Yoga for symptom management in oncology: A review of the evidence base and future directions for research. *Cancer* **2019**, *125*, 1979–1989. [CrossRef]

7. Matchim, Y.; Armer, J.M.; Stewart, B.R. Mindfulness-based stress reduction among breast cancer survivors: A literature review and discussion. *Oncol. Nurs. Forum.* **2011**, *38*, E61–E71. [CrossRef]

8. Chang, Y.C.; Yeh, T.L.; Chang, Y.M.; Hu, W.Y. Short-term Effects of Randomized Mindfulness-Based Intervention in Female Breast Cancer Survivors: A Systematic Review and Meta-analysis. *Cancer Nurs.* **2021**, *44*, E703–E714. [CrossRef]

9. Tsimberidou, A.M.; Fountzilas, E.; Nikanjam, M.; Kurzrock, R. Review of precision cancer medicine: Evolution of the treatment paradigm. *Cancer Treat. Rev.* **2020**, *86*, 102019. [CrossRef]

100. Malfliet, A.; Kregel, J.; Meeus, M.; Danneels, L.; Cagnie, B.; Roussel, N.; Nijs, J. Patients With Chronic Spinal Pain Benefit From Pain Neuroscience Education Regardless the Self-Reported Signs of Central Sensitization: Secondary Analysis of a Randomized Controlled Multicenter Trial. *Phys. Med. Rehabil.* **2018**, *10*, 1330–1343. [CrossRef]

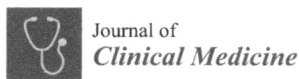

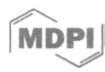

Review

Towards a Real-Life Understanding of the Altered Functional Behaviour of the Default Mode and Salience Network in Chronic Pain: Are People with Chronic Pain Overthinking the Meaning of Their Pain?

Elin Johansson [1,2,3], Huan-Yu Xiong [1], Andrea Polli [1,3,4], Iris Coppieters [1,2,5] and Jo Nijs [1,6,7,*]

[1] Pain in Motion Research Group (PAIN), Department of Physiotherapy, Human Physiology and Anatomy, Faculty of Physical Education and Physiotherapy, Vrije Universiteit Brussel, 1090 Brussels, Belgium; elin.johansson@vub.be (E.J.); huanyu.xiong@vub.be (H.-Y.X.); andrea.polli@vub.be (A.P.); iris.coppieters@vub.be (I.C.)
[2] Laboratory for Brain-Gut Axis Studies (LaBGAS), Translational Research in Gastrointestinal Disorders (TARGID), Department of Chronic Diseases and Metabolism (CHROMETA), Katholieke Universiteit Leuven, 3000 Leuven, Belgium
[3] Flanders Research Foundation-FWO, 1000 Brussels, Belgium
[4] Department of Public Health and Primary Care, Centre for Environment and Health, Katholieke Universiteit Leuven, 3000 Leuven, Belgium
[5] The Experimental Health Psychology Research Group, Faculty of Psychology and Neuroscience, Maastricht University, 6200 Maastricht, The Netherlands
[6] Chronic Pain Rehabilitation, Department of Physical Medicine and Physiotherapy, University Hospital Brussels, 1090 Brussel, Belgium
[7] Department of Health and Rehabilitation, Unit of Physiotherapy, Institute of Neuroscience and Physiology, Sahlgrenska Academy, University of Gothenburg, 405 30 Gothenburg, Sweden
* Correspondence: jo.nijs@vub.be

Citation: Johansson, E.; Xiong, H.-Y.; Polli, A.; Coppieters, I.; Nijs, J. Towards a Real-Life Understanding of the Altered Functional Behaviour of the Default Mode and Salience Network in Chronic Pain: Are People with Chronic Pain Overthinking the Meaning of Their Pain? *J. Clin. Med.* 2024, *13*, 1645. https://doi.org/10.3390/jcm13061645

Academic Editor: Markus W. Hollmann

Received: 5 February 2024
Revised: 10 March 2024
Accepted: 12 March 2024
Published: 13 March 2024

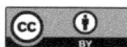

Abstract: Chronic pain is a source of substantial physical and psychological suffering, yet a clear understanding of the pathogenesis of chronic pain is lacking. Repeated studies have reported an altered behaviour of the salience network (SN) and default mode network (DMN) in people with chronic pain, and a majority of these studies report an altered behaviour of the dorsal ventromedial prefrontal cortex (vmPFC) within the anterior DMN. In this topical review, we therefore focus specifically on the role of the dorsal vmPFC in chronic pain to provide an updated perspective on the cortical mechanisms of chronic pain. We suggest that increased activity in the dorsal vmPFC may reflect maladaptive overthinking about the meaning of pain for oneself and one's actions. We also suggest that such overthinking, if negative, may increase the personal "threat" of a given context, as possibly reflected by increased activity in, and functional connectivity to, the anterior insular cortex within the SN.

Keywords: chronic pain; default mode network; salience network; ventromedial prefrontal cortex

1. Introduction

Acute pain plays an important role in warning us of actual or impending tissue harm [1]. However, when pain persists beyond the natural course of healing, it tends to lose many of its otherwise protective features, rather becoming a source of both physical and psychological suffering [2]. Many studies have tried to improve our understanding of chronic pain by exploring it from the perspective of the brain [3], and much progress has been made in the last decade concerning the understanding of how specific patterns of brain activity influence the pain experience [4]. One area of interest has been to interpret chronic pain through established, functional resting-state networks, with the salience network (SN) and default mode network (DMN) having gained much of the spotlight in previous chronic pain models [5–10]. The SN is centred around the anterior insular cortex (AIC) and the dorsal anterior cingulate cortex (ACC; Figure 1). It activates in response to personal salience [11,12] of both positive and negative valence [13–16]; that is, events that "stand out" in the personal environment [17], including acute pain [18,19], but it is also engaged during autonomic [20,21] and emotional regulation [14,22–24]. Furthermore, both the AIC and dorsal ACC are also included in the ventral attention network [25], which together with the dorsal attention network controls attentional relocation [26,27]. In contrast, the DMN was first discovered as a network of regions showing high metabolic activity during rest, whereby it became recognized as a network representative of the brain's "default state" [28]. Today, activation of the DMN is known to reflect complex mentation processes [29,30], such as autobiographical memory retrieval and prospection [31–33], as well as self-generated spontaneous thought [34–36]. Its core regions include the posterior cingulate cortex extending to the precuneus, and the dorsal aspect of the ventromedial prefrontal cortex (vmPFC), with especially prominent intrinsic connectivity to the more posterior aspect of the dorsal vmPFC in and around the pregenual ACC (pgACC; Figure 1) [37], and in contrast to the SN, these regions normally exhibit significant deactivation in response to acute pain [19].

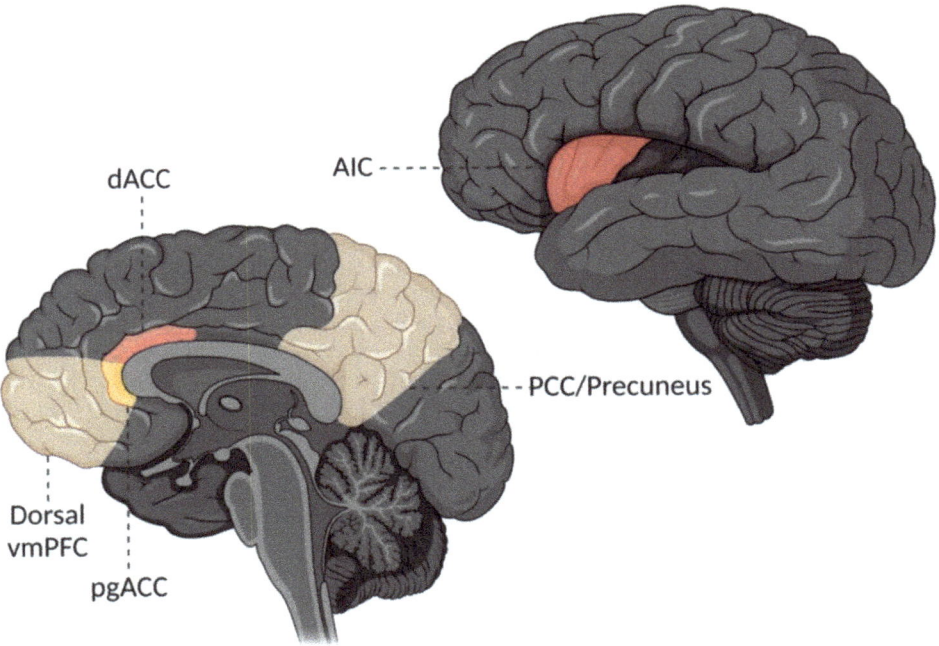

Figure 1. Core regions of the default mode network (orange) and salience network (pink). vmPFC = ventromedial prefrontal cortex; pgACC = pregenual anterior cingulate cortex; dACC = dorsal anterior cingulate cortex; PCC = posterior cingulate cortex; AIC = anterior insular cortex.

In people with chronic pain, meta-analyses have found no difference in acute experimental (stimulus-induced) pain-evoked DMN activity when compared to healthy, pain-free individuals, whereas inconsistent results have been reported for the SN [38–40]. However, many studies show increased functional connectivity between the AIC and the dorsal vmPFC [41–48], as well as altered functional connectivity between the dorsal vmPFC and the posterior DMN [41,44–46,49,50], in people with chronic pain when they experience spontaneous pain (i.e., pain experienced in the absence of external stimuli). Spontaneous pain has also been associated with altered oscillatory power frequencies within the dorsal vmPFC itself in people with chronic pain [41,42,50,51], and reduced deactivation of the dorsal vmPFC has been reported during both simple visuo-motor tasks [52–54] and attention-demanding cognitive tasks [55,56] in people with chronic pain when compared to healthy controls. We recently proposed a model in which we try to explain these functional changes in terms of an aberrant appraisal of threat in people with chronic pain [10]. We also highlight the possible importance of the vmPFC because of its frequent involvement in these changes. In this topical review, we therefore take a more regional standpoint, with a specific focus on altered activity in the dorsal vmPFC, as well as the altered functional connectivity between the dorsal vmPFC and the AIC observed in people with chronic pain. We aim to provide an updated model for what these cortical changes may represent, thereby hoping to extend the current perspective of the cortical mechanisms of chronic pain.

2. Possible Causes of Altered Dorsal Ventromedial Prefrontal Cortex Behaviour in People with Chronic Pain

2.1. Pain Versus No Pain during Scanning

There is an ongoing discussion about whether the observed differences in dorsal vmPFC activity and functional connectivity between people with chronic pain and healthy, pain-free individuals simply reflect the presence of pain itself [10,48,50]. Critically, blunted differences in functional connectivity between people with chronic pain and healthy controls have been observed when the presence of pain is experimentally controlled [48,50], and, in some studies, altered resting-state functional connectivity is only evident following pain exacerbation [45–47]. Furthermore, similar functional connectivity alterations to those observed in people with chronic pain, when they experience spontaneous pain in a resting state, have been observed in healthy individuals exposed to tonic experimental pain [50,57,58]. Although still to be confirmed, these results suggest that the altered behaviour of the dorsal vmPFC observed in people with chronic pain might be dependent on the presence of pain during scanning.

2.2. Inter-Individual Differences in Pain Processing

Most healthy, pain-free individuals display decreasing activity in the dorsal vmPFC during experimental pain [59], with the level of deactivation mediating subjective pain intensity [60]. However, a large-scale study of just over 400 healthy participants recently found that a substantial proportion (~36%) exhibits increased pain-evoked activity in the dorsal vmPFC in response to experimental, stimulus-induced pain [59]. Similarly, Mayr et al. recently showed that the same inter-individual variability in dorsal vmPFC activity, as well as functional connectivity, was present in people with chronic low back pain and migraine when they continuously rated their fluctuations in spontaneous pain intensity [61,62]. This may imply that an altered functional behaviour of the dorsal vmPFC may not reflect the state of chronic pain per se, but possibly inter-individual differences in pain processing. For instance, independent research showed that increased functional connectivity between the dorsal vmPFC and the nucleus accumbens predicted the transition from subacute to chronic low back pain [52,63,64], suggesting that the behaviour of the dorsal vmPFC may already at an early stage of pain increase the susceptibility of developing chronic symptoms in some individuals. Alternatively, the transition from (sub)acute to chronic pain may in itself be associated with increasing activity in the dorsal vmPFC [52]. The latter observation was reported in an early longitudinal study of people who transitioned from subacute to chronic low back pain [52]. However, as this study has not been replicated, the support for a shift in dorsal vmPFC activity during the transition to chronic pain is limited.

3. Revisiting Previous Models of Altered Dorsal Ventromedial Prefrontal Cortex Behaviour in People with Chronic Pain

In the following sections, we discuss the strengths and limitations of our own, as well as some of the most well-cited previous models which try to explain the altered dorsal vmPFC activity and functional connectivity in people with chronic pain. For more in-depth reading, we refer the reader to earlier publications specifically dedicated to each model [5–10].

3.1. Increased Emotional Processing of Pain

An early, well-recognized explanatory model for the altered behaviour of the dorsal vmPFC in people with chronic pain suggested a shift from mainly somatosensory, to mainly emotional cortical processing of pain [6,7]. One of the main functional domains of the dorsal vmPFC is indeed the regulation of emotion and affect [14,22–24,65,66]. Accordingly, human lesions to the vmPFC are associated with both apathy and blunted affect, as well as a lack of empathy [67]. Many of the cortical regions engaged during the experience of pain are also engaged during the expression of emotion [68], and experimentally induced negative emotion has been found to increase spinal reflexes (an index of spinal nociception) via increased activation of both the dorsal and ventral aspect of the vmPFC [69]. However, despite the established role of the dorsal vmPFC in emotional and affective regulation, its complete functional spectrum is highly multidimensional and also includes domains such as valence and reward processing [13,15,16,65,70,71], decision-making [65,72–75], memory retrieval and prospection [65,73], and self-referential processing [76–78]. Accordingly, in addition to emotional dysregulation, individuals with vmPFC lesions also exhibit behavioural changes characterized by increased impulsivity and irresponsibility [67], as well as an impaired or blunted ability to adapt their behaviour to previous experiences and environmental cues [67,79], including in contexts of pain [80]. Hence, increased emotional processing of pain may serve as a partial explanation for the altered behaviour of the dorsal vmPFC, but does it provide the complete explanation?

3.2. Aberrant Appraisal of Threat in the Context of Pain

The experience of pain is, by definition, "associated with, or resembling that associated with, potential tissue damage" [81]. Given the wide spectrum of functions of the dorsal vmPFC, another track of conceptual thought expressed across multiple models [8–10] has therefore been that chronic pain might resemble a more general misperception of pain and its contextual environment as potentially "dangerous", even when the reality is "safe". Similar to experimental pain, the experience of experimentally induced fear evokes similar deactivation of the dorsal vmPFC and activation of the SN [82]. As aforementioned, people with chronic pain are frequently found to show an impaired ability to deactivate the dorsal vmPFC during both simple and complex attention-demanding tasks while experiencing spontaneous pain [52–56]. However, in contrast to the heterogeneous responsiveness of the dorsal vmPFC observed in the context of pain outlined in previous sections, fear and threat learning are consistently associated with distinct deactivation of the dorsal vmPFC [83–86], whereas increased activation of this area is observed during fear and threat extinction [83,86–88]. Furthermore, although recent studies suggest that the vmPFC may not solely constitute a "safety hub" [79,89], such opposing activity responses are concentrated to the more ventral/posterior aspects of the vmPFC [89]. Accordingly, inactivation of the cortical equivalent to the dorsal vmPFC in non-human primates (i.e., area 32) increased behavioural fear responses during fear learning, while impairing fear extinction, whereas the opposite pattern was observed for inactivation of the more ventral/posterior aspect of the vmPFC (i.e., area 25) [90]. Thus, although it is tempting to suggest that chronic pain might be accompanied by a shift in the threat/safety profile of the dorsal vmPFC, is this plausible?

3.3. Increased Internal Attention to Pain

A third explanatory model for the altered behaviour of the dorsal vmPFC in people with chronic pain was presented by Kucyi and Davis, who suggested that it reflected increased internal attention to pain, which might disrupt the top-down endogenous pain modulatory pathway [5]. Specifically, Kucyi and Davis performed a series of experiments [91,92] in which they first observed that healthy individuals exposed to experimental, stimulus-induced pain exhibited an increased activation of the dorsal vmPFC, as well as an increased functional connectivity between the dorsal vmPFC and the periaqueductal gray (PAG) when they spontaneously attended away from pain (i.e., spontaneous non-pain-related mind wandering). Conversely, individuals who spontaneously directed their attention to the experimental pain exhibited reduced dorsal vmPFC activation, as well as an expected increased activation of the ventral attention network, including the core regions of the SN [92]. During a second experiment in people with chronic temporomandibular pain, an increased resting-state functional connectivity between the dorsal vmPFC and PAG was associated with pain rumination, as well as an increased functional connectivity between the dorsal vmPFC and the posterior cingulate cortex/precuneus [91]. Given the established role of the PAG in top-down endogenous pain modulation [93,94], the authors suggested that people with chronic pain who exhibit an altered functional behaviour of the dorsal vmPFC might be more likely to spontaneously ruminate about pain, which in turn may disrupt the communication between the dorsal vmPFC and the anti-nociceptive system [5]. However, given the results observed in the healthy participants [92], increased attention to pain would be expected to reduce the activity in the dorsal vmPFC, as well as the remaining regions of the DMN, possibly explaining the increased functional connectivity between the dorsal vmPFC and the posterior cingulate cortex/precuneus observed in the people with chronic temporomandibular pain [91]. In other words, it is contradictory to the increased activity in the dorsal vmPFC that is frequently reported in people with chronic pain during spontaneous pain [52–56].

4. An Updated Perspective on the Meaning of Altered Dorsal Ventromedial Prefrontal Cortex Behaviour in People with Chronic Pain

4.1. Shared Mechanisms with Placebo Analgesia

Recent findings suggest that a similar response heterogeneity of the dorsal vmPFC as that observed during acute experimental (i.e., stimulus-induced) [59] and chronic spontaneous pain [61] can also present during certain types of endogenous pain modulation. Contradictory to what might be expected given the frequently reported increased activity in the dorsal vmPFC in people with chronic pain [52–56], the vast majority of endogenous pain modulation trials in which healthy individuals exhibit increased activity in the dorsal vmPFC also report an associated reduction in subjective pain intensity and/or unpleasantness. This includes, for instance, relative pain relief (i.e., the pain relief experienced when a moderate-intensity stimulus is presented following a stimulus of high intensity) [95,96], positive reappraisal of pain [97,98], distraction analgesia [99,100], and when pain intensity is expected to be low [101,102] or reduced [103,104]. Increased activity in the dorsal vmPFC has also been found to encode pain-specific, positive reinforcement learning [105,106], and there is even an increased pain-evoked activation of the dorsal vmPFC if a painful stimulus has been accepted on behalf of one's romantic partner [107].

There are, however, critical exceptions to this trend [102,108–113], with one of the main examples being the recent results of Zunhammer et al. concerning placebo analgesia [114]. In accordance with the common trend, early meta-analyses of placebo analgesia report increased pain-evoked activity in the dorsal vmPFC [103,104]. Yet, there are also well-designed studies which report the inverse pattern; that is, reduced activity associated with a greater placebo effect [109,110]. As recently raised by Zunhammer and colleagues, a major limitation of earlier meta-analyses is their reliance on published activation peaks rather than full activation maps, as this inherently increases the risk of biased results [115]. To get around this problem, the authors performed a meta-analysis of single-participant, whole-brain images across 20 independent studies, by which they intriguingly identified a great between-study heterogeneity in the response of the dorsal vmPFC [114]. This implies that a similar response heterogeneity of the dorsal vmPFC as that observed during acute experimental [59] and chronic spontaneous pain [61] is also present during placebo analgesia.

4.2. The Possible Role of the Pregenual Anterior Cingulate Cortex and Independence of Afferent Nociception

Importantly, placebo analgesia typically engages the pgACC subregion of the dorsal vmPFC [103,104], which not only resembles an important functional hub within both the DMN [37], but which also exhibits strong functional connections to the PAG [116]. Critically, the pgACC also resembles one of the areas most frequently reported to exhibit altered activity and/or functional connectivity in people with chronic pain [44,45,47,51,53–56,61,117]. Activity in the pgACC (among other regions) has been found to predict the experience of experimental pain independent of stimulus intensity [118], and data from patients with lesions to the vmPFC, including the pgACC, showed no difference in neither thermal pain threshold nor tolerance compared to healthy controls [80]. Thus, although nociceptive transmission is often facilitated in people with chronic pain via sensitization of peripheral and/or central nociceptive neurons [119–121], such afferent nociceptive mechanisms may not explain the altered functional behaviour of the pgACC in people with chronic pain.

Conversely, experimental pain-evoked activation of the pgACC has been more closely related to the expected value of pain rather than the factual stimulus-evoked pain experience itself [101–103,105,106,110,122]. Expectations are well-known to be able to shape the experience of pain [123], as well as other sensory perceptions [124], and expectations resemble one of the most well-established contributors to the placebo analgesic effect [123,125–127]. However, recent results by Atlas et al. showed that expectations of pain intensity were associated with different pain-evoked activity responses in the pgACC depending on how the cue that caused the expectations had been learned [102]. If the meaning of an auditory cue preceding a painful stimulus had been learned via uninstructed learning (i.e., learning by experience), expectations of high pain were associated with a significant pain-evoked deactivation of the pgACC. In contrast, if the meaning of the cues had been learned through explicit verbal instructions, expectations of high pain were rather associated with increased pain-evoked activation of the pgACC [102]. These results suggest that the altered behaviour of the pgACC observed in people with chronic pain may not be related to the expectations of pain per se. Yet, as instructed learning is a conscious way of learning [123], pgACC hyperactivity in people with chronic pain may reflect a conscious mentation process that covaries with expectations of pain.

4.3. Overthinking about the Meaning of Pain for Oneself and One's Actions

Recently, Zhang and colleagues suggested that activity within the pgACC may encode the level of uncertainty related to pain [128]. The authors exposed healthy individuals to a tonic painful heat stimulus, during which they had to learn, via trial and error, which out of two buttons was associated with a short period of pain relief. Interestingly, the higher the uncertainty about which button to press, the higher the activity in the pgACC [128]. However, other studies found no involvement of the pgACC during uncertainty when there was no motor task performed [129–131], which suggests that the uncertainty component observed by the group of Zhang and colleagues most likely does not reflect uncertainty as to whether the tonic pain would be relieved or not, but to which choice to make to achieve pain relief. Similarly, a series of rigorous studies by Kolling et al. outside the context of pain have shown that the pgACC is activated during decision making but does not encode factual decision value [73,132]. In contrast, pgACC activity was suggested to reflect prospective consequential thinking, irrespective of the factual value of the participant's final decision [73]. Together with the results by Zhang et al. [128], these findings suggest that activity in the pgACC might reflect the conscious weighing of the potential future consequences of one's behavioural choices. However, repeated meta-analyses have found that the pgACC also increases in activity when individuals are actively reflecting or making judgements related to the self in general [76–78]. Altogether, this may imply that individuals with chronic pain who exhibit increased pain-evoked activity in the pgACC may be more likely to reflect on what their pain means for them and their actions (Figure 2). If negative, overthinking of such character may, at least in part, explain some of the common psychosocial characteristics of many people with chronic pain, such as trouble falling asleep and/or maintaining sleep, emotional distress (e.g., anxiety, depression), and/or avoidant behaviours (e.g., physical inactivity, social isolation) [2].

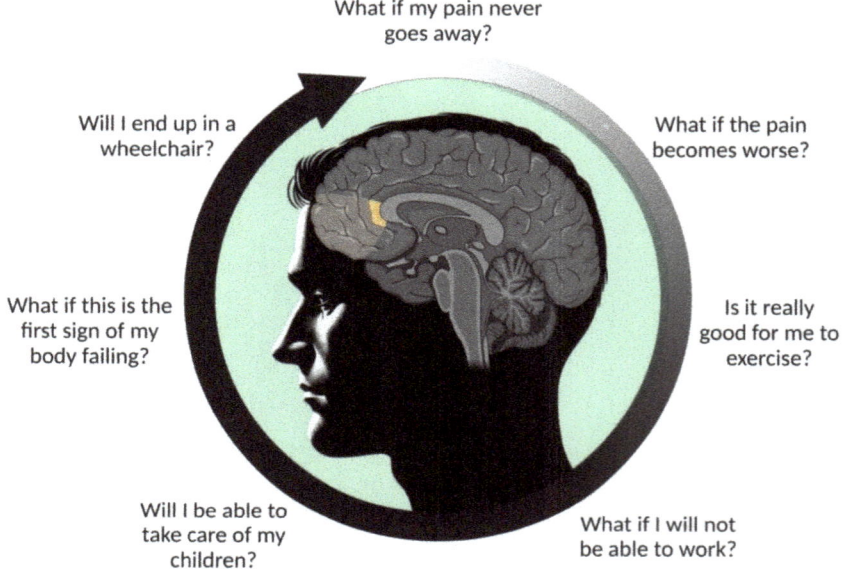

Figure 2. Examples of thoughts in people with chronic pain that might be associated with activation of the pregenual anterior cingulate cortex (bright orange) within the dorsal ventromedial prefrontal cortex (transparent orange).

5. Anterior Insula Hyper-Connectivity to the Dorsal Ventromedial Prefrontal Cortex

No brain region works in isolation, and as mentioned in the introduction, one of the most frequently reported functional connectivity deviations in people with chronic pain is an increased functional connectivity between the dorsal vmPFC and the AIC [41–48]. In addition to its consistent activation in response to salience, the AIC has also been recognized as a region critical for interoception [11,12,133,134]; that is, the cortical processes underlying our ability to feel internal signals arising within our own body (e.g., nociception) [133,134]. In accordance, increasing AIC activity has been found to track increases in spontaneous pain intensity in people with chronic pain [53,61] and to predict subjective experimental pain intensity in healthy individuals [60,135]. Furthermore, activation of the AIC was recently found to mediate the relationship between actual stimulus intensity and subjective pain intensity [60].

However, similar to the dorsal vmPFC, activation of the AIC can also be modulated independent of stimulus intensity. For example, pain-evoked AIC activity was increased when contextual circumstances induced an increased subjective pain intensity or unpleasantness, such as when expectations of high or reduced pain were inferred [101–103,122,136], when a painful stimulus of moderate intensity was presented following a low-intensity stimulus [95], or when participants engaged in cognitive downregulation of pain [97]. Furthermore, AIC activity can also increase during the anticipation of pain [137], and if a given stimulus is more painful than expected, activation of the AIC has been found to increase further both during and anticipatory to the subsequent stimulus [105,106]. These observations suggest that activity in the AIC might be related to the perceived intensity of pain. However, given the prominent effect of contextual modulation on the level of AIC activity, this relationship may not rely solely on afferent nociception. In the context of pain,

AIC activity may thus possibly reflect a more general type of pain-related processing, such as the level of personal "threat" of a given context [9,10].

If our previously suggested role of the pgACC in (chronic) pain processing holds true, increased functional connectivity between the pgACC and AIC, as often observed in people with chronic pain [41–48], may thus possibly reflect a process by which negative overthinking about the meaning of pain for oneself and one's actions might increase the personal "threat" of a given context. This may in turn increase the likelihood of "harmless" afferent signals from the body to be interpreted as "potentially harmful", thereby increasing the susceptibility of experiencing pain in the absence of ongoing tissue damage (Figure 3).

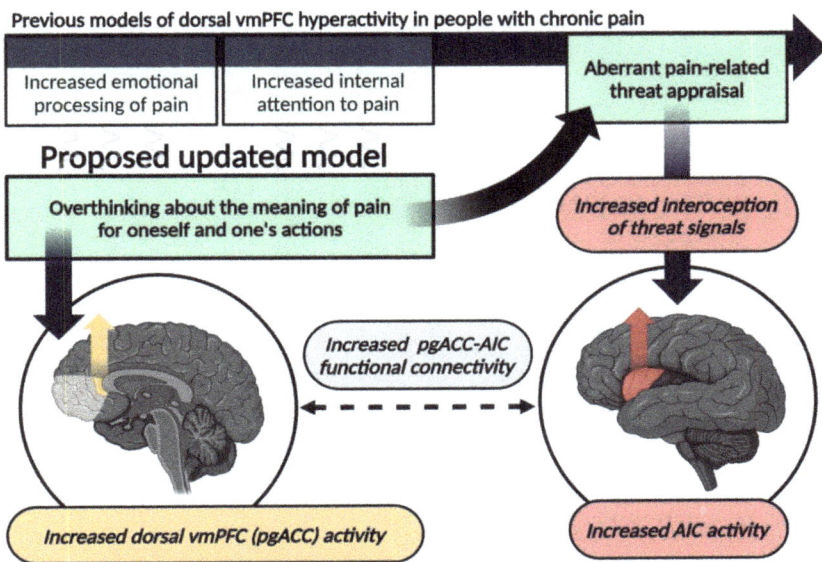

Figure 3. A proposed updated model for the meaning of the altered behaviour of the pregenual anterior cingulate cortex (pgACC), within the dorsal ventromedial prefrontal cortex (vmPFC), in people with chronic pain. Overthinking about the meaning of pain is suggested to be associated with increased activation of the pgACC within the dorsal vmPFC. This cognitive behaviour may subsequently lead to an aberrant appraisal of threat in the context of pain via increased interoception of threat signals (e.g., nociception) processed in the anterior insular cortex (AIC). The simultaneous increased activation in the pgACC and AIC may present as an increased functional connectivity between the two cortical regions.

6. Conclusions

In the present review, we discuss the altered functional behaviour within DMN and SN in people with chronic pain, with a special focus on the dorsal vmPFC and its functional connections to the AIC. By integrating previous theoretical models with novel research findings, we suggest an updated model of what both the altered activity in and functional connectivity to the dorsal vmPFC may represent in people with chronic pain. We suggest that increased dorsal vmPFC activity may reflect a tendency to overthink the meaning of pain for oneself and one's actions. This may in turn increase the personal threat of a given context and thereby increase the susceptibility to experience pain, which we suggest might be reflected by an increased functional connectivity between the dorsal vmPFC and the AIC.

Author Contributions: Conceptualization, J.N. and E.J.; methodology, E.J.; writing—original draft preparation, E.J.; writing—review and editing, E.J., H.-Y.X., A.P., I.C. and J.N.; visualization, E.J.; supervision, J.N. and I.C.; All authors have read and agreed to the published version of the manuscript.

Funding: This research was funded by Research Foundation—Flanders (FWO), which provides a PhD fellowship to Elin Johansson [Grant number: FWOTM1187] and a post-doctoral fellowship to Andrea Polli [Grant number: FWOTM1051].

Institutional Review Board Statement: Not applicable.

Informed Consent Statement: Not applicable.

Data Availability Statement: Not applicable.

Conflicts of Interest: Jo Nijs and the Vrije Universiteit Brussel received lecturing/teaching fees from various professional associations and educational organizations.

References

1. Tracey, I. Why pain hurts. *Trends Cogn. Sci.* **2022**, *26*, 1070–1072. [CrossRef]
2. Cohen, S.P.; Vase, L.; Hooten, W.M. Chronic pain: An update on burden, best practices, and new advances. *Lancet* **2021**, *397*, 2082–2097. [CrossRef]
3. Reddan, M.C.; Wager, T.D. Brain systems at the intersection of chronic pain and self-regulation. *Neurosci. Lett.* **2019**, *702*, 24–33. [CrossRef]
4. van der Miesen, M.M.; Lindquist, M.A.; Wager, T.D. Neuroimaging-based biomarkers for pain: State of the field and current directions. *Pain Rep.* **2019**, *4*, e751. [CrossRef]
5. Kucyi, A.; Davis, K.D. The dynamic pain connectome. *Trends Neurosci.* **2015**, *38*, 86–95. [CrossRef]
6. Apkarian, V.A.; Hashmi, J.A.; Baliki, M.N. Pain and the brain: Specificity and plasticity of the brain in clinical chronic pain. *Pain* **2011**, *152* (Suppl. S3), S49–S64. [CrossRef] [PubMed]
7. Baliki, M.N.; Apkarian, A.V. Nociception, Pain, Negative Moods, and Behavior Selection. *Neuron* **2015**, *87*, 474–491. [CrossRef] [PubMed]
8. Koban, L.; Gianaros, P.J.; Kober, H.; Wager, T.D. The self in context: Brain systems linking mental and physical health. *Nat. Rev. Neurosci.* **2021**, *22*, 309–322. [CrossRef] [PubMed]
9. Pinto, A.M.; Geenen, R.; Wager, T.D.; Lumley, M.A.; Hauser, W.; Kosek, E.; Ablin, J.N.; Amris, K.; Branco, J.; Buskila, D.; et al. Emotion regulation and the salience network: A hypothetical integrative model of fibromyalgia. *Nat. Rev. Rheumatol.* **2023**, *19*, 44–60. [CrossRef] [PubMed]
10. Johansson, E.; Coppieters, I.; Nijs, J. The default mode of chronic pain: What does it mean and how should we frame it to our patients? *J. Spine Pract.* **2023**, *2*, 32–42. [CrossRef]
11. Seeley, W.W. The Salience Network: A Neural System for Perceiving and Responding to Homeostatic Demands. *J. Neurosci.* **2019**, *39*, 9878–9882. [CrossRef]
12. Seeley, W.W.; Menon, V.; Schatzberg, A.F.; Keller, J.; Glover, G.H.; Kenna, H.; Reiss, A.L.; Greicius, M.D. Dissociable intrinsic connectivity networks for salience processing and executive control. *J. Neurosci.* **2007**, *27*, 2349–2356. [CrossRef] [PubMed]
13. Bartra, O.; McGuire, J.T.; Kable, J.W. The valuation system: A coordinate-based meta-analysis of BOLD fMRI experiments examining neural correlates of subjective value. *Neuroimage* **2013**, *76*, 412–427. [CrossRef]
14. Lindquist, K.A.; Satpute, A.B.; Wager, T.D.; Weber, J.; Barrett, L.F. The Brain Basis of Positive and Negative Affect: Evidence from a Meta-Analysis of the Human Neuroimaging Literature. *Cereb. Cortex* **2016**, *26*, 1910–1922. [CrossRef] [PubMed]
15. Fouragnan, E.; Retzler, C.; Philiastides, M.G. Separate neural representations of prediction error valence and surprise: Evidence from an fMRI meta-analysis. *Hum. Brain Mapp.* **2018**, *39*, 2887–2906. [CrossRef]
16. Lee, S.A.; Jae-Joong, L.; Han, J.; Choi, M.; Wager, T.D.; Woo, C.W. Brain representations of affective valence and intensity of in sustained pleasure and pain. *bioRxiv* 2023. [CrossRef]
17. Uddin, L.Q. Salience processing and insular cortical function and dysfunction. *Nat. Rev. Neurosci.* **2015**, *16*, 55–61. [CrossRef]
18. Eccleston, C.; Crombez, G. Pain demands attention: A cognitive-affective model of the interruptive function of pain. *Psychol. Bull.* **1999**, *125*, 356–366. [CrossRef]
19. Wager, T.D.; Atlas, L.Y.; Lindquist, M.A.; Roy, M.; Woo, C.W.; Kross, E. An fMRI-based neurologic signature of physical pain. *N. Engl. J. Med.* **2013**, *368*, 1388–1397. [CrossRef]
20. Beissner, F.; Meissner, K.; Bar, K.J.; Napadow, V. The autonomic brain: An activation likelihood estimation meta-analysis for central processing of autonomic function. *J. Neurosci.* **2013**, *33*, 10503–10511. [CrossRef] [PubMed]
21. Ferraro, S.; Klugah-Brown, B.; Tench, C.R.; Bazinet, V.; Bore, M.C.; Nigri, A.; Demichelis, G.; Bruzzone, M.G.; Palermo, S.; Zhao, W.; et al. The central autonomic system revisited—Convergent evidence for a regulatory role of the insular and midcingulate cortex from neuroimaging meta-analyses. *Neurosci. Biobehav. Rev.* **2022**, *142*, 104915. [CrossRef] [PubMed]
22. Kragel, P.A.; LaBar, K.S. Multivariate neural biomarkers of emotional states are categorically distinct. *Soc. Cogn. Affect. Neurosci.* **2015**, *10*, 1437–1448. [CrossRef] [PubMed]

3. Wager, T.D.; Kang, J.; Johnson, T.D.; Nichols, T.E.; Satpute, A.B.; Barrett, L.F. A Bayesian model of category-specific emotional brain responses. *PLoS Comput. Biol.* **2015**, *11*, e1004066. [CrossRef]
4. Ceko, M.; Kragel, P.A.; Woo, C.W.; Lopez-Sola, M.; Wager, T.D. Common and stimulus-type-specific brain representations of negative affect. *Nat. Neurosci.* **2022**, *25*, 760–770. [CrossRef]
25. Yeo, B.T.; Krienen, F.M.; Sepulcre, J.; Sabuncu, M.R.; Lashkari, D.; Hollinshead, M.; Roffman, J.L.; Smoller, J.W.; Zöllei, L.; Polimeni, J.R.; et al. The organization of the human cerebral cortex estimated by intrinsic functional connectivity. *J. Neurophysiol.* **2011**, *106*, 1125–1165. [PubMed]
26. Corbetta, M.; Patel, G.; Shulman, G.L. The reorienting system of the human brain: From environment to theory of mind. *Neuron* **2008**, *58*, 306–324. [CrossRef]
27. Fox, M.D.; Snyder, A.Z.; Vincent, J.L.; Corbetta, M.; Van Essen, D.C.; Raichle, M.E. The human brain is intrinsically organized into dynamic, anticorrelated functional networks. *Proc. Natl. Acad. Sci. USA* **2005**, *102*, 9673–9678. [CrossRef]
28. Raichle, M.E.; MacLeod, A.M.; Snyder, A.Z.; Powers, W.J.; Gusnard, D.A.; Shulman, G.L. A default mode of brain function. *Proc. Natl. Acad. Sci. USA* **2001**, *98*, 676–682. [CrossRef]
29. Menon, V. 20 years of the default mode network: A review and synthesis. *Neuron* **2023**, *111*, 2469–2487. [CrossRef]
30. Raichle, M.E. The brain's default mode network. *Annu. Rev. Neurosci.* **2015**, *38*, 433–447. [CrossRef]
31. Spreng, R.N.; Mar, R.A.; Kim, A.S. The common neural basis of autobiographical memory, prospection, navigation, theory of mind, and the default mode: A quantitative meta-analysis. *J. Cogn. Neurosci.* **2009**, *21*, 489–510. [CrossRef]
32. Schacter, D.L.; Addis, D.R.; Buckner, R.L. Remembering the past to imagine the future: The prospective brain. *Nat. Rev. Neurosci.* **2007**, *8*, 657–661. [CrossRef]
33. Warren, K.N.; Hermiller, M.S.; Nilakantan, A.S.; O'Neil, J.; Palumbo, R.T.; Voss, J.L. Increased fMRI activity correlations in autobiographical memory versus resting states. *Hum. Brain Mapp.* **2018**, *39*, 4312–4321. [CrossRef]
34. Fox, K.C.; Spreng, R.N.; Ellamil, M.; Andrews-Hanna, J.R.; Christoff, K. The wandering brain: Meta-analysis of functional neuroimaging studies of mind-wandering and related spontaneous thought processes. *Neuroimage* **2015**, *111*, 611–621. [CrossRef]
35. Kucyi, A.; Davis, K.D. Dynamic functional connectivity of the default mode network tracks daydreaming. *Neuroimage* **2014**, *100*, 471–480. [CrossRef] [PubMed]
36. Christoff, K.; Irving, Z.C.; Fox, K.C.; Spreng, R.N.; Andrews-Hanna, J.R. Mind-wandering as spontaneous thought: A dynamic framework. *Nat. Rev. Neurosci.* **2016**, *17*, 718–731. [CrossRef] [PubMed]
37. Andrews-Hanna, J.R.; Reidler, J.S.; Sepulcre, J.; Poulin, R.; Buckner, R.L. Functional-anatomic fractionation of the brain's default network. *Neuron* **2010**, *65*, 550–562. [CrossRef] [PubMed]
38. Ferraro, S.; Klugah-Brown, B.; Tench, C.R.; Yao, S.; Nigri, A.; Demichelis, G.; Pinardi, C.; Bruzzone, M.G.; Becker, B. Dysregulated anterior insula reactivity as robust functional biomarker for chronic pain-Meta-analytic evidence from neuroimaging studies. *Hum. Brain Mapp.* **2022**, *43*, 998–1010. [CrossRef] [PubMed]
39. Jensen, K.B.; Regenbogen, C.; Ohse, M.C.; Frasnelli, J.; Freiherr, J.; Lundstrom, J.N. Brain activations during pain: A neuroimaging meta-analysis of patients with pain and healthy controls. *Pain* **2016**, *157*, 1279–1286. [CrossRef] [PubMed]
40. Xu, A.; Larsen, B.; Henn, A.; Baller, E.B.; Scott, J.C.; Sharma, V.; Adebimpe, A.; Basbaum, A.I.; Corder, G.; Dworkin, R.H. Brain Responses to Noxious Stimuli in Patients With Chronic Pain: A Systematic Review and Meta-analysis. *JAMA Netw. Open* **2021**, *4*, e2032236. [CrossRef]
41. Baliki, M.N.; Mansour, A.R.; Baria, A.T.; Apkarian, A.V. Functional reorganization of the default mode network across chronic pain conditions. *PLoS ONE* **2014**, *9*, e106133. [CrossRef]
42. Baliki, M.N.; Baria, A.T.; Apkarian, A.V. The cortical rhythms of chronic back pain. *J. Neurosci.* **2011**, *31*, 13981–13990. [CrossRef]
43. Napadow, V.; LaCount, L.; Park, K.; As-Sanie, S.; Clauw, D.J.; Harris, R.E. Intrinsic brain connectivity in fibromyalgia is associated with chronic pain intensity. *Arthritis Rheum.* **2010**, *62*, 2545–2555. [CrossRef]
44. Tu, Y.; Jung, M.; Gollub, R.L.; Napadow, V.; Gerber, J.; Ortiz, A.; Lang, C.; Mawla, I.; Shen, W.; Chan, S.-T.; et al. Abnormal medial prefrontal cortex functional connectivity and its association with clinical symptoms in chronic low back pain. *Pain* **2019**, *160*, 1308–1318. [CrossRef]
45. Loggia, M.L.; Kim, J.; Gollub, R.L.; Vangel, M.G.; Kirsch, I.; Kong, J.; Wasan, A.D.; Napadow, V. Default mode network connectivity encodes clinical pain: An arterial spin labeling study. *Pain* **2013**, *154*, 24–33. [CrossRef]
46. Kim, J.; Mawla, I.; Kong, J.; Lee, J.; Gerber, J.; Ortiz, A.; Kim, H.; Chan, S.-T.; Loggia, M.L.; Wasan, A.D.; et al. Somatotopically specific primary somatosensory connectivity to salience and default mode networks encodes clinical pain. *Pain* **2019**, *160*, 1594–1605. [CrossRef]
47. Ichesco, E.; Puiu, T.; Hampson, J.P.; Kairys, A.E.; Clauw, D.J.; Harte, S.E.; Peltier, S.; Harris, R.; Schmidt-Wilcke, T. Altered fMRI resting-state connectivity in individuals with fibromyalgia on acute pain stimulation. *Eur. J. Pain* **2016**, *20*, 1079–1089. [CrossRef]
48. Ceko, M.; Frangos, E.; Gracely, J.; Richards, E.; Wang, B.; Schweinhardt, P.; Bushnell, M.C. Default mode network changes in fibromyalgia patients are largely dependent on current clinical pain. *Neuroimage* **2020**, *216*, 116877. [CrossRef] [PubMed]
49. Bolwerk, A.; Seifert, F.; Maihofner, C. Altered resting-state functional connectivity in complex regional pain syndrome. *J. Pain* **2013**, *14*, 1107–1115.e8. [CrossRef] [PubMed]
50. Alshelh, Z.; Marciszewski, K.K.; Akhter, R.; Di Pietro, F.; Mills, E.P.; Vickers, E.R.; Peck, C.; Murray, G.; Henderson, L. Disruption of default mode network dynamics in acute and chronic pain states. *Neuroimage Clin.* **2018**, *17*, 222–231. [CrossRef] [PubMed]

51. Otti, A.; Guendel, H.; Wohlschlager, A.; Zimmer, C.; Noll-Hussong, M. Frequency shifts in the anterior default mode network and the salience network in chronic pain disorder. *BMC Psychiatry* **2013**, *13*, 84. [CrossRef]
52. Hashmi, J.A.; Baliki, M.N.; Huang, L.; Baria, A.T.; Torbey, S.; Hermann, K.M.; Schnitzer, T.J.; Apkarian, A.V. Shape shifting pain: Chronification of back pain shifts brain representation from nociceptive to emotional circuits. *Brain* **2013**, *136 Pt 9*, 2751–2768. [CrossRef]
53. Baliki, M.N.; Chialvo, D.R.; Geha, P.Y.; Levy, R.M.; Harden, R.N.; Parrish, T.B.; Apkarian, A.V. Chronic pain and the emotional brain: Specific brain activity associated with spontaneous fluctuations of intensity of chronic back pain. *J. Neurosci.* **2006**, *26*, 12165–12173. [CrossRef]
54. Baliki, M.N.; Geha, P.Y.; Apkarian, A.V.; Chialvo, D.R. Beyond feeling: Chronic pain hurts the brain, disrupting the default-mode network dynamics. *J. Neurosci.* **2008**, *28*, 1398–1403. [CrossRef] [PubMed]
55. Ceko, M.; Gracely, J.L.; Fitzcharles, M.A.; Seminowicz, D.A.; Schweinhardt, P.; Bushnell, M.C. Is a Responsive Default Mode Network Required for Successful Working Memory Task Performance? *J. Neurosci.* **2015**, *35*, 11595–11605. [CrossRef]
56. Weissman-Fogel, I.; Moayedi, M.; Tenenbaum, H.C.; Goldberg, M.B.; Freeman, B.V.; Davis, K.D. Abnormal cortical activity in patients with temporomandibular disorder evoked by cognitive and emotional tasks. *Pain* **2011**, *152*, 384–396. [CrossRef] [PubMed]
57. Alhajri, N.; Boudreau, S.A.; Graven-Nielsen, T. Decreased Default Mode Network Connectivity Following 24 Hours of Capsaicin-induced Pain Persists During Immediate Pain Relief and Facilitation. *J. Pain* **2023**, *24*, 796–811. [CrossRef]
58. Makovac, E.; Dipasquale, O.; Jackson, J.B.; Medina, S.; O'Daly, O.; O'Muircheartaigh, J.; Rubio, A.d.L.; Williams, S.C.R.; McMahon, S.B.; Howard, M.A. Sustained perturbation in functional connectivity induced by cold pain. *Eur. J. Pain* **2020**, *24*, 1850–1861. [CrossRef] [PubMed]
59. Kohoutova, L.; Atlas, L.Y.; Buchel, C.; Buhle, J.T.; Geuter, S.; Jepma, M.; Koban, L.; Krishnan, A.; Lee, D.H.; Lee, S.; et al. Individual variability in brain representations of pain. *Nat. Neurosci.* **2022**, *25*, 749–759. [CrossRef]
60. Geuter, S.; Reynolds Losin, E.A.; Roy, M.; Atlas, L.Y.; Schmidt, L.; Krishnan, A.; Koban, L.; Wager, T.D.; Lindquist, M.A. Multiple Brain Networks Mediating Stimulus-Pain Relationships in Humans. *Cereb. Cortex* **2020**, *30*, 4204–4219. [CrossRef]
61. Mayr, A.; Jahn, P.; Stankewitz, A.; Deak, B.; Winkler, A.; Witkovsky, V.; Eren, O.; Straube, A.; Schulz, E. Patients with chronic pain exhibit individually unique cortical signatures of pain encoding. *Hum. Brain Mapp.* **2022**, *43*, 1676–1693. [CrossRef]
62. Mayr, A.; Jahn, P.; Deak, B.; Stankewitz, A.; Devulapally, V.; Witkovsky, V.; Dietrich, O.; Schulz, E. Individually unique dynamics of cortical connectivity reflect the ongoing intensity of chronic pain. *Pain* **2022**, *163*, 1987–1998. [CrossRef]
63. Baliki, M.N.; Petre, B.; Torbey, S.; Herrmann, K.M.; Huang, L.; Schnitzer, T.J.; Fields, H.L.; Apkarian, A.V. Corticostriatal functional connectivity predicts transition to chronic back pain. *Nat. Neurosci.* **2012**, *15*, 1117–1119. [CrossRef] [PubMed]
64. Loffler, M.; Levine, S.M.; Usai, K.; Desch, S.; Kandic, M.; Nees, F.; Flor, H. Corticostriatal circuits in the transition to chronic back pain: The predictive role of reward learning. *Cell Rep. Med.* **2022**, *3*, 100677. [CrossRef] [PubMed]
65. de la Vega, A.; Chang, L.J.; Banich, M.T.; Wager, T.D.; Yarkoni, T. Large-Scale Meta-Analysis of Human Medial Frontal Cortex Reveals Tripartite Functional Organization. *J. Neurosci.* **2016**, *36*, 6553–6562. [CrossRef] [PubMed]
66. Kragel, P.A.; Kano, M.; Van Oudenhove, L.; Ly, H.G.; Dupont, P.; Rubio, A.; Delon-Martin, C.; Bonaz, B.L.; Manuck, S.B.; Gianaros, P.J.; et al. Generalizable representations of pain, cognitive control, and negative emotion in medial frontal cortex. *Nat. Neurosci.* **2018**, *21*, 283–289. [CrossRef] [PubMed]
67. Schneider, B.; Koenigs, M. Human lesion studies of ventromedial prefrontal cortex. *Neuropsychologia* **2017**, *107*, 84–93. [CrossRef] [PubMed]
68. Gilam, G.; Gross, J.J.; Wager, T.D.; Keefe, F.J.; Mackey, S.C. What Is the Relationship between Pain and Emotion? Bridging Constructs and Communities. *Neuron* **2020**, *107*, 17–21. [CrossRef] [PubMed]
69. Roy, M.; Piche, M.; Chen, J.I.; Peretz, I.; Rainville, P. Cerebral and spinal modulation of pain by emotions. *Proc. Natl. Acad. Sci. USA* **2009**, *106*, 20900–20905. [CrossRef]
70. Morelli, S.A.; Sacchet, M.D.; Zaki, J. Common and distinct neural correlates of personal and vicarious reward: A quantitative meta-analysis. *Neuroimage* **2015**, *112*, 244–253. [CrossRef]
71. Smith, D.V.; Hayden, B.Y.; Truong, T.K.; Song, A.W.; Platt, M.L.; Huettel, S.A. Distinct value signals in anterior and posterior ventromedial prefrontal cortex. *J. Neurosci.* **2010**, *30*, 2490–2495. [CrossRef]
72. Koban, L.; Lee, S.; Schelski, D.S.; Simon, M.C.; Lerman, C.; Weber, B.; Kable, J.W.; Plassmann, H. An fMRI-Based Brain Marker of Individual Differences in Delay Discounting. *J. Neurosci.* **2023**, *43*, 1600–1613. [CrossRef] [PubMed]
73. Kolling, N.; Scholl, J.; Chekroud, A.; Trier, H.A.; Rushworth, M.F.S. Prospection, Perseverance, and Insight in Sequential Behavior. *Neuron* **2018**, *99*, 1069–1082.e7. [CrossRef] [PubMed]
74. Kolling, N.; Wittmann, M.; Rushworth, M.F.S. Multiple neural mechanisms of decision making and their competition under changing risk pressure. *Neuron* **2014**, *81*, 1190–1202. [CrossRef]
75. Wittmann, M.K.; Kolling, N.; Akaishi, R.; Chau, B.K.; Brown, J.W.; Nelissen, N.; Rushworth, M.F.S. Predictive decision making driven by multiple time-linked reward representations in the anterior cingulate cortex. *Nat. Commun.* **2016**, *7*, 12327. [CrossRef]
76. Denny, B.T.; Kober, H.; Wager, T.D.; Ochsner, K.N. A meta-analysis of functional neuroimaging studies of self- and other-judgments reveals a spatial gradient for mentalizing in medial prefrontal cortex. *J. Cogn. Neurosci.* **2012**, *24*, 1742–1752. [CrossRef]

7. Murray, R.J.; Schaer, M.; Debbane, M. Degrees of separation: A quantitative neuroimaging meta-analysis investigating self-specificity and shared neural activation between self- and other-reflection. *Neurosci. Biobehav. Rev.* **2012**, *36*, 1043–1059. [CrossRef] [PubMed]

8. Qin, P.; Northoff, G. How is our self related to midline regions and the default-mode network? *Neuroimage* **2011**, *57*, 1221–1233. [CrossRef]

9. Battaglia, S.; Garofalo, S.; di Pellegrino, G.; Starita, F. Revaluing the Role of vmPFC in the Acquisition of Pavlovian Threat Conditioning in Humans. *J. Neurosci.* **2020**, *40*, 8491–8500. [CrossRef]

10. Motzkin, J.C.; Hiser, J.; Carroll, I.; Wolf, R.; Baskaya, M.K.; Koenigs, M.; Atlas, L.Y. Human ventromedial prefrontal cortex lesions enhance the effect of expectations on pain perception. *Cortex* **2023**, *166*, 188–206. [CrossRef]

11. Raja, S.N.; Carr, D.B.; Cohen, M.; Finnerup, N.B.; Flor, H.; Gibson, S.; Keefe, F.J.; Mogil, J.S.; Ringkamp, M.; Sluka, K.A.; et al. The revised International Association for the Study of Pain definition of pain: Concepts, challenges, and compromises. *Pain* **2020**, *161*, 1976–1982. [CrossRef] [PubMed]

12. Zhou, F.; Zhao, W.; Qi, Z.; Geng, Y.; Yao, S.; Kendrick, K.M.; Wager, T.D.; Becker, B. A distributed fMRI-based signature for the subjective experience of fear. *Nat. Commun.* **2021**, *12*, 6643. [CrossRef]

13. Savage, H.S.; Davey, C.G.; Wager, T.D.; Garfinkel, S.N.; Moffat, B.A.; Glarin, R.K.; Harrison, B.J. Neural mediators of subjective and autonomic responding during threat learning and regulation. *Neuroimage* **2021**, *245*, 118643. [CrossRef]

14. Fullana, M.A.; Harrison, B.J.; Soriano-Mas, C.; Vervliet, B.; Cardoner, N.; Avila-Parcet, A.; Radua, J. Neural signatures of human fear conditioning: An updated and extended meta-analysis of fMRI studies. *Mol. Psychiatry* **2016**, *21*, 500–508. [CrossRef] [PubMed]

15. Savage, H.S.; Davey, C.G.; Fullana, M.A.; Harrison, B.J. Clarifying the neural substrates of threat and safety reversal learning in humans. *Neuroimage* **2020**, *207*, 116427. [CrossRef]

16. Marstaller, L.; Burianova, H.; Reutens, D.C. Adaptive contextualization: A new role for the default mode network in affective learning. *Hum. Brain Mapp.* **2017**, *38*, 1082–1091. [CrossRef]

17. Harrison, B.J.; Fullana, M.A.; Via, E.; Soriano-Mas, C.; Vervliet, B.; Martinez-Zalacain, I.; Pujol, J.; Davey, C.G.; Kircher, T.; Straube, B.; et al. Human ventromedial prefrontal cortex and the positive affective processing of safety signals. *Neuroimage* **2017**, *152*, 12–18. [CrossRef]

18. Milad, M.R.; Wright, C.I.; Orr, S.P.; Pitman, R.K.; Quirk, G.J.; Rauch, S.L. Recall of fear extinction in humans activates the ventromedial prefrontal cortex and hippocampus in concert. *Biol. Psychiatry* **2007**, *62*, 446–454. [CrossRef]

19. Tashjian, S.M.; Zbozinek, T.D.; Mobbs, D. A Decision Architecture for Safety Computations. *Trends Cogn. Sci.* **2021**, *25*, 342–354. [CrossRef] [PubMed]

20. Wallis, C.U.; Cardinal, R.N.; Alexander, L.; Roberts, A.C.; Clarke, H.F. Opposing roles of primate areas 25 and 32 and their putative rodent homologs in the regulation of negative emotion. *Proc. Natl. Acad. Sci. USA* **2017**, *114*, E4075–E4084. [CrossRef] [PubMed]

21. Kucyi, A.; Moayedi, M.; Weissman-Fogel, I.; Goldberg, M.B.; Freeman, B.V.; Tenenbaum, H.C.; Davis, K.D. Enhanced medial prefrontal-default mode network functional connectivity in chronic pain and its association with pain rumination. *J. Neurosci.* **2014**, *34*, 3969–3975. [CrossRef]

22. Kucyi, A.; Salomons, T.V.; Davis, K.D. Mind wandering away from pain dynamically engages antinociceptive and default mode brain networks. *Proc. Natl. Acad. Sci. USA* **2013**, *110*, 18692–18697. [CrossRef] [PubMed]

23. Chen, Q.; Heinricher, M.M. Shifting the Balance: How Top-Down and Bottom-Up Input Modulate Pain via the Rostral Ventrome-dial Medulla. *Front. Pain Res.* **2022**, *3*, 932476. [CrossRef] [PubMed]

24. Fields, H. State-dependent opioid control of pain. *Nat. Rev. Neurosci.* **2004**, *5*, 565–575. [CrossRef]

25. Leknes, S.; Berna, C.; Lee, M.C.; Snyder, G.D.; Biele, G.; Tracey, I. The importance of context: When relative relief renders pain pleasant. *Pain* **2013**, *154*, 402–410. [CrossRef] [PubMed]

26. Leknes, S.; Lee, M.; Berna, C.; Andersson, J.; Tracey, I. Relief as a reward: Hedonic and neural responses to safety from pain. *PLoS ONE* **2011**, *6*, e17870. [CrossRef] [PubMed]

27. Woo, C.W.; Roy, M.; Buhle, J.T.; Wager, T.D. Distinct brain systems mediate the effects of nociceptive input and self-regulation on pain. *PLoS Biol.* **2015**, *13*, e1002036. [CrossRef] [PubMed]

28. Schulz, E.; Stankewitz, A.; Witkovsky, V.; Winkler, A.M.; Tracey, I. Strategy-dependent modulation of cortical pain circuits for the attenuation of pain. *Cortex* **2019**, *113*, 255–266. [CrossRef] [PubMed]

29. Valet, M.; Sprenger, T.; Boecker, H.; Willoch, F.; Rummeny, E.; Conrad, B.; Erhard, P.; Tolle, T.R. Distraction modulates connectivity of the cingulo-frontal cortex and the midbrain during pain—An fMRI analysis. *Pain* **2004**, *109*, 399–408. [CrossRef]

100. Bantick, S.J.; Wise, R.G.; Ploghaus, A.; Clare, S.; Smith, S.M.; Tracey, I. Imaging how attention modulates pain in humans using functional MRI. *Brain* **2002**, *125 Pt 2*, 310–319. [CrossRef]

101. Atlas, L.Y.; Bolger, N.; Lindquist, M.A.; Wager, T.D. Brain mediators of predictive cue effects on perceived pain. *J. Neurosci.* **2010**, *30*, 12964–12977. [CrossRef]

102. Atlas, L.Y.; Dildine, T.C.; Palacios-Barrios, E.E.; Yu, Q.; Reynolds, R.C.; Banker, L.A.; Grant, S.S.; Pine, D.S. Instructions and experiential learning have similar impacts on pain and pain-related brain responses but produce dissociations in value-based reversal learning. *eLife* **2022**, *11*, e73353. [CrossRef]

103. Atlas, L.Y.; Wager, T.D. A meta-analysis of brain mechanisms of placebo analgesia: Consistent findings and unanswered questions. *Handb. Exp. Pharmacol.* **2014**, *225*, 37–69.
104. Amanzio, M.; Benedetti, F.; Porro, C.A.; Palermo, S.; Cauda, F. Activation likelihood estimation meta-analysis of brain correlates of placebo analgesia in human experimental pain. *Hum. Brain Mapp.* **2013**, *34*, 738–752. [CrossRef]
105. Jepma, M.; Koban, L.; van Doorn, J.; Jones, M.; Wager, T.D. Behavioural and neural evidence for self-reinforcing expectancy effects on pain. *Nat. Hum. Behav.* **2018**, *2*, 838–855. [CrossRef] [PubMed]
106. Roy, M.; Shohamy, D.; Daw, N.; Jepma, M.; Wimmer, G.E.; Wager, T.D. Representation of aversive prediction errors in the human periaqueductal gray. *Nat. Neurosci.* **2014**, *17*, 1607–1612. [CrossRef] [PubMed]
107. Lopez-Sola, M.; Koban, L.; Wager, T.D. Transforming Pain With Prosocial Meaning: A Functional Magnetic Resonance Imaging Study. *Psychosom. Med.* **2018**, *80*, 814–825. [CrossRef] [PubMed]
108. Bingel, U.; Rose, M.; Glascher, J.; Buchel, C. fMRI reveals how pain modulates visual object processing in the ventral visual stream. *Neuron* **2007**, *55*, 157–167. [CrossRef]
109. Eippert, F.; Bingel, U.; Schoell, E.D.; Yacubian, J.; Klinger, R.; Lorenz, J.; Büchel, C. Activation of the opioidergic descending pain control system underlies placebo analgesia. *Neuron* **2009**, *63*, 533–543. [CrossRef]
110. Wager, T.D.; Atlas, L.Y.; Leotti, L.A.; Rilling, J.K. Predicting individual differences in placebo analgesia: Contributions of brain activity during anticipation and pain experience. *J. Neurosci.* **2011**, *31*, 439–452. [CrossRef]
111. Salomons, T.V.; Johnstone, T.; Backonja, M.M.; Davidson, R.J. Perceived controllability modulates the neural response to pain. *J. Neurosci.* **2004**, *24*, 7199–7203. [CrossRef] [PubMed]
112. Salomons, T.V.; Johnstone, T.; Backonja, M.M.; Shackman, A.J.; Davidson, R.J. Individual differences in the effects of perceived controllability on pain perception: Critical role of the prefrontal cortex. *J. Cogn. Neurosci.* **2007**, *19*, 993–1003. [CrossRef]
113. Lopez-Sola, M.; Geuter, S.; Koban, L.; Coan, J.A.; Wager, T.D. Brain mechanisms of social touch-induced analgesia in females. *Pain* **2019**, *160*, 2072–2085. [CrossRef] [PubMed]
114. Zunhammer, M.; Spisak, T.; Wager, T.D.; Bingel, U.; Placebo Imaging, C. Meta-analysis of neural systems underlying placebo analgesia from individual participant fMRI data. *Nat. Commun.* **2021**, *12*, 1391. [CrossRef] [PubMed]
115. Kober, H.; Wager, T.D. Meta-analysis of neuroimaging data. *Wiley Interdiscip. Rev. Cogn. Sci.* **2010**, *1*, 293–300. [CrossRef] [PubMed]
116. Kong, J.; Tu, P.C.; Zyloney, C.; Su, T.P. Intrinsic functional connectivity of the periaqueductal gray, a resting fMRI study. *Behav. Brain Res.* **2010**, *211*, 215–219. [CrossRef]
117. Baliki, M.N.; Geha, P.Y.; Fields, H.L.; Apkarian, A.V. Predicting value of pain and analgesia: Nucleus accumbens response to noxious stimuli changes in the presence of chronic pain. *Neuron* **2010**, *66*, 149–160. [CrossRef]
118. Woo, C.W.; Schmidt, L.; Krishnan, A.; Jepma, M.; Roy, M.; Lindquist, M.A.; Atlas, L.Y.; Wager, T.D. Quantifying cerebral contributions to pain beyond nociception. *Nat. Commun.* **2017**, *8*, 14211. [CrossRef]
119. Gold, M.S.; Gebhart, G.F. Nociceptor sensitization in pain pathogenesis. *Nat. Med.* **2010**, *16*, 1248–1257. [CrossRef]
120. Basbaum, A.I.; Bautista, D.M.; Scherrer, G.; Julius, D. Cellular and molecular mechanisms of pain. *Cell* **2009**, *139*, 267–284. [CrossRef]
121. Nijs, J.; George, J.; Clauw, D.; Fernández-de-las-Peñas, C.; Kosek, E.; Ickmans, K.; Fernández-Carnero, J.; Polli, A.; Kapreli, E.; Huysmans, E.; et al. Central sensitisation in chronic pain conditions: Latest discoveries and their potential for precision medicine. *Lancet Rheumatol.* **2021**, *3*, E383–E392. [CrossRef] [PubMed]
122. Tinnermann, A.; Geuter, S.; Sprenger, C.; Finsterbusch, J.; Buchel, C. Interactions between brain and spinal cord mediate value effects in nocebo hyperalgesia. *Science* **2017**, *358*, 105–108. [CrossRef] [PubMed]
123. Atlas, L.Y. How Instructions, Learning, and Expectations Shape Pain and Neurobiological Responses. *Annu. Rev. Neurosci.* **2023**, *46*, 167–189. [CrossRef] [PubMed]
124. de Lange, F.P.; Heilbron, M.; Kok, P. How Do Expectations Shape Perception? *Trends Cogn. Sci.* **2018**, *22*, 764–779. [CrossRef]
125. Wager, T.D.; Atlas, L.Y. The neuroscience of placebo effects: Connecting context, learning and health. *Nat. Rev. Neurosci.* **2015**, *16*, 403–418. [CrossRef]
126. Atlas, L.Y. A social affective neuroscience lens on placebo analgesia. *Trends Cogn. Sci.* **2021**, *25*, 992–1005. [CrossRef]
127. Geuter, S.; Koban, L.; Wager, T.D. The Cognitive Neuroscience of Placebo Effects: Concepts, Predictions, and Physiology. *Annu. Rev. Neurosci.* **2017**, *40*, 167–188. [CrossRef]
128. Zhang, S.; Mano, H.; Lee, M.; Yoshida, W.; Kawato, M.; Robbins, T.W.; Seymour, B. The control of tonic pain by active relief learning. *eLife* **2018**, *7*, e31949. [CrossRef]
129. Yoshida, W.; Seymour, B.; Koltzenburg, M.; Dolan, R.J. Uncertainty increases pain: Evidence for a novel mechanism of pain modulation involving the periaqueductal gray. *J. Neurosci.* **2013**, *33*, 5638–5646. [CrossRef]
130. Seidel, E.M.; Pfabigan, D.M.; Hahn, A.; Sladky, R.; Grahl, A.; Paul, K.; Kraus, C.; Küblböck, M.; Kranz, G.S.; Hummer, A.; et al. Uncertainty during pain anticipation: The adaptive value of preparatory processes. *Hum. Brain Mapp.* **2015**, *36*, 744–755. [CrossRef]
131. Willems, A.L.; Van Oudenhove, L.; Vervliet, B. Omissions of threat trigger subjective relief and reward prediction error-like signaling in the human reward system. *bioRxiv* **2023**. [CrossRef]
132. Kolling, N.; Behrens, T.E.; Mars, R.B.; Rushworth, M.F. Neural mechanisms of foraging. *Science* **2012**, *336*, 95–98. [CrossRef] [PubMed]

33. Craig, A.D. How do you feel? Interoception: The sense of the physiological condition of the body. *Nat. Rev. Neurosci.* **2002**, *3*, 655–666. [CrossRef] [PubMed]

34. Craig, A.D. Interoception: The sense of the physiological condition of the body. *Curr. Opin. Neurobiol.* **2003**, *13*, 500–505. [CrossRef] [PubMed]

35. Petre, B.; Kragel, P.; Atlas, L.Y.; Geuter, S.; Jepma, M.; Koban, L.; Krishnan, A.; Lopez-Sola, M.; Losin, E.A.R.; Roy, M.; et al. A multistudy analysis reveals that evoked pain intensity representation is distributed across brain systems. *PLoS Biol.* **2022**, *20*, e3001620. [CrossRef]

36. Fazeli, S.; Buchel, C. Pain-Related Expectation and Prediction Error Signals in the Anterior Insula Are Not Related to Aversiveness. *J. Neurosci.* **2018**, *38*, 6461–6474. [CrossRef]

37. Palermo, S.; Benedetti, F.; Costa, T.; Amanzio, M. Pain anticipation: An activation likelihood estimation meta-analysis of brain imaging studies. *Hum. Brain Mapp.* **2015**, *36*, 1648–1661. [CrossRef]

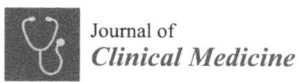

Journal of
Clinical Medicine

Article

Sex Differences in Opioid Response Linked to *OPRM1* and *COMT* genes DNA Methylation/Genotypes Changes in Patients with Chronic Pain

Laura Agulló [1,2], Javier Muriel [1], César Margarit [3], Mónica Escorial [1,2], Diana Garcia [4], María José Herrero [5], David Hervás [6], Juan Sandoval [4,*] and Ana M. Peiró [1,2,*]

1 Pharmacogenetic Unit, Alicante Institute for Health and Biomedical Research (ISABIAL), Dr. Balmis General University Hospital, Pintor Baeza, 12, 03010 Alicante, Spain
2 Clinical Pharmacology, Toxicology and Chemical Safety Unit, Institute of Bioengineering, Miguel Hernández University, Avda. de la Universidad s/n, 03202 Elche, Spain
3 Pain Unit, Department of Health of Alicante, Dr. Balmis General University Hospital, c/Pintor Baeza, 12, 03010 Alicante, Spain
4 Epigenomics Core Facility, La Fe Health Research Institute, Ave. Fernando Abril Martorell, 106, 46026 Valencia, Spain
5 Pharmacogenetics Unit, La Fe Health Research Institute, Ave. Fernando Abril Martorell, 106, 46026 Valencia, Spain
6 Department of Applied Statistics and Operations Research and Quality, Universitat Politècnica de Valéncia, 46022 Valencia, Spain
* Correspondence: epigenomica@iislafe.es (J.S.); peiro_ana@gva.es (A.M.P.); Tel.: +34-96-1246-709 (J.S.); +34-96-591-3868 (A.M.P.)

Citation: Agulló, L.; Muriel, J.; Margarit, C.; Escorial, M.; Garcia, D.; Herrero, M.J.; Hervás, D.; Sandoval, J.; Peiró, A.M. Sex Differences in Opioid Response Linked to *OPRM1* and *COMT* genes DNA Methylation/ Genotypes Changes in Patients with Chronic Pain. *J. Clin. Med.* 2023, 12, 3449. https://doi.org/10.3390/jcm12103449

Academic Editors: Jo Nijs and Polli Andrea

Received: 27 March 2023
Revised: 10 May 2023
Accepted: 10 May 2023
Published: 13 May 2023

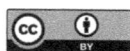
Abstract: Analgesic-response variability in chronic noncancer pain (CNCP) has been reported due to several biological and environmental factors. This study was undertaken to explore sex differences linked to *OPRM1* and *COMT* DNA methylation changes and genetic variants in analgesic response. A retrospective study with 250 real-world CNCP outpatients was performed in which data from demographic, clinical, and pharmacological variables were collected. DNA methylation levels (CpG island) were evaluated by pyrosequencing, and their interaction with the *OPRM1* (A118G) and *COMT* (G472A) gene polymorphisms was studied. A priori-planned statistical analyses were conducted to compare responses between females and males. Sex-differential *OPRM1* DNA methylation was observed to be linked to lower opioid use disorder (OUD) cases for females ($p = 0.006$). Patients with lower *OPRM1* DNA methylation and the presence of the mutant G-allele reduced opioid dose requirements ($p = 0.001$), equal for both sexes. Moreover, *COMT* DNA methylation levels were negatively related to pain relief ($p = 0.020$), quality of life ($p = 0.046$), and some adverse events (probability > 90%) such as constipation, insomnia, or nervousness. Females were, significantly, 5 years older with high anxiety levels and a different side-effects distribution than males. The analyses demonstrated significant differences between females and males related to *OPRM1* signalling efficiency and OUD, with a genetic–epigenetic interaction in opioid requirements. These findings support the importance of sex as a biological variable to be factored into chronic pain-management studies.

Keywords: sex differences; chronic pain; epigenetics; DNA methylation; pharmacogenetics

1. Introduction

Some inherent biological differences contribute to sex differences in chronic noncancer pain (CNCP) [1,2], where females are more vulnerable to maintaining musculoskeletal pain with greater psychological distress [3,4]. Traditionally, it has been thought that such differences are largely due to the endogenous opioid system and hormonal regulation [5,6], but there are also genetic and epigenetic factors (i.e., DNA methylation, noncoding RNA expression, or histone modifications) [7,8] that could contribute as they do in other autoimmune disorders or neuropsychiatric diseases [9].

Current research suggests that there are significant differences between males and females in the genetics and epigenetics associated with chronic pain [10,11]. Some studies have identified specific genes and signalling pathways that are involved in pain sensation and perception [12], and these genes may be expressed differently in males and females [13]. In addition, epigenetics, which is the study of how environmental factors may influence gene expression, also appears to play an important role in sex differences in chronic pain [14].

In recent years, some genetic markers have been linked with interindividual differences in analgesic response [15,16], such as μ-opioid receptor 1 (*OPRM1*, A118G, rs1799971-G allele, 11–17% in the Caucasian population). This variant has been associated with higher doses of opioid requirements [17], and being more predisposed to compulsive behaviours and opioid dependence compared to rs1799971-A carriers [18,19]. In the same way, variants of the gene that encodes enzyme catechol-O-methyltransferase (*COMT*, G472A, and rs4680-A allele) are linked with a lesser capacity to metabolise monoamines and, thus, higher dopamine levels arise. Here, a lower pain threshold and increased vulnerability to chronic pain have been observed compared to the rs4680-G ancestral allele, and even more when combined with the *OPRM1* variant genotypes [20]. However, scientific evidence for the effect of these gene variants is not complete enough to explain the wide variability observed in the real world.

Hence, the possible involvement of a sex-mediated genetic–epigenetic interaction could be considered a modulator factor [21,22]. The aim of this study was to explore sex differences linked to DNA methylation/genotype changes that may affect the expression of the genes *OPRM1* and *COMT* by conditioning a different analgesic response.

2. Materials and Methods

2.1. Study Design

A retrospective study (EPA-OD) was designed and conducted at the Pain Unit of the Alicante Health Department, Dr. Balmis General University Hospital, in Spain, from March 2021 to March 2022. The study was approved by the Ethics Committee (Protocol Code 2020-158). Written informed consent was waived due to the retrospective nature of the study. In any case, all the patients had already given informed consent to participate in previous observational studies done in the same setting [23,24]. The last study ended early due to the COVID-19 pandemic, as seen in Figure A1.

2.2. Participants and Data Collection

All the samples taken from the candidates in the present study ($n = 250$) were obtained from Biobank (Alicante Institute for Health and Biomedical Research (ISABIAL), Spain). This study adhered to the Spanish National Biobanks Network. Data were collected from original databases and completed from patients' electronic health records. The inclusion criteria were patients aged $\geq$18 years old, CNCP (moderate or severe pain lasting at least 6 months) with long-term opioids ($\geq$3 months), and with available DNA samples previously donated to Biobank. Patients under 18 years old, with oncologic pain or any psychiatric disorders that could interfere with the proper development of the study were excluded. Other chronic-pain syndromes of unclear pathophysiologies, such as fibromyalgia or neuropathic pain, such as painful polyneuropathy, postherpetic neuralgia, trigeminal neuralgia, and poststroke pain, were not included.

2.2.1. Clinical Outcomes

A Global Pain State questionnaire [25], which qualitatively measures pain intensity and relief, was collected at the time that each patient was included in the study using the Visual Analogue Scale (VAS). This consists of a horizontal line ranging from 0 (lowest) to

100 mm (highest), where the patient points on the line the intensity of the pain or relief that he/she feels, respectively. Quality of life was evaluated through the EuroQol-5D-3L scale that consists of a VAS vertical line from 0 (the worst imaginable health status) to 100 mm (the best imaginable) where the patient indicates his/her actual health status. The patient's diagnosis and demographic characteristics, such as age, sex, and employment status (active, retired, or work disability) were also registered. Psychological status was calculated with the Hospital Anxiety and Depression Scale: HADS, 0–21 scores, classified as normal (<7), probable (8–10) and case (>11 scores) [26].

2.2.2. Pharmacology and Hospital Resources Use

Pharmacological variables such as the main opioid (i.e., tramadol, fentanyl, tapentadol, buprenorphine, oxycodone, and morphine) was registered (Table A2). In different opioid combinations, oral morphine equivalent daily dose (MEDD) was estimated using available references [27]; the number of adverse events was collected with a list of the most frequent analgesic side effects from the Summary of Product Characteristics frequency as "very common" or "common", and a blank field to add any other adverse event was developed. Opioid use disorder (OUD) was diagnosed by a psychiatrist according to DSM-5 as part of an established opioid tapering procedure followed since 2018 [17].

2.3. Genetic/Epigenetic Data

At the time of enrolment in the original study, patient samples were collected for the pharmacogenetic analysis. Approximately 2 mL of saliva were collected in tubes containing 5 mL of PBS. Once the saliva sample was taken, it was stored at −80 °C until its processing. Genomic DNA was isolated using an E.N.Z.A. forensic DNA kit (Omega Bio-Tek Inc., Norcross, GA, USA) in accordance with the manufacturer's instructions. In the present study, samples were provided by the Alicante BioBank and processed following standard operating procedures.

2.3.1. Genotypes Analysis

The following gene variants were genotyped at the ISABIAL Molecular Biology Laboratory (Alicante GVA, Spain): *OPRM1* (rs1799971) and *COMT* (rs4680) using the realtime PCR rotor gene Q system (Qiagen, Hilden DE-NW, Germany), through the use of specific TaqMan MGB® probes (Applied Biosystems, Pleasanton, CA, USA). Amplification parameters were as follows: pre-PCR for 10 min at 95 °C, 40 cycles for 15 s denaturation at 92 °C, and 1 min final extension at 60 °C.

2.3.2. DNA Methylation Analysis

The Epigenomics Core Facility of the Health Research Institute La Fe performed the methylation analysis. Before this, a DNA integrity quality control was performed to ensure that DNA met standard quality measurements. All the DNA samples were assessed for purity using a NanoDrop 2000c (Thermo Fisher Scientific, Wilmington, DE, USA) with 260/280 and 260/230 ratio measurements and quantified by the fluorometric method (Quan-iT PicoGreen DsDNA Assay, Life Technologies, Carlsbad, CA, USA). Agarose gels at 1.5% were performed to assess DNA integrity. The obtained high-quality DNA samples (500 ng) were selected for bisulphite conversion using the EZ DNA Methylation kit (Zymo Research Corp., Irvine, CA, USA) following the manufacturer's recommendations.

A triplet of primers was designed for each promoter region of genes *OPRM1* and *COMT* using Qiagen's PyroMark Assay Design 2.0 software to hybridise to CpG-free sites to ensure methylation-independent amplification and pyrosequencing steps. Primers sequences are listed in Table A1 (all given as 5′ > 3′). Briefly, the PCR was performed under standard conditions with biotinylated primers. Pyrosequencing reactions and the DNA methylation quantification of *OPRM1* and *COMT* CpG sites located at their promoter regions were performed in a PyroMark Q24 System, version 2.0.7 (Qiagen), using appropriate reagents and recommended protocols. Samples were repeated if pyrosequencing runs did not pass the pyrosequencer quality checks or if the internal bisulphite conversion controls failed.

As shown in Figure 1, the CpG island we studied in the *OPRM1* gene (chr6: 154039512-154039571) is located between nucleotides −35 and +27 (relative to the adenine of the ATG translation start site). We examined five CpG dinucleotides located at nucleotides −32, −25, −18, −14, −10, and +12. The CpG dinucleotides −18 and −14 are located at a potential Sp1 binding site, and the CpG +12 site at a second binding site. The selection of these CpG sites was based on the previous study conducted by Nielsen et al. [28]. As for the *COMT* gene, seven CpG sites located between nucleotides −97 and −50 (chr22:19929354-19929398) of the MB-*COMT* promoter region were selected based on the work of Zhong et al. [29]. The MB-*COMT* promoter is part of a complex regulatory region that includes multiple enhancers and silencers that regulate the expression of the *COMT* gene.The seven specific CpG dinucleotides are located at nucleotides −89, −86, −84, −75, −72, −67, and −62.

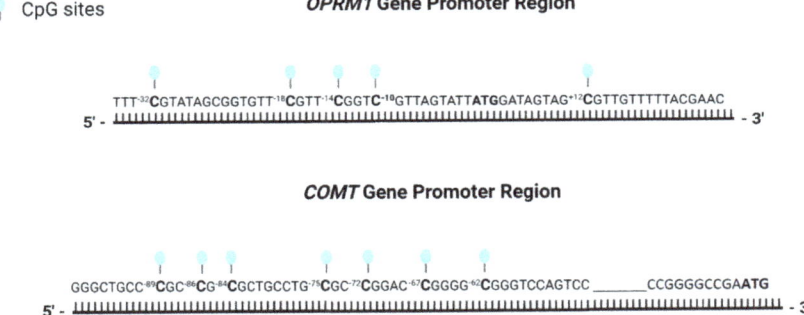

Figure 1. The *OPRM1* (μ-opioid receptor 1) and *COMT* (catechol-O-methyltransferase) gene promoter region. The locations of the CpG sites are represented by knobs and translation start sites (ATG) are shown in bold.

2.4. Statistical Analysis

A convenient sample size of 250 participants (stratified by sex: 1:1 men/women) was defined due to the number of biological samples available at Biobank (ISABIAL, Spain). Data distribution was analysed by the Kolmogorov–Smirnov test following the Lilliefors correction method. A descriptive analysis of continuous quantitative variables (i.e., pain intensity, relief, and quality of life) was presented as the mean ± standard deviation (SD) while discrete variables (i.e., HADS scores and adverse events) are shown using their median and interquartile range (IQR). Categorical data (sex, employment status, anxiety and depression groups, and pharmacological prescription) were expressed by percentages (%).

The demographic, clinical, pharmacological, and epigenetic/genetic factors were compared using χ2 or Fisher's exact test for the categorical variables, and the t-test or Mann–Whitney U test for the continuous variables depending on their distribution. When more than two groups were involved, ANOVA/Kruskal–Wallis or chi-square tests were used for continuous or categorical variables, respectively.

After performing the pyrosequencing technique, we obtained the methylation percentages of the *OPRM* and *COMT* genes. These values were used to carry out the analysis of the possible associations between the DNA methylation level and the selected variables, by means of a linear mixed-regression model using logarithmic transformation for the absolute values. A Bayesian regression analysis was also performed to analyse the association between DNA methylation and the presence of all the different adverse events. The probability of the effect of the variable being negative (higher methylation values, lower risk) or positive (higher methylation values, higher risk) is reported. An ordinal regression model was used to explain the DNA methylation-*OPRM1/COMT* genotypes interaction for clinical variables. Given the high correlation between the different methylation values of the CpG sites selected at the gene promoter region, only one CpG site per gene was selected to carry out the regression model (*COMT*-CpG6 and *OPRM1*-CpG2). Specifically, the selection of the CpG site was based on the degree of variability (the site with the highest variability was selected for each gene). Averaging the methylation values of the different CpGs of the region might introduce a bias since the average is not an observed variable. Nevertheless, the methylation values were so similar that the results would have been almost the same if including another CpG or even using the average in this case. The variable sex was included as a possible confounding factor. Statistical analyses were performed using the R software (v 4.0.3, Auckland, CA, USA). A $p < 0.05$ was considered to be statistically significant.

3. Results

A total of 250 candidates, 125 females and 125 males, were included after excluding patients who were duplicated between studies or did not meet the inclusion criteria. All included participants (Figure S1) were referred to our Pain Unit for routine pain management, mostly due to nonspecific low back pain (83%).

The sample's mean age was 62 ± 14 years, 59% were retired, and all the participants were Caucasian residents of Spain. The mean for moderate pain intensity (67 ± 21 mm), pain relief (32 ± 27 mm), and quality of life (43 ± 23 mm) was equal for both sexes.

3.1. Sex Differences in the Demographic and Clinical Data

Females were a significant mean of 5 years older (64 ± 14 vs. 59 ± 14 years old, $p < 0.05$), have significantly higher nonspecific low back pain (95%, $p < 0.001$), significantly higher 4 anxiety scores (9 [5,13] vs. 5 [2,11] scores, $p < 0.05$), showed 15% more dry skin (31 vs. 16%, $p < 0.05$) and 17% more weight changes (33 vs. 16%, $p < 0.05$) compared to males. In contrast, males presented 9% higher OUD (26 vs.15%, $p < 0.05$) and 13% higher sexually adverse events (33 vs. 20%, $p < 0.05$) than females. Demographic and clinical data are shown in Table 1.

Table 1. Demographic and clinical data in the total population according to sex. Values are %, mean (standard deviation), or median [interquartile range].

	Total $n = 250$	Females $n = 125$	Males $n = 125$
Age	62 (14)	**64 (14) ***	59 (14)
Employment status (%)			
At work	10	10	10
Retired	59	68	52
Work Disability	31	22	38
Diagnosis (%)			
Nonspecific low back pain	83	**95 ****	65
Other pain	17	5	35
Pain intensity (0–100 mm)	67 (21)	68 (22)	66 (20)
Relief (0–100 mm)	32 (27)	34 (26)	30 (28)
Quality of life (0–100 mm)	43 (23)	40 (22)	46 (23)
HAD-Anxiety (0–21 scores)	8 [3, 12]	**9 [5, 13] ***	5 [2, 11]
HAD-Depression (0–21 scores)	7 [4, 12]	8 [5, 13]	7 [3, 11]

Table 1. *Cont.*

	Total $n = 250$	Females $n = 125$	Males $n = 125$
MEDD (mg/day)	106 (99)	104 (99)	109 (98)
Total Adverse Events	3 [1, 6]	3 [1, 6]	3 [1, 5]
Opioid use disorder (%)	21	15	**26 ***
Adverse Events (%)			
Dry Mouth	45	53	41
Constipation	41	46	42
Insomnia	28	34	26
Dry Skin	22	**31 ***	16
Nervousness	26	30	26
Dizziness	26	32	23
Sexual disturbance	25	20	**33 ***
Weight changes	23	**33 ***	16
Lack of appetite	13	17	11
Red skin	11	27	13

HAD: Hospital Anxiety and Depression Scale; MEDD: Morphine Equivalent Daily Dose. * Denotes $p < 0.05$ and ** denotes $p < 0.01$ when comparing females to males. The highest value is shown in bold.

3.2. DNA Methylation/Genotypes and Analgesic Response

The DNA methylation values obtained in the seven selected CpG sites of the *COMT* gene (sites 1–7) showed low variability, with values close to 0 (0.54–1.52%). However, the five selected CpG sites of the *OPRM1* gene (sites 1–5) were methylated to a larger extent with typical dynamic ranges between 8.2% and 16.6%. DNA methylation values at the selected CpG sites and the variability level appear in Table 2 and Figure 2, respectively.

Table 2. DNA Methylation (%) as the mean (standard deviation) at the CpG sites selected in genes *OPRM1* (sites 1–5) and *COMT* (sites 1–7) (counted from the adenine of the start codon).

Code	CpG Sites	Total $n = 250$	Female $n = 125$	Male $n = 125$	p-Value
		OPRM1 DNA Methylation (%)			
CpG 1	−32	8.2 (3.8)	8.3 (3.6)	8.1 (4.1)	0.3
CpG 2	−18	16.6 (6.2)	16.6 (5.8)	16.7 (6.7)	0.8
CpG 3	−14	14.2 (5.5)	14.2 (5.0)	14.2 (6.1)	0.5
CpG 4	−10	10.1 (3.9)	10.2 (3.5)	10.0 (4.3)	0.4
CpG 5	+12	8.3 (4.0)	8.3 (3.5)	8.3 (4.5)	0.4
		COMT DNA Methylation (%)			
CpG 1	−89	1.5 (1.0)	1.5 (0.8)	1.5 (1.1)	0.1
CpG 2	−86	0.9 (1.0)	0.8 (0.6)	0.9 (1.2)	0.1
CpG 3	−84	0.7 (0.9)	0.7 (0.7)	0.7 (1.1)	0.05
CpG 4	−75	1.5 (0.9)	1.5 (0.7)	1.5 (1.1)	0.3
CpG 5	−72	0.8 (0.9)	0.7 (0.6)	0.8 (1.1)	0.06
CpG 6	−67	1.1 (1.5)	1.1 (1.6)	1 (1.4)	0.07
CpG 7	−62	0.5 (0.8)	0.5 (0.5)	0.6 (1.0)	0.1

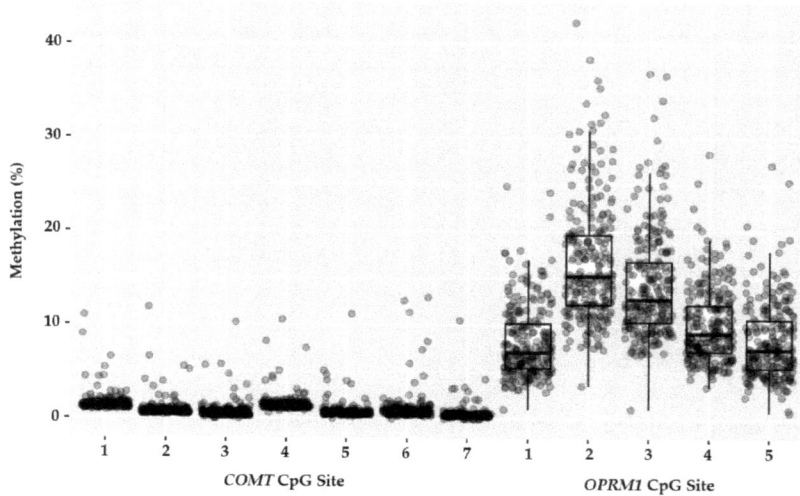

Figure 2. Distribution of methylation values (%) at each CpG site of the *COMT* (sites 1–7) and *OPRM1* (sites 1–5) genes.

As already mentioned in the statistical analysis section, the level of association between the different CpG sites located in each of the genes was high, and they were almost identical and provided hardly any additional information. The degree of association between the methylation value of the different CpG sites is depicted in Figure A2. Therefore, only one CpG site was selected from each gene (*COMT*-CpG6 and *OPRM1*-CpG2) and the percentages obtained were used to perform the regression analysis.

The obtained genotypic frequencies were equally distributed by sex in genes *OPRM1* (AA = 67; AG = 30; GG = 3%) and *COMT* (GG = 22; GA = 54; AA = 24%). Sex differences observed for the influence of *OPRM1* and *COMT* DNA methylation on clinical outcomes are shown in Table 3.

Table 3. Sex differences in the association between *OPRM1* and *COMT* DNA methylation and analgesic response.

		Estimate	SD	*p*-Value
Pain intensity				
OPRM1		−0.079	0.250	0.751
COMT		0.717	1.114	0.520
	Sex	−0.521	3.023	0.863
Relief				
OPRM1		0.248	0.294	0.400
COMT		−3.149 *	1.344	**0.020**
	Sex	3.326	3.65	0.363
Quality of life				
OPRM1		0.190	0.238	0.425
COMT		−2.069 *	1.028	**0.046**
	Sex	−2.108	2.83	0.457

Table 3. *Cont.*

		Estimate	SD	*p*-Value
HAD-Anxiety				
OPRM1		−0.178 *	0.088	**0.046**
COMT		0.228	0.273	0.404
	Sex	**1.869 ***	0.891	**0.039**
HAD-Depression				
OPRM1		−0.072	0.081	0.378
COMT		−0.011	0.251	0.965
	Sex	0.78	0.821	0.345
Opioid Use Disorder				
OPRM1		**−0.165 ****	0.036	**<0.001**
COMT		0.018	0.104	0.859
	Sex	**−2.123 ****	0.772	**0.006**
	OPRM1: Sex	**0.099 ***	0.05	**0.047**
MEDD (mg/day)				
OPRM1 G-allele		**−0.914 ****	0.24	**<0.001**
OPRM1		**−0.023 ****	0.008	**0.005**
OPRM1: OPRM1 G-allele		**0.046 ****	0.014	**0.001**
	Sex	0.009	0.081	0.908

OPRM1 (CpG2 site), COMT (CpG6 site); HAD: Hospital Anxiety and Depression Scale; MEDD: Morphine Equivalent Daily Dose * Denotes $p < 0.05$ and ** denotes $p < 0.01$, *p*-value <0.05 is shown in bold.

3.2.1. Associations Linked to *OPRM1* DNA Methylation

Linear-regression models show that anxiety and OUD were negatively related to *OPRM1* DNA methylation levels ($\beta = -0.178$, $p = 0.046$ and $\beta = -0.165$ $p < 0.001$, respectively); furthermore, females had a lower OUD prevalence ($\beta = -2.123$, $p = 0.006$) but higher anxiety impact scores appeared ($\beta = 1.869$, $p = 0.039$). A sex interaction with *OPRM1* DNA methylation levels was observed due to OUD ($\beta = 0.099$, $p = 0.047$). Females with lower *OPRM1* DNA methylation levels presented fewer OUD prevalence than males, as shown in Figure 3.

Additionally, an ordinal regression model has been used to explain the association between *OPRM1* DNA methylation and genotype. The results show that the MEDD requirements were impacted by the *OPRM1*-G-allele ($\beta = -0.914$, $p < 0.001$), *OPRM1* DNA methylation ($\beta = -0.023$, $p = 0.005$), and their genotype/epigenetic interaction ($\beta = 0.046$, $p = 0.001$). The data suggest a MEDD reduction with the presence of mutant G-allele/lower *OPRM1* DNA methylation. In contrast, for higher *OPRM1* DNA methylation, no reducing effect of the G allele was observed, as shown in Table 3.

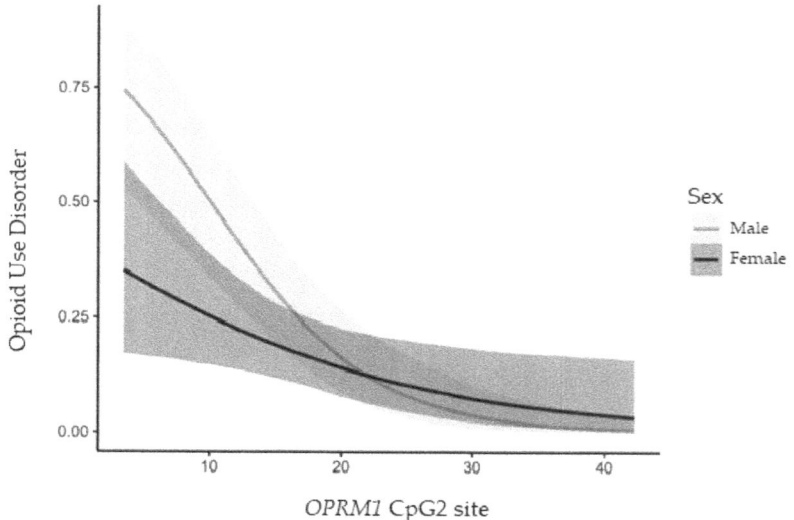

Figure 3. Effect of *OPRM1* DNA methylation (%) on opioid use disorder per sex according to male (M) or female (F).

3.2.2. Associations Linked to *COMT* DNA Methylation

The data show that when DNA *COMT* methylation increased, both pain relief ($\beta = -3.15$, $p = 0.020$) and quality of life ($\beta = -2.07$, $p = 0.046$) decreased. Furthermore, a positive correlation between pain relief and quality of life was found (Spearman r = 0.31, $p < 0.001$). Regarding the different adverse events, an inverse correlation of *COMT* was noted in relation to constipation, insomnia, dry mouth, dry skin, lack of appetite, red skin, and nervousness (probability > 90%). This means that a lower *COMT* DNA methylation level would imply a higher risk of these individual adverse events appearing. On the contrary, a positive correlation between *COMT* (the greater methylation, the higher the appearance risk) was observed for dizziness, as seen in Table 4.

Table 4. Probability (%) of the DNA methylation effect on the different adverse events.

Adverse Event	Estimate	SD	− Effect Prob.	+ Effect Prob.
Constipation				
OPRM1	0.035	0.022	0	25.5
COMT	−0.299	0.17	**95.84**	0.36
Insomnia				
OPRM1	0.02	0.024	0.37	14.43
COMT	−1.145	0.494	**99.92**	0
Dry mouth				
OPRM1	0.009	0.022	0.32	2.99
COMT	−0.416	0.215	**98.66**	0.08
Dry skin				
OPRM1	0.006	0.026	3.66	8.88
COMT	−0.648	0.381	**98.16**	0.37

Table 4. *Cont.*

Adverse Event	Estimate	SD	− Effect Prob.	+ Effect Prob.
Lack of appetite				
OPRM1	−0.03	0.035	42.15	2.37
COMT	−1.191	0.636	**98.89**	0.44
Red skin				
OPRM1	0.045	0.035	2.2	68.85
COMT	−0.765	0.56	**95.24**	2.6
Nervousness				
OPRM1	−0.05	0.027	58.74	0.01
COMT	−0.341	0.253	**91.11**	2.35
Dizziness				
OPRM1	−0.056	0.028	66.16	0
COMT	0.211	0.104	0.53	**95.4**

OPRM1-CpG2 site, *COMT*-CpG6 site; (−) or (+) Effect probabilities >90% are shown in bold.

4. Discussion

Our data showed significant sex differences related to *OPRM1* signalling efficiency in OUD, with an *OPRM1*-G allele interaction for the opioid dose requirement. A lower OUD probability appeared for females with decreased *OPRM1* DNA methylation. Additionally, sex conditioned a different anxiety level together with 5-years older females and a different side-effects pattern than males. These findings support the importance of sex as a biological variable to be factored into opioid management studies. Moreover, once data validation is performed, this information could be useful for developing predictive models of OUD based on sex and DNA methylation level, as well as for adjusting required opioid doses based on the genetic/epigenetic profile in clinical practice.

DNA methylation is a dynamic process that can change depending on different factors such as age, exposure to toxic substances, diet, and lifestyle. According to previous studies, a region of the genome is considered to be hypomethylated when the methylation level is less than 20%, while a region is considered to be hypermethylated when the methylation level is greater than 80% [30]. Both stages can affect gene expression and are related to various diseases and biological processes. However, these methylation thresholds are only a guide and should not be taken as absolute values to classify DNA methylation in all cases. It is important to keep in mind that reference values for normal DNA methylation should be considered in a broader context to understand its biological and clinical significance. For this reason, in this study, we have studied the associations between DNA methylation level and clinical, pharmacological and safety variables, but we have not categorized the methylation values obtained.

4.1. OPRM1 DNA Methylation and Opioid Use Disorder

Epigenetic mechanisms provide a platform that represents the convergence between the combined effect of biological and environmental influences on sex differences. However, data must be carefully interpreted for making gene-regulation predictions, which can vary in life spans based on DNA methylation changes at a few CpG sites. Conversely to our results, the literature shows that a lower *OPRM1* gene expression may condition higher OUD rates in patients with long-term opioid use, such as cancer-pain patients [31], subjects in methadone programmes [32], or former heroin addicts [28]. An increase in DNA methylation of CpG sites in the *OPRM1* promoter may block the binding of Sp1 and other transcription factors, which can reduce protein and mRNA expression and final *OPRM1* silencing [33]. New hypotheses arise about the possibility of a sex difference DNA methylation pattern in patients as a consequence of long-term opioid use history and/or of the presence of OUD. For potent drugs such as opioids, initial exposure is a crucial phase on the path to dependence and addiction, and it is reasonable to expect some epigenome modifications to occur during the first few exposures [34]. The question is whether epigenetic changes are induced after repeated opioid exposures or if, on the contrary, these are indicators of early epigenomic and potentially transcriptomic responses This should be profoundly explored together with sex differences in the methylation pattern.

Similarly, the limited but growing literature based on human studies has demonstrated that DNA methylation changes occur in response to environmental stress or lifestyle factors, such as physical activity. Exercise is a commonly prescribed treatment for chronic low-back pain, and sex-specific epigenetic mRNA gene expression adaptation, in response to endurance exercise, has been reported. Yet it is uncertain why global DNA methylation after exercise is similar between males and females despite the difference in mRNA expression of the epigenetic regulatory genes [35]. This may support the notion that dysregulated histone acetylation can be an important mechanism for memories of life stress that occurred early in life and can increase visceral pain in adulthood [1,36] or different gene networks function in the peripheral nervous systems that may contribute to sex differences in pain with rats after nerve injury [37]. Understanding the underlying biological mechanism of this different health risk may help to shed light on a possible sexually dimorphic risk for, or resilience from, developing OUD [38]. Therefore, although we have described the potential role of DNA methylation in OUD prevalence, further research is needed to unravel the role of the interaction among the different epigenetic factors in this regulatory context.

4.2. OPRM1 Methylation-Genotype Interaction in MEDD

Our data indicated that *OPRM* 118-G allele carriers were associated with a lower requirement of MEDD to achieve analgesia. Previous data suggest that the presence of homozygous ancestral-natural-type AA alleles of SNP *OPRM1* (A118G/dbSNP rs1799971-G) protects against pain perception and reduces problems that derive from pain perception, which preserves mobility, improves self-care, reduces anxiety-related problems in patients, and diminishes activities of daily living-related problems. Conversely to our results, patients who are G-allele carriers have been associated with higher opioid-dose requirements, as they are usually more sensitive to pain, and are more predisposed to compulsive behaviours and opioid dependence compared to rs1799971-A carriers [18,19]. In addition, in this work we have studied the effect of the interaction of G allele–DNA methylation, and the data show that as the *OPRM1* methylation increased, a decrease in the G-allele-reducing MEDD was observed. In line with our result, a previous study on *OPRM1* methylation of 22 CpG sites (including the five selected sites) analyzed 133 adolescents and reported that hypermethylation of the gene leads to a decreased response to opioids with an increased experience of pain [39].

4.3. COMT Methylation and Analgesic Response

Our results showed low variability and methylation values close to zero (0.54–1.52%) in the *COMT* promoter region. However, despite the low values, a negative association between pain relief and quality of life was found and patients were more likely to present different adverse events. According to the literature, higher *COMT* expression could increase dopamine degradation in the brain while being more sensitive to pain relief, but different adverse events appeared [40] as in our study. In fact, the *COMT* gene plays a critical role in the synaptic catabolism of neurotransmitters in the prefrontal cortex, where dopamine is crucial and involved in the pharmacological mechanisms of psychostimulant effects [41]. Furthermore, some sex-specific differences have been observed in the response of dopamine neurons in the attenuating pain of female rats [42,43], and in relation to the variability of behavioural and physiological correlates of cognitive control [44,45]. There are accumulating and sometimes compelling data showing that *COMT* has marked sexually dimorphic effects on brain function and its dysfunction in psychiatric disorders [46]. However, our results did not evidence of any sex influence.

Finally, it is well-known that age, sex, psychological status, disabilities, and cultural expectations may influence individual responses to chronic pain [47]. In our study, sex differences were related to significantly older age and higher anxiety levels in females. They should be closely analysed in terms of biopsychosocial mechanisms by adjusting for other confounding factors, such as gender bias due to pain normalisation in females, which may underlie these sex differences [48,49]. Furthermore, females have been described to report being prescribed more anxiolytics, sedatives, or hypnotics which could contribute to OUD [50]. However, our data suggested greater OUD behaviour for males, which agrees with other clinical evidence [51]. All this information needs to undergo a multidimensional approach to assess its impact, plus the epigenetic/genetic influence, on CNCP analgesic response.

4.4. Limitations

This study has some limitations that need to be acknowledged. Due to its retrospective design, the data collection of some variables could have been limited by lacking some information reported by clinicians. Additionally, as patients were on concomitant medication to treat other pathologies, unmeasured factors could have contributed to the observed differences. They could have independently contributed to the observed adverse events and differences in pain care [52,53]. The sample size was limited to DNA samples available from a single pain unit but included subjects from different trials, which could add heterogeneity. So, the relatively high OUD incidence in our setting could have affected the results, which need to be replicated in a more diverse population. In addition, it should be noted that some other important factors, such as pain duration, body-mass index, testosterone/estrogen levels, or other lifestyle influences were not controlled in this study. All these factors could introduce a mediated bias that could be more relevant than the pain itself. Therefore, it would be necessary to replicate this analysis, including other factors that could influence our results, in order to reach more accurate conclusions. Nevertheless, one of the strengths of our study lies in the fact that the data was obtained from real-world outpatients. Finally, some analytical limitations have also emerged. We have found evidence of an association between *COMT* gene methylation values and the level of relief and quality of life. Interestingly, the *COMT* promoter site shows methylation values close to zero and with very little variability, so the findings of these analyses should be taken with caution as they may be due to other uncontrolled factors.

5. Conclusions

Sex differences in *OPRM1* DNA methylation that impact OUD were proposed and discussed. In addition, we have also found an *OPRM1* genotype/methylation interaction with MEDD, plus an association of *COMT* DNA methylation with pain relief and quality of life in real-world outpatients with CNCP. The study of new factors such as sex and DNA methylation could lead to the identification of new biomarkers to improve analgesic response as a fundamental step towards precision medicine.

Author Contributions: Conceptualization, A.M.P. and J.M.; Data curation, L.A.; Formal analysis, L.A. and D.H.; Funding acquisition, A.M.P. and J.M.; Investigation, L.A. and M.E.; Methodology, L.A., D.G. and J.S.; Project administration, L.A., J.M., and A.M.P.; Resources, A.M.P. and C.M.; Supervision, A.M.P. and J.S.; Visualization, L.A.; Writing—original draft, L.A. and A.M.P.; Writing—review & editing, L.A., J.M., C.M., M.E., D.G., M.J.H., D.H., J.S., and A.M.P. All authors have read and agreed to the published version of the manuscript.

Funding: This work was funded by the Instituto de Salud Carlos III (ISCIII, Madrid, Spain) through a grant to Independent Clinical Research Projects of the Strategic Action in Health 2017–2020 (AES, ICI20/00146), and co-financed by the European Union, through FEDER funds. Publication funded by the Instituto de Investigación Sanitaria y Biomédica de Alicante (ISABIAL).

Institutional Review Board Statement: This study was approved by the Spanish Agency of Medicines and Medical Devices (AEMPS) with its registered protocol and is identified by EudraCT Number: 2021-001238-21. The study conforms to the Declaration of Helsinki as regards research involving human subjects and was approved by the Ethics Committee Board of the Alicante University General Hospital (Code: 2020-158).

Informed Consent Statement: Informed consent was obtained from all subjects involved in the study. Written informed consent has been obtained from the patients to publish this paper.

Data Availability Statement: The data presented in this study are available on request from the corresponding author. The data are not publicly available because they contain clinical data of patients.

Acknowledgments: We wish to thank the Department of Health of the Dr. Balmis Alicante General Hospital, Alicante, Spain: Pain Unit Nursery (BSc. Alicia López, Fernanda Jiménez), and anaesthesiologists (Drs. Panadero, Eiden, Sastre and Gómez). Special thanks go to Jordi Barrachina for his help in data collection.

Conflicts of Interest: The authors declare no conflict of interest. The funders had no role in the design of the study; in the collection, analyses, or interpretation of data; in the writing of the manuscript; or in the decision to publish the results.

Appendix A

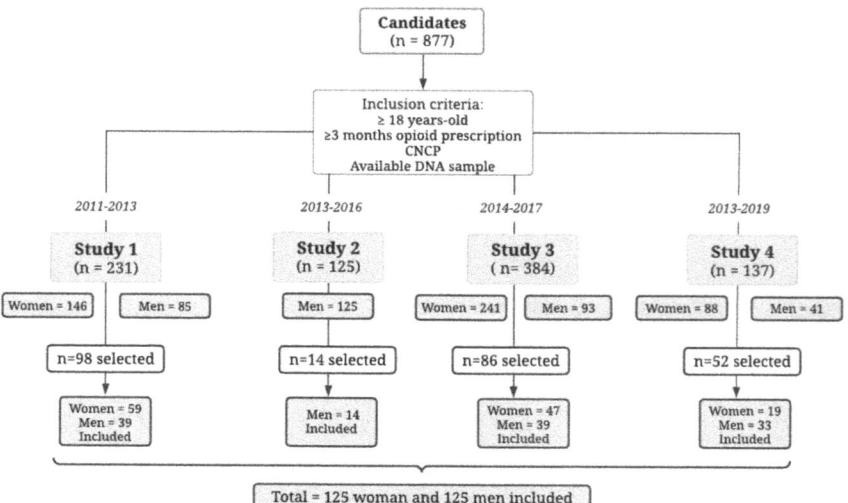

Figure A1. Flow chart of the included patients and their studies of provenance. CNCP, chronic noncancer pain.

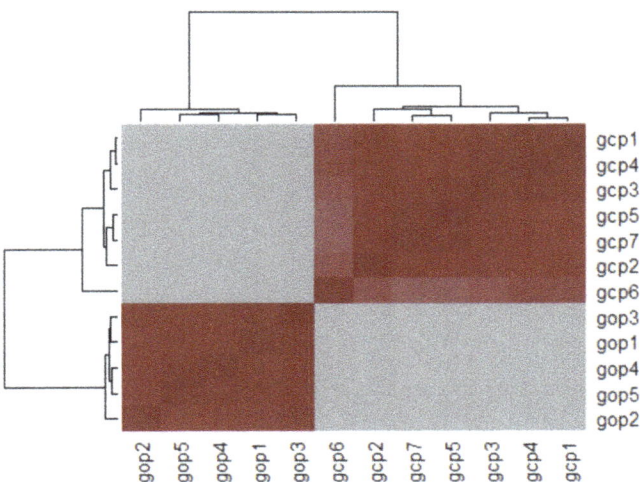

Figure A2. Degree of association between the methylation value of the different sites of OPRM1 (gene OPRM1 position, gop 1 to 5) and COMT (gene COMT position, gcp 1 to 7) genes. The intense garnet colours correspond to very high degrees of association.

Table A1. Primers used in the pyrosequencing assay.

Primer	Sequence	CpG sites
OPRM1_F1	5′-GGATTGGTTTTTGTAAGAAATAGTAGG-3′	
OPRM1_R1	5′-ATACRCCAAAACATCAATACAATTACTAAC-3′	
OPRM1_S1	5′-AAGTTTYGGTGTTTTTGGTTA-3′	CpG 7–11
COMT_F1	5′-GTGGGGTTTTTGGGGTAGT-3′	
COMT _R1	5′-ATCTAACCAACRCTCTCACCTCTCCC-3′	
COMT _S1	5′-GGGTTTTTGGGGTAGTTA-3′	CpG 37–42

Table A2. Pharmacological data in the total population according to sex.

	Total n = 250	Females n = 125	Males n = 125
Main opioid (%)			
Buprenorphine	5	2	9
Fentanyl	24	26	22
Morphine	8	5	11
Oxycodone	19	25	13
Tapentadol	31	29	33
Tramadol	12	14	11

References

1. Louwies, T.; Greenwood-Van Meerveld, B. Sex Differences in the Epigenetic Regulation of Chronic Visceral Pain Following Unpredictable Early Life Stress. *Neurogastroenterol. Motil.* **2020**, *32*, e13751. [CrossRef] [PubMed]
2. Kubota, T. Epigenetic Effect of Environmental Factors on Neurodevelopmenal Disorders. *Jpn. J. Hyg.* **2016**, *71*, 200–207. [CrossRef]
3. Sorge, R.E.; Totsch, S.K. Sex Differences in Pain. *J. Neurosci. Res.* **2017**, *95*, 1271–1281. [CrossRef]
4. Osborne, V.; Serdarevic, M.; Crooke, H.; Striley, C.; Cottler, L.B. Non-Medical Opioid Use in Youth: Gender Differences in Risk Factors and Prevalence. *Addict. Behav.* **2017**, *72*, 114–119. [CrossRef]

5. Nasser, S.A.; Afify, E.A. Sex Differences in Pain and Opioid Mediated Antinociception: Modulatory Role of Gonadal Hormones. *Life Sci.* **2019**, *237*, 116926. [CrossRef]
6. Pieretti, S.; Di Giannuario, A.; Di Giovannandrea, R.; Marzoli, F.; Piccaro, G.; Minosi, P.; Aloisi, A.M. Gender Differences in Pain and Its Relief. *Ann. Dell'istituto Super. Di Sanita* **2016**, *52*, 184–189. [CrossRef]
7. Pisanu, C.; Franconi, F.; Gessa, G.L.; Mameli, S.; Pisanu, G.M.; Campesi, I.; Leggio, L.; Agabio, R. Sex Differences in the Response to Opioids for Pain Relief: A Systematic Review and Meta-Analysis. *Pharmacol. Res.* **2019**, *148*, 104447. [CrossRef] [PubMed]
8. Oertel, B.G.; Doehring, A.; Roskam, B.; Kettner, M.; Hackmann, N.; Ferreirós, N.; Schmidt, P.H.; Lötsch, J. Genetic-Epigenetic Interaction Modulates μ-Opioid Receptor Regulation. *Hum. Mol. Genet.* **2012**, *21*, 4751–4760. [CrossRef] [PubMed]
9. Chlamydas, S.; Markouli, M.; Strepkos, D.; Piperi, C. Epigenetic Mechanisms Regulate Sex-Specific Bias in Disease Manifestations. *J. Mol. Med.* **2022**, *100*, 1111–1123. [CrossRef] [PubMed]
10. Fillingim, R.B.; King, C.D.; Ribeiro-Dasilva, M.C.; Rahim-Williams, B.; Riley, J.L. Sex, Gender, and Pain: A Review of Recent Clinical and Experimental Findings. *J. Pain* **2009**, *10*, 447–485. [CrossRef]
11. Mogil, J.S.; Bailey, A.L. Sex and Gender Differences in Pain and Analgesia. *Prog. Brain Res.* **2010**, *186*, 140–157. [CrossRef]
12. Diatchenko, L.; Slade, G.D.; Nackley, A.G.; Bhalang, K.; Sigurdsson, A.; Belfer, I.; Goldman, D.; Xu, K.; Shabalina, S.A.; Shagin, D.; et al. Genetic Basis for Individual Variations in Pain Perception and the Development of a Chronic Pain Condition. *Hum. Mol. Genet.* **2005**, *14*, 135–143. [CrossRef]
13. Bartley, E.J.; Fillingim, R.B. Sex Differences in Pain: A Brief Review of Clinical and Experimental Findings. *Br. J. Anaesth.* **2013**, *111*, 52–58. [CrossRef] [PubMed]
14. Bagot, R.C.; Meaney, M.J. Epigenetics and the Biological Basis of Gene × Environment Interactions. *J. Am. Acad. Child Adolesc. Psychiatry* **2010**, *49*, 752–771. [CrossRef]
15. Owusu Obeng, A.; Hamadeh, I.; Smith, M. Review of Opioid Pharmacogenetics and Considerations for Pain Management. *Pharmacotherapy* **2017**, *37*, 1105–1121. [CrossRef]
16. Yoshida, K.; Nishizawa, D.; Ide, S.; Ichinohe, T.; Fukuda, K.I.; Ikeda, K. A Pharmacogenetics Approach to Pain Management. *Neuropsychopharmacol. Rep.* **2018**, *38*, 2–8. [CrossRef]
17. Muriel, J.; Margarit, C.; Barrachina, J.; Ballester, P.; Flor, A.; Morales, D.; Horga, J.F.; Fernández, E.; Peiró, A.M. Pharmacogenetics and Prediction of Adverse Events in Prescription Opioid Use Disorder Patients. *Basic Clin. Pharmacol. Toxicol.* **2019**, *124*, 439–448. [CrossRef]
18. Sia, A.T.; Lim, Y.; Lim, E.C.P.; Ocampo, C.E.; Lim, W.Y.; Cheong, P.; Tan, E.C. Influence of Mu-Opioid Receptor Variant on Morphine Use and Self-Rated Pain Following Abdominal Hysterectomy. *J. Pain* **2013**, *14*, 1045–1052. [CrossRef] [PubMed]
19. Somogyi, A.A.; Coller, J.K.; Barratt, D.T. Pharmacogenetics of Opioid Response. *Clin. Pharmacol. Ther.* **2015**, *97*, 125–127. [CrossRef]
20. Crews, K.R.; Monte, A.A.; Huddart, R.; Caudle, K.E.; Kharasch, E.D.; Gaedigk, A.; Dunnenberger, H.M.; Leeder, J.S.; Callaghan, J.T.; Samer, C.F.; et al. Clinical Pharmacogenetics Implementation Consortium Guideline for CYP2D6, OPRM1, and COMT Genotypes and Select Opioid Therapy. *Clin. Pharmacol. Ther.* **2021**, *110*, 888–896. [CrossRef] [PubMed]
21. Swiergiel, A.H.; Juszczak, G.R.; Stankiewicz, A.M. Genetic and Epigenetic Mechanisms Linking Pain and Psychiatric Disorders. *Pain Psychiatr. Disord.* **2015**, *30*, 120–137.
22. Polli, A.; Ickmans, K.; Godderis, L.; Nijs, J. When Environment Meets Genetics: A Clinical Review of the Epigenetics of Pain, Psychological Factors, and Physical Activity. *Arch. Phys. Med. Rehabil.* **2019**, *100*, 1153–1161. [CrossRef] [PubMed]
23. Planelles, B.; Margarit, C.; Ajo, R.; Sastre, Y.; Muriel, J.; Inda, M.-D.; Esteban, M.D.; Peiró, A.M. Health Benefits of an Adverse Events Reporting System for Chronic Pain Patients Using Long-Term Opioids. *Acta Anaesthesiol. Scand.* **2019**, *63*, 248–258. [CrossRef] [PubMed]
24. Margarit, C.; Roca, R.; Inda, M.D.; Muriel, J.; Ballester, P.; Moreu, R.; Conte, A.L.; Nunez, A.; Morales, D.; Peiro, A.M. Genetic Contribution in Low Back Pain: A Prospective Genetic Association Study. *Pain Pract.* **2019**, *19*, 836–847. [CrossRef]
25. Barrachina, J.; Muriel, J.; Margarit, C.; Planelles, B.; Ballester, P.; Richart-Martínez, M.; Cutillas, E.; Zandonai, T.; Morales, D.; Peiró, A.M. Global Pain State Questionnaire: Reliability, Validity, and Gender Gap. *Arch. Intern. Med. Res.* **2021**, *4*, 91–113. [CrossRef]
26. Snaith, R.P. The Hospital Anxiety And Depression Scale. *Health Qual Life Outcomes.* **2003**, *1*, 29. [CrossRef]
27. Pergolizzi, J.; Böger, R.H.; Budd, K.; Dahan, A.; Erdine, S.; Hans, G.; Kress, H.G.; Langford, R.; Likar, R.; Raffa, R.B.; et al. Opioids and the Management of Chronic Severe Pain in the Elderly: Consensus Statement of an International Expert Panel with Focus on the Six Clinically Most Often Used World Health Organization Step III Opioids (Buprenorphine, Fentanyl, Hydromorphone, Methadone, Morphine, Oxycodone). *Pain Pract.* **2008**, *8*, 287–313. [CrossRef]
28. Nielsen, D.A.; Yuferov, V.; Hamon, S.; Jackson, C.; Ho, A.; Ott, J.; Kreek, M.J. Increased OPRM1 DNA Methylation in Lymphocytes of Methadone-Maintained Former Heroin Addicts. *Neuropsychopharmacology* **2009**, *34*, 867–873. [CrossRef] [PubMed]
29. Zhong, J.; Chen, X.; Wu, N.; Shen, C.; Cui, H.; Du, W.; Zhang, Z.; Feng, M.; Liu, J.; Lin, S.; et al. Catechol-O-Methyltransferase Promoter Hypomethylation Is Associated with the Risk of Coronary Heart Disease. *Exp. Ther. Med.* **2016**, *12*, 3445–3449. [CrossRef]
30. Kulis, M.; Esteller, M. Chapter 2—DNA Methylation and Cancer. *Adv. Genet.* **2010**, *70*, 27–56. [CrossRef]
31. Viet, C.T.; Dang, D.; Aouizerat, B.E.; Miaskowski, C.; Ye, Y.; Viet, D.T.; Ono, K.; Schmidt, B.L. OPRM1 Methylation Contributes to Opioid Tolerance in Cancer Patients. *J. Pain* **2017**, *18*, 1046–1059. [CrossRef] [PubMed]

32. Ebrahimi, G.; Asadikaram, G.; Akbari, H.; Nematollahi, M.H.; Abolhassani, M.; Shahabinejad, G.; Khodadadnejad, L.; Hashemi, M. Elevated Levels of DNA Methylation at the OPRM1 Promoter Region in Men with Opioid Use Disorder. *Am. J. Drug Alcohol Abus.* **2018**, *44*, 193–199. [CrossRef] [PubMed]
33. Nielsen, R.; Korneliussen, T.; Albrechtsen, A.; Li, Y.; Wang, J. SNP Calling, Genotype Calling, and Sample Allele Frequency Estimation from New-Generation Sequencing Data. *PLoS ONE* **2012**, *7*, e37558. [CrossRef] [PubMed]
34. Sandoval-Sierra, J.V.; Salgado García, F.I.; Brooks, J.H.; Derefinko, K.J.; Mozhui, K. Effect of Short-Term Prescription Opioids on DNA Methylation of the OPRM1 Promoter. *Clin. Epigenetics* **2020**, *12*, 76. [CrossRef]
35. Kawarai, Y.; Jang, S.H.; Lee, S.; Millecamps, M.; Kang, H.M.; Gregoire, S.; Suzuki-Narita, M.; Ohtori, S.; Stone, L.S. Exercise Attenuates Low Back Pain and Alters Epigenetic Regulation in Intervertebral Discs in a Mouse Model. *Spine J.* **2021**, *21*, 1938–1949. [CrossRef] [PubMed]
36. Grégoire, S.; Jang, S.H.; Szyf, M.; Stone, L.S. Prenatal Maternal Stress Is Associated with Increased Sensitivity to Neuropathic Pain and Sex-Specific Changes in Supraspinal MRNA Expression of Epigenetic- and Stress-Related Genes in Adulthood. *Behav. Brain Res.* **2020**, *380*, 112396. [CrossRef] [PubMed]
37. Stephens, K.E.; Zhou, W.; Ji, Z.; Chen, Z.; He, S.; Ji, H.; Guan, Y.; Taverna, S.D. Sex Differences in Gene Regulation in the Dorsal Root Ganglion after Nerve Injury. *BMC Genom.* **2019**, *20*, 147. [CrossRef]
38. Uddin, M.; Sipahi, L.; Li, J.; Koenen, K.C. Sex Differences in Dna Methylation May Contribute to Risk of PTSD and Depression: A Review of Existing Evidence. *Depress Anxiety* **2013**, *30*, 1151–1160. [CrossRef] [PubMed]
39. Chidambaran, V.; Zhang, X.; Martin, L.J.; Ding, L.; Weirauch, M.T.; Geisler, K.; Stubbeman, B.L.; Sadhasivam, S.; Ji, H. Dna Methylation at the Mu-1 Opioid Receptor Gene (OPRM1) Promoter Predicts Preoperative, Acute, and Chronic Postsurgical Pain after Spine Fusion. *Pharm. Pers. Med.* **2017**, *10*, 157–168. [CrossRef]
40. Tammimäki, A.; Männistö, P.T. Catechol-O-Methyltransferase Gene Polymorphism and Chronic Human Pain: A Systematic Review and Meta-Analysis. *Pharm. Genom.* **2012**, *22*, 673–691. [CrossRef]
41. Fageera, W.; Chaumette, B.; Fortier, M.È.; Grizenko, N.; Labbe, A.; Sengupta, S.M.; Joober, R. Association between COMT Methylation and Response to Treatment in Children with ADHD. *J. Psychiatr. Res.* **2021**, *135*, 86–93. [CrossRef]
42. Liu, P.; Xing, B.; Chu, Z.; Liu, F.; Lei, G.; Zhu, L.; Gao, Y.; Chen, T.; Dang, Y.H. Dopamine D3 Receptor Knockout Mice Exhibit Abnormal Nociception in a Sex-Different Manner. *J. Neurosci. Res.* **2017**, *95*, 1438–1445. [CrossRef] [PubMed]
43. Hagiwara, H.; Funabashi, T.; Akema, T.; Kimura, F. Sex-Specific Differences in Pain Response by Dopamine in the Bed Nucleus of the Stria Terminalis in Rats. *Neuroreport* **2013**, *24*, 181–185. [CrossRef] [PubMed]
44. Mione, V.; Canterini, S.; Brunamonti, E.; Pani, P.; Donno, F.; Fiorenza, M.T.; Ferraina, S. Both the COMT Val158Met Single-Nucleotide Polymorphism and Sex-Dependent Differences Influence Response Inhibition. *Front. Behav. Neurosci.* **2015**, *9*, 127. [CrossRef] [PubMed]
45. Papaleo, F.; Erickson, L.; Liua, G.; Chena, J.; Weinberger, D.R. Effects of Sex and COMT Genotype on Environmentally Modulated Cognitive Control in Mice. *Proc. Natl. Acad. Sci. USA* **2012**, *109*, 20160–20165. [CrossRef] [PubMed]
46. Tunbridge, E.M.; Harrison, P.J. Importance of the COMT Gene for Sex Differences in Brain Function and Predisposition to Psychiatric Disorders. *Biol. Basis Sex Differ. Psychopharmacol.* **2011**, *8*, 119–140. [CrossRef]
47. Roberto, K.A.; Reynolds, S.G. Older Women's Experiences with Chronic Pain: Daily Challenges and Self-Care Practices. *J. Women Aging* **2002**, *14*, 5–23. [CrossRef]
48. Votaw, V.R.; McHugh, R.K.; Witkiewitz, K. Alcohol Use Disorder and Motives for Prescription Opioid Misuse: A Latent Class Analysis. *Subst. Use Misuse* **2019**, *54*, 1558–1568. [CrossRef]
49. McLean, C.P.; Anderson, E.R. Brave Men and Timid Women? A Review of the Gender Differences in Fear and Anxiety. *Clin. Psychol. Rev.* **2009**, *29*, 496–505. [CrossRef]
50. Peltier, M.R.; Sofuoglu, M.; Petrakis, I.L.; Stefanovics, E.; Rosenheck, R.A. Sex Differences in Opioid Use Disorder Prevalence and Multimorbidity Nationally in the Veterans Health Administration. *J. Dual Diagn.* **2021**, *17*, 124–134. [CrossRef]
51. Moran, L.M.; Kowalczyk, W.J.; Phillips, K.A.; Vahabzadeh, M.; Lin, J.L.; Mezghanni, M.; Epstein, D.H.; Preston, K.L. Sex Differences in Daily Life Stress and Craving in Opioid-Dependent Patients. *Am. J. Drug Alcohol Abus.* **2018**, *44*, 512–523. [CrossRef] [PubMed]
52. Ruiz-Cantero, M.T.; Blasco-Blasco, M.; Chilet-Rosell, E.; Peiró, A.M. Gender Bias in Therapeutic Effort: From Research to Health Care. *Farm. Hosp.* **2020**, *44*, 109–113. [PubMed]
53. Schäfer, G.; Prkachin, K.M.; Kaseweter, K.A.; Williams, A.C.D.C. Health Care Providers' Judgments in Chronic Pain: The Influence of Gender and Trustworthiness. *Pain* **2016**, *157*, 1618–1625. [CrossRef] [PubMed]

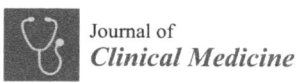

Journal of
Clinical Medicine

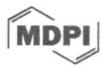

Article

Current Evidence for Biological Biomarkers and Mechanisms Underlying Acute to Chronic Pain Transition across the Pediatric Age Spectrum

Irina T. Duff [1], Kristen N. Krolick [2], Hana Mohamed Mahmoud [2] and Vidya Chidambaran [2,*]

[1] Department of Neurosurgery, Johns Hopkins University, Baltimore, MD 21218, USA; iduff.md@gmail.com
[2] Department of Anesthesia, Cincinnati Children's Hospital, Cincinnati, OH 45242, USA;
kristen.krolick@cchmc.org (K.N.K.); hmmahmou@purdue.edu (H.M.M.)
[*] Correspondence: vidya.chidambaran@cchmc.org; Tel.: +1-15136368021

Abstract: Chronic pain is highly prevalent in the pediatric population. Many factors are involved in the transition from acute to chronic pain. Currently, there are conceptual models proposed, but they lack a mechanistically sound integrated theory considering the stages of child development. Objective biomarkers are critically needed for the diagnosis, risk stratification, and prognosis of the pathological stages of pain chronification. In this article, we summarize the current evidence on mechanisms and biomarkers of acute to chronic pain transitions in infants and children through the developmental lens. The goal is to identify gaps and outline future directions for basic and clinical research toward a developmentally informed theory of pain chronification in the pediatric population. At the outset, the importance of objective biomarkers for chronification of pain in children is outlined, followed by a summary of the current evidence on the mechanisms of acute to chronic pain transition in adults, in order to contrast with the developmental mechanisms of pain chronification in the pediatric population. Evidence is presented to show that chronic pain may have its origin from insults early in life, which prime the child for the development of chronic pain in later life. Furthermore, available genetic, epigenetic, psychophysical, electrophysiological, neuroimaging, neuroimmune, and sex mechanisms are described in infants and older children. In conclusion, future directions are discussed with a focus on research gaps, translational and clinical implications. Utilization of developmental mechanisms framework to inform clinical decision-making and strategies for prevention and management of acute to chronic pain transitions in children, is highlighted.

Keywords: chronic pain; chronification of pain; molecular markers; biomarkers; mechanisms; pediatric pain; developmental; peripheral sensitization; central sensitization; neuroimaging of pain; genetics and epigenetics of pain; neurophysiological markers; EEG; QST

Citation: Duff, I.T.; Krolick, K.N.; Mahmoud, H.M.; Chidambaran, V. Current Evidence for Biological Biomarkers and Mechanisms Underlying Acute to Chronic Pain Transition across the Pediatric Age Spectrum. *J. Clin. Med.* **2023**, *12*, 5176. https://doi.org/10.3390/jcm12165176

Academic Editors: Andrea Polli and Jo Nijs

Received: 5 July 2023
Revised: 1 August 2023
Accepted: 5 August 2023
Published: 9 August 2023

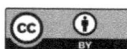

1. Introduction

Acute pain in children (postsurgical, inflammatory, posttraumatic pain or due to other pathologies) is typically protective, subsiding within 14 days, depending on the extent of injury. However, acute to chronic pain transitions are increasingly being described in literature. Chronic pain as a continuum that develops earlier in life is suggested by the evidence that 17% of adults with chronic pain report onset of pain in childhood [1]. In fact, about 20–40% of acute pediatric pain has the potential to transition into chronic pain in children and adolescents [2–6]. Studying chronic pain transitions in the pediatric age group is of utmost importance because (a) children experiencing chronic pain have a ≈3- to 6-fold higher risk of developing chronic pain and disability in adulthood, such that 40–60% of children with chronic pain continue to experience pain as adults [7]; (b) chronic pain in children has greater socioeconomic consequences with a high financial burden [8], stemming from psychosocial and physical disabilities [9,10], impacting quality of life and development of children negatively; and (c) maturational development of the pain connectome is a dynamic process [11], emphasizing neurodevelopmental differences between children, adolescents, and adults' nociception [12].

In fact, secondary chronic pain such as chronic post-surgical pain has been recognized as an independent entity by being included as a diagnosis under the 11th version of the International Classification of Diseases (ICD-11) [13]. However, the need remains for pediatric specifications for primary pain diagnoses in the ICD-11 [14]. Chronic pain is known to be a complex experience with biological, psychological, and social components. While psychosocial aspects of pain chronification have received much consideration, the biological biomarkers and mechanisms in the pediatric age group have received less attention in the literature, although they are very interrelated. The biological components of pain include sensory and autonomic components of the peripheral and the central nervous system. Neuroendocrine, immune, and genomic mechanisms also participate in injury-induced pain response and chronification of acute pain. This article is stratified by age, and sex as a biological variable has been included in relevant sections.

Currently, there are conceptual models proposed for pain chronification in the pediatric population [15,16], but there exists a need for an integrated theory explaining the mechanisms of acute to chronic pediatric pain transition, factoring in the stages of child development. For example, the narrative for mechanisms of chronic pain development and maintenance has shifted from nociception to mesolimbic circuitry in the brain [11,17]. Thus, clinical practice would be better guided by objective biomarkers with the potential to capture the pathological stages of pain chronification. In this article, we review current evidence on mechanisms and biomarkers of acute to chronic pain transitions in infants, children, and adolescents. The available evidence is reviewed in a way that clinicians can integrate the evidence into their daily clinical practice. In addition, this state-of-the-art review article also serves researchers to build upon the best evidence for designing and developing future innovative trials and implementation studies rooted in regarding the biology of chronic pain. Our goal is to help identify gaps and outline future directions for basic and clinical research towards a developmentally informed theory of pain chronification in the pediatric population. We start by outlining the importance of objective biomarkers for chronification of pain in children. Next, we summarize current evidence on the mechanisms of acute to chronic pain transition in adults to draw the contrast with the current evidence on biomarkers of pain chronification in infants, children, and adolescents. Finally, we present a detailed summary of the multifaceted evidence informing developmentally informed mechanisms for transitioning of acute pediatric pain into a chronic state. We conclude our review by discussing future directions, gaps, and clinical implications.

2. State-of-the-Art Review

2.1. Importance of Objective Biomarkers

In 2006, the Initiative on Methods, Measurement, and Pain Assessment in Clinical Trials (PedIMMPACT) identified eight core outcome domains for clinical trials of pain interventions in children, which included pain intensity, physical functioning, symptoms/adverse events, global satisfaction with treatment, emotional functioning, role functioning, sleep, and economic factors [18]. In 2021, this core set of outcome measures was updated, with biomarkers identified as an emerging priority [19]. Biomarkers are objective measures of biological or pathological processes, or a pharmacological response to therapeutic intervention [20]. A joint FDA-NIH working group for developing biomarker endpoints and other tools identified seven distinct biomarker categories that could be applied across all areas of biological research [20]. Three categories of biomarkers that could be of special importance in chronic pain development in children are predictive, prognostic, and susceptibility/risk biomarkers. Susceptibility/risk and prognostic biomarkers would identify the likelihood (risk stratification) and progression of chronic pain development in children, respectively. Examples are genetic tests, neurophysiological measures, and quantitative sensory tests. Predictive biomarkers would help clinicians to identify patients with a higher chance of responding either favorably or unfavorably to pain treatment. An example is microRNA, *miR-548d*, levels for response to intravenous ketamine in complex regional pain syndrome [21].

Biomarkers for pediatric acute to chronic pain transition are still in the discovery stage. Examples of genetic biomarkers are gene expression changes, single-nucleotide polymorphisms (SNPs), patterns of open or closed chromatin, or polygenic risk scores (PRS). For example, PRS from a panel of 20 variants has been proposed for chronic post-surgical pain (CPSP) in children undergoing spine fusion [5]. Following validation across different cohorts and use of laboratory techniques, genetic biomarkers could be useful for personalizing pain management. Due to use of selective cases and controls for genome-wide association studies (GWAS) [22], PRS score use may not be generalizable across all patient populations. Moreover, pediatric populations and people of non-European descent are not well represented in research studies or within large databases such as the UK Biobank [23], making large-scale studies difficult. In addition, epigenetic changes, such as DNA methylation, can arise from environmental impacts and be passed on mitotically [24], leading to long-term alterations in the regulation of genes with long-term impacts on disease phenotypes [25]. For this reason, the study of DNA methylation or other epigenetic processes in blood for use as biomarkers of acute to chronic pain transition is relevant. For example, DNA methylation levels of 5′-cytosine-phosphate-guanine (CpG) sites in major stress genes in patients aged 18–65 years-old revealed distinct methylation differences predictive of chronic pain symptoms 6 months after injury [26]. In general, pediatric -omics big data are not currently available to conduct large-scale research in pediatric phenotypes. One way to circumvent such handicaps may be the use of systems biology approaches to understand functional pathways associated with CPSP, leveraging evidence from already available animal and human literature [27].

Altered functional connectivity has been identified as a neuroimaging biomarker of chronic pain after acute brain injury in adults - reduced negative functional connectivity of the nucleus accumbens (NAc) with a primary motor cortex region was reported in those who developed chronic pain [28]. Adult patient-specific immune biomarkers, assessed by mass cytometry for single-type specific intracellular signaling molecules, were also predictive of patients' speed of recovery from surgical pain [29]. As these previous examples were performed in adults, pediatric-population-specific biomarkers are needed. In later sections, we discuss any evidence available from the pediatric literature. It is important to recognize that chronic pain is a complex disease, and utilization of several distinct biomarkers together, such as neuroimaging combined with PRS, may better represent the variable etiology and sub-phenotypes of chronic pain.

2.2. Developmental Mechanisms of Pain Chronification

Peripheral and central mechanisms of chronification of pain in adults have been described previously [30,31]. A diagrammatic presentation of these mechanisms is presented in Figure 1. While we acknowledge the pediatric literature remains scarce compared to adults, with gaps in understanding, we present a visual basis of known mechanisms of chronification of pain with pediatric developmental context (from animal/human studies) denoted in blue font in Figure 1, overlaid on the known mechanisms in adults (black lettered headings). The evidence from pediatric studies may be mixed or even contradictory, depending on context, but a detailed description of such nuances is beyond the scope of this review. For example, the direction of connectivity between specific brain regions within the default mode network is different within the same pain condition (for example: lower resting-state connectivity between the posterior cingulate and insula, but greater functional connectivity between the thalamus and posterior cingulate in children with irritable bowel syndrome) or opposite between pain conditions (for example, connectivity was higher, not lower, in complex regional pain syndrome) [32].

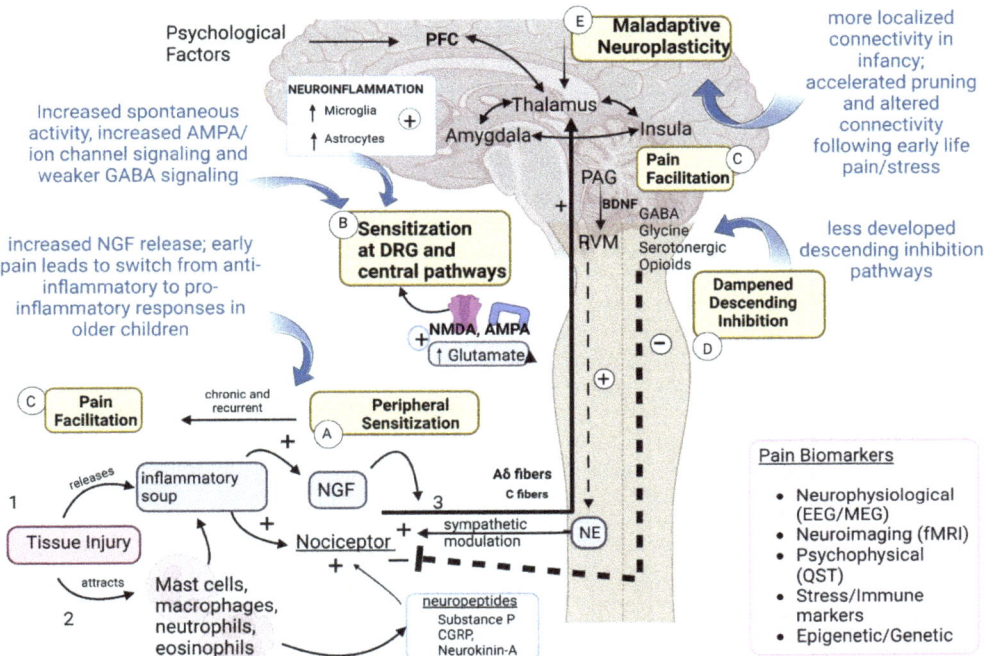

Figure 1. Peripheral and central mechanisms associated with chronification of pain with relevance to the pediatric population (based on animal studies). The main adult mechanisms are mentioned in bold black color denoted by letters, with pediatric-specific features that contribute to pain chronification overlaid in blue-colored text. Figure depicts (1) tissue injury as an acute injury, which then (2) recruits mast cells, macrophages, neutrophils, and eosinophils to the area. Both these cells and tissue injury all contribute to release of the inflammatory soup (proinflammatory cytokines, prostaglandins, histamine, nitric oxide, serotonin, and NGF), which increases NGF. (3) NGF binds to TrkA at peripheral ends of the sensory nerve fibers (C-fiber and A-δ fibers), leading to upregulation and stimulation of Na$^+$ channels and causes peripheral sensitization (A). When NGF binds to TrkA on afferent inputs inside the dorsal root ganglion of the spinal cord, it prolongs their stimulation and increases glutamate release onto NMDA and AMPA receptors, resulting in central sensitization at the level of the spinal cord dorsal root ganglion (B), while neuroinflammation due to increased microglia and astrocyte responses leads to central sensitization (B). This is also facilitated by weaker GABA signaling and increased spontaneous firing. Chronic/recurrent stimulation and activation of PAG results in release of BDNF into the RVM, and BDNF-TrkB signaling leads to pain facilitation (C). Decreases in GABA, glycine, serotonergic, and opioid responses, leading to decreased inhibitory sympathetic output, contributing to pain sensitization, also known as decreased descending inhibition (D). Lastly, maladaptive neuroplasticity (E) takes place, contributing to central sensitization of pain. Pediatric developmental context from available studies is shown in blue: For example, increased growth factor release by tissue injury in neonatal rats [33], nerve injury in neonatal rats produces more anti-inflammatory responses and descending inhibition is not developed [34–36], earlier synaptic pruning, altered pain connectivity and myelination [32]. Abbreviations: α-amino-3-hydroxy-5-methylisoxazole-4-propionic acid (AMPA), brain-derived neurotrophic factor (BDNF), calcitonin gene-related peptide (CGRP), dorsal root ganglion (DRG), electroencephalography (EEG), functional magnetic resonance imaging (fMRI), γ-aminobutyric acid (GABA), magnetoencephalography (MEG), nerve growth factor (NGF), N-methyl-D-aspartic acid (NMDA), norepinephrine (NE), periaqueductal gray (PAG), prefrontal cortex (PFC), quantitative sensory testing (QST), rostral ventromedial medulla (RVM), tropomyosin-related kinase A (TrkA). Created with BioRender.com.

Also, the bulk of the literature on developmental mechanisms are from animal studies. The reader is referred to a recent review published by our team [37] for a comprehensive understanding of animal models that currently exist to study acute to chronic pain transition in the pediatric population and the limitations of such models. Briefly, the following rodent models exist for studying pain: local or systemic injections of inflammatory agents into hindpaw or intraperitoneally to model local and systemic inflammation respectively (e.g., see [38–40]); transient compression of cervical nerve [41] and spared nerve injury [42,43] models to study neuropathic pain; neonatal manipulations such as repetitive needle pricks [44], injections [45,46], and nonpainful tactile stimulation [47] with or without maternal separation to model and study the stressors neonates experience in the NICU; and hindpaw incision [48,49], which can be used to model pain after surgery [50]. However, as mentioned in our last review, few of these models have been used to study acute to chronic pain transition, with even fewer modeling pediatric age ranges. It is promising though that for adult age ranges, similar genetic and epigenetic findings between humans who experience chronic pain and rodent models are beginning to be found [37].

Animal studies have shown us that the consequences of early life injury vary depending on the type of injury, the sensory modality, and the timing of injury. For instance, repetitive needle pricking of the paw during the first week after birth can result in heat hypersensitivity several weeks later [51]. However, neonatal hindpaw inflammation has a significant impact on behavioral responses and dorsal horn cell activity during a subsequent inflammatory challenge in adulthood [52], but does not induce prolonged heat or mechanical hypersensitivity beyond the first week [53]. Thus, hindpaw inflammation leads to a generalized and slowly developing reduction in baseline sensitivity throughout the body in response to mechanical and thermal stimuli with an increased chance for inflammation later in life. Early life injury can also have the opposite effect. Repetitive formalin injections into neonatal paws can result in generalized heat hypoalgesia in adulthood [54]. These early onset inflammatory hyperalgesia and later-onset baseline hypoalgesia occur only if the original inflammatory stimulus is applied within the first 10 days of life, and both responses persist into adulthood. Long-term hypoalgesia affecting the entire body likely arises from changes in stress response, as exposure to stress during the perinatal period is known to influence nociceptive behavior in adulthood [55]. This adaptation could be seen as a useful response to early trauma. Any long-term sensitization occurring at the segmental level may remain masked and require a strong stimulus, such as second inflammation, to uncover it. In contrast, chemical or mechanical irritation of the colon in rats aged P8–21 leads to persistent visceral hypersensitivity in adulthood [56]. Neuropathic pain development after early life nerve injury presents a different picture—while partial peripheral nerve damage in adult rodents leads to significant and prolonged neuropathic pain behavior characterized by marked allodynia, this does not occur in rat pups up to P21 [34]. Tight ligation of the fifth and sixth lumbar spinal nerves during the first two postnatal weeks produces only transient mechanical allodynia [35], and no changes in sensitivity occur in the spared nerve injury and chronic constriction injury models until P28 [34].

There are several explanations for these findings, including one that it takes time for ascending and descending pathways to form (Figure 1). Also, infant nerve injury triggers an ani-inflammatory immune response in the dorsal horn of the spinal cord (increased interleukin (IL)-4 and IL-10), which is protective. However, after adolescence (post-natal day 25–30), the immune profile of the dorsal horn switches to producing tumor necrosis factor (TNF) and BDNF, pro-inflammatory factors associated with late onset neuropathic pain behavior [36] (Figure 1). Thus, while the neonatal brain and nervous system protect from developing neuropathic pain at this period of time, they still prime it for reactivation later in life if a second injury takes place [36]. Neonatal rats also experience much higher concentrations of growth factors (Figure 1) released by tissue injuries compared to adults, which can influence the development of peripheral nociceptors in various ways [33]. Thus, nerve growth factor (NGF) signaling through trkA receptors leads to enhanced glutamatergic transmission after neonatal incision during a critical time window (first post-natal week) characterized by higher spontaneous signaling and highly sensitive somatosensory circuits, unlike in adults [57–59]. Similarly, in the first 2 weeks after birth, neonatal incision increases calcium-permeable AMPA receptors and other ion channel signaling, leading to spike timing-dependent long-term potentiation of responses [60]. Inhibitory synaptic signaling mediated by GABA or glycine is thus weaker at early ages in the spinal cord dorsal horn [61].

Normal maturation of nociceptive circuits requires input from tactile receptors, which guide the nociceptive synaptic organization during the critical stage of development mentioned above [62]. As discussed, intrinsically driven spontaneous activity is prevalent in developing nociceptive circuits which makes them particularly susceptible to permanent reorganization (pruning, altered synaptic connectivity), influenced by altered neuroimmune/endocrine functions in response to early exposure to nociceptive stimuli [63,64]. While the central mechanisms behind the long-term changes in pain behavior are not fully understood, potential mechanisms include alterations in synaptic connectivity and signaling within postnatal nociceptive pathways, as well as shifts in the balance between inhibition and excitation. Descending modulation of spinal nociceptive signaling is immature early in life (Figure 1), and importantly, it favors greater nociceptive transmission [65]. In fact, adult modulatory responses are also modified by early exposure to nociceptive stimuli. Also, in rats, the first postnatal week represented a critical period as incision during that stage (P3-6) increases hyperalgesia following repeat surgery two weeks later. Importantly, use of repeat nerve blocks decreased this hyperalgesic response [66]. This has potential clinical implications for the use of regional analgesia for neonatal surgery.

Furthermore, use of functional magnetic resonance imaging (fMRI) revealed differences in infant cerebral processing of pain perception compared to adults [67]. Interestingly, hyperconnectivity of brain regions seen in chronic pain in adults mirror those involved in neuro-affective disorders in childhood [68,69]. Thus, it has been postulated that "speed-up processes" of neural development through childhood involving increased myelin production and selective pruning might facilitate increased early subcortical–cortical connectivity after early life injury, stress, and pain [32,70]. In addition, pain connectomes are more localized (Figure 1) at younger ages [71], defined more by anatomical proximity, which transition into more specialized neural networks with a more distributed architecture by young adulthood. There may also be a role for "microglial priming" and neuro–glial interactions in the spinal cord and brain in chronic, persistent pain. Microglia in the brain monitor the interstitial fluid and in the presence of threat, resulting in exaggerated neuroinflammatory responses with loss of gray matter (GM) and synaptic pruning. These changes may also have an epigenetic basis. In this context, "neonatal nociceptive priming" is a term coined for increased vulnerability to pain sensitivity to injury in later life, due to early life injury. Neuroimmune interactions related to growth hormone signaling have been elucidated in animal models [72]. There is evidence from animal studies for long-lasting epigenetic remodeling of macrophages that might influence pain memory. For example, the p75 neurotrophic factor was found to regulate inflammatory profile and responses in rodent models and may be a mechanism involved in pain chronification in infants [73].

Thus, neurobiological mechanisms underlying pain chronification may be different in children and adolescents compared with adults. Future studies at the intersection of these different mechanistic processes are needed to quantify the pain dose response, critical development periods, and factors involved in the chronification of pediatric pain [74].

2.3. Acute to Chronic Pain Transitions in Infants

2.3.1. Does Neonatal Pain Lead to Chronic Pain Later in Life?

As discussed in the previous section, studies in animals suggest neurotoxic effects of early exposure to pain. An important question remains whether the evidence in animal studies translates to humans. Preterm newborns are known to undergo many potentially painful procedures, including heel sticks, tracheal suctioning, surgeries, etc. On average, it is estimated they are subjected to about 10 daily stress/pain events [75]. In 2005, authors of a cross-sectional study in 164 infants evaluated pain, opioid use, and norepinephrine levels in a subsequent surgery among infants who had major surgery in their first three months of life and compared them to controls. The authors found that, compared to controls, surgery in early infancy led to higher pain as well as higher norepinephrine and opioid requirements when subsequent surgery involved the same dermatomal levels of prior tissue damage [76]. This supports spinal mechanisms of sensitization that could be potentially decreased by use of regional analgesia, as mentioned previously [66]. A stunning statistic revealed by another study evaluating long-term neurobiological, neuropsychological, and sensory development effects of prematurity, procedural pain, and opioids in early neonatal life was that up to 68.4% of children who spend time in the neonatal intensive care unit experienced pain over the 3 months before their visit and 15.8% had chronic pain by ten years of age [77].

An important difference between animal nociceptive studies and neonatal experience is that neonates in the ICU are exposed to not only pain, but also opioids, anesthetics, and other drugs [75,78]. Animal studies on exposure to opioids in early life show opioids were neuroprotective if administrated in the presence of pain and in specific situations [79,80]. A recent meta-analysis showed that a higher number of neonatal pain events, but not opioid administration, in rodents was associated with increased neuronal cell death, increased anxiety, and depressant-like behavior [81]. However, studies in humans show mixed results, which are elucidated in an excellent narrative review [82]. Of note, a longitudinal study found no major effects of neonatal pain nor opioid or anesthetic exposure in the early life in children and young adults (8–19 years of age), using thermal detection, pain thresholds, and high-resolution structural and task-based fMRI during pain. They reported potential neuropsychological effects in the groups with the highest opioid exposure [83], which needs further follow up. Similarly, the study mentioned in the prior paragraph also did not find associations of morphine administration during neonatal life with neurocognitive performance or thermal sensitivity later in childhood [77]. While this is heartening, the authors discuss limitations of sample size and selection bias in their study. In the following sections, we present mechanistic evidence from human studies investigating early pain and stress.

2.3.2. Mechanistic Evidence and Biomarkers for Pain Chronification in INFANTS

(a) Neuroimaging evidence

Neuroplasticity plays a crucial role in the formation of neural circuits and the development of GM, white matter (WM), and RS-FC throughout developmental stages, influencing pain perception [84–86]. Factors such as pain-related stressors, painful procedures, and exposure to morphine in the NICU are associated with lower global brain volumes and reduced GM throughout the brain during childhood [77]. Smaller brain volumes in general are correlated with lower gestational age, a higher number of painful procedures in the first 14 days of life, and higher exposure to morphine in the first 28 days of life [77]. Abnormalities in the microstructure of white matter are linked to a higher number of invasive procedures by the age of 7 and lower cognitive function [87]. The authors of one study compared cerebral pain response in children and adolescents (11–16 years) using fMRI between groups with experience in a NICU after preterm (≤31 weeks gestational age) and full-term birth (≥37 weeks gestational age) with full term control children without early hospitalization. Compared to controls, significant activations in the thalamus, anterior cingulate cortex, cerebellum, basal ganglia, and periaquaeductal gray were found in the NICU groups, as well as higher activations in primary somatosensory cortex, anterior cingulate cortex, and insula in preterm infants [88]. Also, the authors of a different, longitudinal study in children born very preterm (24–32 weeks gestational age) found that neonatal-pain-related stress was associated with a thinner cortex in multiple (21/66) brain regions at school age (mean 7.9 years), independent of other neonatal risk factors [89]. These findings suggest that the developing brain is both adaptable and susceptible, and changes in pain processing circuits in response to nociceptive stimuli can result in long-term anatomical and functional alterations that contribute to lifelong chronic pain. Structural MRI scans and RS-FC functional brain imaging can reveal signs of neonatal injury, surgery, or inflammation, which could serve as biomarkers for preventive medical treatment of postsurgical/posttraumatic pain in adolescence or adulthood, depending on the timing of secondary insult.

(b) Electrophysiological evidence

A wide range of electrophysiological methods are employed to study infant pain processing and the effects of noxious stimulation in both healthy full-term infants and premature infants undergoing multiple procedures in the NICU. These methods include electroencephalography (EEG), magnetoencephalography (MEG), and near-infrared spectroscopy.

Infants who experience stress, multiple medical procedures, or illness exhibit different responses to noxious stimuli. Slater et al. [90] used EEG to determine that noxious-evoked potentials following medically necessary heel lances were larger in ex-premature infants at term-corrected age who had experienced painful procedures in neonatal units, compared to age-matched term-born infants. Jones et al. [91] reported that stress, as measured by salivary cortisol levels, increases noxious-evoked brain activity without a proportional increase in behavioral response. This finding aligns with evidence in adults that stress enhances pain sensitivity [92]. The authors postulated that this disconnect with pain behavior may imply that observation of pain behavior may not be a reliable indicator of pain stress in neonates. Ozawa et al. [93] also demonstrated that prior pain disrupts the relationship between cortical and behavioral measures of pain, emphasizing the need to consider previous experiences when assessing neonatal pain. Prior pain experience from heel lances in the first 24–36 h after birth was reported to elicit pain anticipation and heightened behavioral pain responses to venipuncture in both premature [94] and term-born infants [95]. Importantly, negative responses were mitigated by the use of sucrose [96] and skin-to-skin care [97] during painful procedures.

Mitigation is very important as effects may persist into childhood and adulthood. Children who have experienced early life pain exhibit increased cerebral responses to pain [88] and pain catastrophizing [98]. Additional evidence was derived from a study measuring functional brain activity using MEG and visual-perceptual abilities in school-age children who were born very prematurely (<32 weeks). They demonstrated alterations in spontaneous cortical oscillatory activity and lower perceptual disabilities correlated with cumulative neonatal pain [99], as well as altered network connectivity across standard theta, alpha, beta, and gamma bands in the middle gyrus [100]. This is in line with the thalamo-cortical dysrhythmia model for chronic pain proposed in adults [101,102]. According to this model, abnormal nociceptive input leads to irregular bursts of theta oscillations in the thalamus. These oscillations are then transmitted to the cerebral cortex, resulting in the disinhibition of neighboring areas. Consequently, gamma frequency oscillations occur in the affected regions, leading to the persistence of ongoing pain.

Research on the chronification of pain in infants using electrophysiological markers is still in its early stages. Of note, abnormal neural synchronization [100], low amygdala volumes [77], and altered sub-cortical connectivity [103] have been shown in neuro-affective disorders such as autism. Questions have been raised regarding the potential association of early life stress/pain and life-long influences on neurobehavioral and neuropsychiatric outcomes [104]. In fact, upon implementation of an opioid protocol for NICU babies, Steinbauer et al. reported that the resulting increased neonatal opiate exposure was a potential risk factor for autism spectrum disorder and withdrawn behavior at preschool age. They recommended vigilant use of opiates [105].

(c) Genetics And Epigenetics

To understand how many studies have been performed on potential genetic and epigenetic mechanisms of pain chronification in the human infant population, a scoping search (see supplementary file for search terms) for all evidence of genetic and epigenetic alterations after an infant or neonate is subjugated to a painful event was performed. Twelve human studies (see below), along with two reviews [106,107], were returned. While none of the infant epigenetic and genetic studies quantified pain again later in life to truly represent acute to chronic pain transition, three of the infant studies followed the effect of painful procedures through to 4 years [108], 7 years [109], and 8 years [110] after skin-breaks in the NICU (Figure 2a).

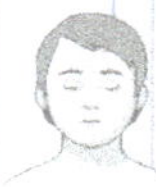

	Author	Year	Age/Sex	Sample Size/ Groups	Gene/ CpG/ SNP Analyzed?	Outcomes
a.	C. M. Chau, M. Ranger, D. Sulistyoningrum, A. M. Devlin, T. F. Oberlander and R. E. Grunau	2014	Male and Female infants	n=61 preterm n = 50 full-term	10 CpG sites of *SLC6A4* promoter . COMT Val158Met and COMT Met/Met genotyped.	Increased methylation in 7/10 CpG sites & increased behavior problems in pre-term born 7-year-olds. Both neontal pain and COMT Met/ Met genotype were associated with increased *SLC6A* methylation.
	L. Provenzi, M. Fumagalli, G. Scotto di Minico, R. Giorda, F. Morandi, I. Sirgiovanni, et al	2020	male and female infants	n=32 preterm n=37 full-term	20 CpG sites of *SLC64A* promotor	Pre-term 4.5 yr olds displayed greater anger in response to an emotional stressor compared to full-term 4.5 yr olds. CpG5 and CpG9m was increased in preterm compared to fullterm. CpG5 and 9 at discharge was significantly associated with increased anger display.
	C.M. Chau, M. Ranger, M. Bichin, M. T. M. Park, R. S.C. Amaral, M. Chakravarty, K. Poskitt, A. R. Synnes, S. P. Miller, and R. E. Grunau	2019	male and female infants	n = 56 total	*COMT*, SLC6A4, and *BDNF* genotyped	COMT 158MetMet and BDNF 66Met allele carriers predicted smaller right hippocampal total and subregional volumes respectively in 8 yr olds..
b.	V. Chidambaran, V. Pilipenko, A. G. Jegga, K. Geisler and L. J. Martin	2021	male and female 10-18 years	n = 53 CPSP; n = 78 non-CPSP spine fusion	Illumina Omni Arrays and previous literature for training set	Twenty variants, annotated to 7 genes: *ATXN1, PRKCA, CACNG2, DRD2, KCNJ3, KCNJ6,* and *KCNK3 made up the PRS for CPSP.*
	V. Chidambaran, X. Zhang, L. Martin, L. Ding, M. Weirauch, K. Geisler, et al	2017	male and female 10-18 years	n= 44 CPSP n=121 non-CPSP spine fusion	22 CpG sites of *OPRM1* promotor	Higher methylation of all sites was associated with higher odds of CPSP. Significant association with nonpromotor sites CpG13 and 22 with CPSP.
	V. Chidambaran, X. Zhang, K. Geisler, B. L. Stubbeman, X. Chen, M. T. Weirauch, et al.	2019	male and mostly female 10-18 years	pilot study n = 15 CPSP n = 40 non-CPSP spine fusion	Human Infinium Methylation Epic microarray	637 CpG sites were differentially methylated in CPSP. Located in genes involved in pathways such as GABA receptor signaling, protein kinase C signaling, dopamine receptor, and cAMP-mediated signaling
	V. Chidambaran, X. Zhang, V. Pilipenko, X. Chen, B. Wronowski, K. Geisler, et al.	2021	male and mostly female 10-18 years	n = 20 CPSP n = 38 non-CPSP spine fusion	Human Omni Arrays for methylation and genotyping	methylation at 127 CpG sites mediated association of 470 methylation quantitative trait (meQTL) with chronic pain. CpG-meQTL in genes: *SLC45A3, NUCKS1, RAB7, RAB7L1, SLC41A1,* and *PM20D1*
	M. Perry, C. B. Sieberg, E. E. Young, K. Baumbauer, V. Singh, C. Wong, et al.	2021	male and mostly female adolescents	n = 13 CPSP n = 23 non-CPSP spine fusion	Whole blood RNA-sequencing	Increased expression of *HLA-DRB3* in CPSP.

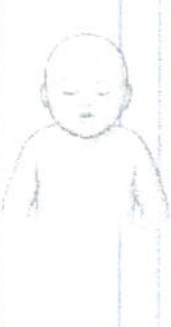

Figure 2. Genetic and epigenetic evidence of acute to chronic pain transition in the pediatric population. Summary of the genetic and epigenetic evidence found for acute to chronic pain transition in the human pediatric population. (**a**) Evidence from infant studies [108–110], and (**b**) from child/adolescent studies [4,5,111–113]. Abbreviations: *Ataxin 1 (ATXN1)*; brain-derived neurotrophic factor (BDNF); chronic postsurgical pain (CPSP); *calcium voltage-gated channel auxiliary subunit gamma 2 (CACNG2); catechol-O-methyltransferase (COMT)*; 5′-cytosine-phosphate-guanine (CpG); *dopamine receptor D2 (DRD2); major histocompatibility complex, class II, DR beta 3 (HLA-DRB3)*; methylation quantitative trait loci (meQTL); *nuclear casein kinase and cyclin-dependent kinase substrate 1 (NUCKS1); opioid receptor mu 1 (OPRM1); peptidase M20 domain-containing 1 (PM20D1)*; polygenic risk score (PRS); *potassium inwardly rectifying channel subfamily J member 3 (KCNJ3); potassium inwardly rectifying channel subfamily J member 6 (KCNJ6); potassium two pore domain channel subfamily K member 3 (KCNK3); protein kinase C alpha (PRKCA); RAB7, member RAS oncogene family (RAB7); RAB7, member RAS oncogene family-like 1 (RAB7L1); solute carrier family 6 member 1 (SLC6A); solute carrier family 41 member 1 (SCL41A1); solute carrier family 45 member 3 (SLC45A3)*. Figure created with BioRender, modified from a template by Ruslan Medzhitov (Creator), Akiko Iwasaki, and Wendy Jiang (See the Supplementary File for details on the search strategy).

Six [108,114–118] out of the twelve human infant studies were by the same team and conducted in Italy between the years of 2015 and 2021. For pre-term infants exposed to high-level, but not low-level, pain-related stress during the NICU stay, as quantified by number of skin break procedures, the methylation of two CpG sites within the *SLC6A4* promotor region increased from birth to discharge [114]. Later, the face-to-face still face paradigm was used as a measure of the mothers' levels of maternal sensitivity. In pre-term infants, and full-term infants of less-sensitive but not sensitive mothers, increased *SLC6A4* methylation at discharge was associated with a higher negative emotionality (stress-response) at 3 months of age [115]. Thus, it was indicated that in full-term but not pre-term infants, maternal sensitivity served as a protective factor against *SLC6A4* epigenetic variations [115]. A limitation of this study was that pain could not be analyzed as a causal factor in pre-term infants, and instead the authors hypothesized that premature separation of mother–infant contact in the NICU could be the cause [115]. In another study, maternal sensitivity as a protective factor was corroborated—low levels of maternal touch intensified the DNA methylation at CpG sites within the *SLC6A4* promotor that were altered by NICU stay [118]. In another study, the authors followed pre-term infants until 4.5 months of age and analyzed their DNA methylation [108]. Pre-term 4.5-year-olds displayed greater anger in response to an emotional stressor compared to full-term 4.5-year-olds. The methylation of two sites, labeled CpG5 and CpG9, was increased in pre-term compared to full-term infants. CpG5 and CpG9 at discharge were significantly associated with increased anger display [115]. Lastly, this group also conducted two studies on pain exposure, as performed in the NICU on very pre-term infants, and telomere length erosion [116,117]. The authors found that preterm infants who experienced high levels of skin-breaking procedures had decreased telomere length from birth to discharge, while preterm infants exposed to low-levels of skin breaking procedures had no significant difference in telomere length [117], and that this decreased telomere length was predictive of a reduced salivary cortisol response to a stressor (still face paradigm) [116].

Three out of the twelve human infant studies were performed by a group located in Canada [109,110,119]. In 2013, they found reduced hair cortisol levels in 7-year-old children born pre-term compared to full-term [119]. Furthermore, the lower cortisol was associated with greater neonatal pain when in the presence of the minor allele, *NFKBIA* rs2233409, in boys but not girls. In 2014, they measured *SLC6A* promoter methylation for children born very pre-term compared to full-term at 7 years of age [109]. The authors found that at 7 years of age, the children born very pre-term had significantly increased child behavioral problems, as measured by the Child Behavior Checklist questionnaire, and they had significantly increased methylation in 7/10 CpG sites in *SLC6A* compared to those children who were born full-term [109]. After correcting for clinical confounders, neonatal pain and the presence of the *COMT* Met/Met genotype were found to be associated with *SLC6A* methylation [109]. In 2019, they found that in the presence of the minor allele *COMT* 158 MetMet, greater neonatal invasive procedures predicted smaller right hippocampal volumes in ≈8-year-old ex-very-pre-term children, and in the presence of the *BDNF* 66Met allele, a greater number of surgeries predicted smaller right hippocampal subregional volumes in ≈8-year-old children born very pre-term [110].

Out of the remaining studies, two were conducted in Pennsylvania, USA, in 2013 [120] and 2018 [121], and one was conducted in Italy in 2020 [122]. In the 2013 study, 16 out of 31 infants undergoing elective surgery were carriers of the MOR 118G allele and exhibited higher basal skin conductance, a measure of pain, compared to non-carriers [120]. In the 2018 study, no difference in levels of methylation in the first exon of *OPRM1* was found; however, the authors pointed out that this was a preliminary study mainly to obtain data on patient retention, and low sample size (n = 12 NICU-admitted infants) could not be ruled out as the reason for why no differences were found [121]. In the 2020 study, in which ≈1000 neonates were enrolled, infants who were homozygous carriers of the G allele of rs1799971 in *OPRM1* had higher pain scores in response to heel lance after dextrose administration [122].

In conclusion, early life painful events were associated with increased methylation in *SLC6A4* promoter CpG sites (up to 7 years of age), decreased telomere length, and adverse behaviors. Variants in *COMT* and *BDNF* interact with *SCL6A4* DNAm changes to influence outcomes. *OPRM1* and *NFKBIA* variants also potentially influence the stress/pain response to early life pain. The interesting sex difference for *NFKBIA* variant association needs follow up. These findings offer potential as biomarkers to identify neonates at risk for adverse long-term outcomes from early life stress.

(d) Neuroendocrine evidence

In utero and perinatal stress might have long-lasting effects on pain processing later in life. The mechanisms underlying the influence of early life stress on pain pathways are mediated by the hypothalamic–pituitary axis (HPA). Prolonged exposure to stress hormones prenatally leads to decreased glucocorticoid receptors in the hippocampus, poorer glucocorticoid feedback sensitivity, and heightened glucocorticoid production in childhood, which manifests as increased anxiety several years later [123]. Neonatal maternal separation, which manifests as stress, has been shown to be associated with reduced sensitivity to noxious heat stimuli [124], as well as visceral hypersensitivity in adult rats [125]. Insufficient nesting material during early life also prolongs muscle hyperalgesia following prostaglandin administration in adulthood, increases the excitability of mature nociceptors innervating the muscle [126], and elevates plasma levels of the pro-inflammatory cytokine interleukin-6 in adulthood [127].

In adults, the HPA axis can directly impact the neurophysiological mechanisms involved in pain perception through brainstem descending pain control pathways [128]. Hypo-responsiveness of the HPA axis in pre-term but not full-term infants has been reported. Specifically, prior neonatal pain exposure (quantified by the number of skin-breaks) was associated with lower plasma cortisol responses to stress in pre-term infants [129]. This corroborates with the evidence presented in above genetics section, where higher number of infant skin-breaks was associated with lower hair cortisol levels in boys 7 years later [119]. Although it is unclear whether the stress response directly influences the development of pain pathways in humans, the immaturity of brainstem descending pain control pathways at birth [65] suggests that increased HPA activity could exert significant modifications. Another important stress axis, the sympathoadrenal system, and its primary mediator, catecholamines, have been implicated in inducing and sustaining the stress-induced maintenance of mechanical hyperalgesia in adults [130], but there is no evidence reported for its involvement in neonatal nociceptive priming.

(e) Sex differences

Animal studies reveal age-dependent sexual dimorphism in susceptibility to develop chronic pain [131]. In rats, younger males were found to be less susceptible to TNFα-induced priming compared to older males, and younger females more susceptible compared to older females. This sexual dimorphism was explained by age-related changes in estrogen levels, which is protective [131]. In another study, specifically, female rats were more vulnerable to the long-term consequences of neonatal inflammatory injury [132]. Neonatally injured females exhibited significantly greater hypoalgesia at P60 (adulthood), as well as enhanced inflammatory hyperalgesia following re-injury compared to neonatally injured males and controls [79]. Specifically, in rats, neonatal nociceptive priming susceptibility was dependent on estrogen action on the estrogen receptor, with a neuroprotective effect [131,133,134]. In human infants, the only genetic/epigenetic study analyzing sex differences was in relation to the *NFKBIA* variant. While no association of neonatal pain and cortisol levels was found in girls, in boys, an interaction with the *NFKBIA* variant was found [119]. Sex differences in the HPA axis responsiveness are well established throughout the literature (e.g., see review [135]), and thus future studies on sex differences in early life stress effects on pain pathways in relation to later-life pain chronicity are warranted.

2.4. Pain Chronification in Children and Adolescents

In the United States, ≈3.9–6 million children undergo surgery annually [136,137], and injury is the leading cause of death among children older than 1 year. With a reported 14.5–38% (median 20%) incidence of CPSP, the impact on children is high.

2.5. Mechanisms and Biomarkers for Pain Chronification in Children and Adolescents

(a) Neuroimaging evidence

Structural and functional MRI studies have revealed several brain networks are involved in chronic pain. In children, lower GM and greater RS-FC within the major pain-associated networks were found in several of the chronic pain conditions studied. While functional hubs are mostly confined locally to sensorimotor networks in the early years, with age, they shift to the posterior cingulate cortex and insula [70]. It was recently demonstrated by Jones at et al. that higher pain intensity during adolescent years is potentially associated with desegregation patterns of cerebellum default mode network connectivity [138]. The central executive (memory), salience (expectation response), and default mode networks (emotional processing) are identifiable at an early age and undergo significant change until the age of about 20 years. Baliki et al. conducted a longitudinal study in adult patients with subacute low back pain followed for 1 year for development of chronic pain and compared imaging signals with controls. They found that the functional connectivity between the medial prefrontal cortex and nucleus accumbens in the brain's emotional learning circuitry was predictive (>80% accuracy) of pain chronification [68]. This connectivity is part of the mesolimbic–prefrontal network, which the authors purported to play a role in reward behavior (with dopaminergic and glutaminergic projections) and addiction potential [139,140]. Interestingly, they found that the prediction was better with longer time lapse between the brain activity measurement and the pain outcomes [141]. The same group also used diffusion tensor imaging and showed that pre-existing brain white matter structural abnormalities were predictive of pain persistence [142]. Readers are referred to an excellent review of a developmental perspective of these networks in pediatrics by Bhatt et al. [32]. Brain imaging research to identify mechanisms of pain chronification in the pediatric age group remains in its infancy. Besides MRI, neural inflammatory markers and neurotransmitters in pain (including creatine, N-acetylaspartate (NAA), myo-inositol, choline, glutamate, glutamine, and gamma-aminobutyric acid (GABA)) may be assessed in vivo by magnetic resonance spectroscopy (MRS) with the advantages of being non-invasive and having no risk of radiation [143]. Neurometabolites detected with MRS have improved the understanding of pathological mechanisms in the pain of fibromyalgia as well as the effectiveness of pharmacologic therapies [144,145]. Another interesting modality is the use of functional near-infrared spectroscopy (fNIRS), a noninvasive optical imaging technique that measures changes in oxygenated and deoxygenated hemoglobin within the brain and has been used in newborns and adults [146]. Using fNIRS, specific changes in the somatosensory cortices are able to be detected (both when patient is or is not undergoing anesthesia), making it a potent and potentially useful technique in evaluating objective pain markers in infants and children [147].

(b) Electrophysiological evidence

EEG can be useful in characterizing the neurological processes underlying pediatric chronic pain transitions. EEG frequency, connectivity, and EEG entropy (a measure of EEG information content describing regularity of continuous EEG time series) have been found to characterize chronic pain in adult studies [148]. In adolescents with chronic musculoskeletal pain, increased resting global delta and beta power, changes in EEG spectral power, peak frequency, permutation entropy, and network functional connectivity at specific frequency bands were described during tonic heat and cold stimulations [149]. Similarly, permutation entropy in the theta frequency band was used to classify the presence and absence of chronic pain in female adolescents, showing potential for a point-of-care biomarker to detect pain in the absence of self-report [150]. While it has promise as a non-invasive, low-cost, clinically accessible biomarker [151], it needs to be evaluated further as a marker for chronic pain transitions in children.

(c) Genetics and Epigenetics

Figure 2b includes a summary of the major findings from the evidence available for genetic and epigenetic contributions to chronic pain in children and adolescents (see the Supplementary File for search terms). Chidambaran et al. (2020) conducted a systematic review and meta-analysis on genetic risk associated with the development of chronic postsurgical pain in humans [152]. Their meta-analysis included 21 full-text articles, of which only one study included pediatric age ranges. They found significant association of variants with chronic post-surgical pain in 26 genes important in neurotransmission, pain signaling, the immune response, neuroactive ligand–receptor interaction, apoptosis signaling, and metabolism and transport [152]. Since not enough genome-wide association studies (GWAS) analyzing chronic postsurgical pain in the pediatric population are available, Chidambaran et al. (2021) used computational biology to develop a PRS predicting the development of chronic pain in the pediatric population. Twenty variants, annotated to seven genes: *ATXN1, PRKCA, CACNG2, DRD2, KCNJ3, KCNJ6,* and *KCNK3,* comprised the PRS predicting risk of development of chronic pain in 10–18-year-olds [5].

DNA methylation is the main epigenetic mechanism investigated for pain chronification in children. Chidambaran et al. (2017) pyro sequenced 22 CpG sites at the *OPRM1* promoter and found the altered methylation of two CpG sites in adolescents exhibiting chronic pain after spine fusion surgery compared to controls with no chronic pain [4]. In a follow-up analysis using methylation array data, Chidambaran et al. (2019) reported differential DNA methylation of 637 CpG sites in spine-fusion patients (n = 56) aged 10–18 years old who developed chronic postsurgical pain compared to those who did not [111]. These sites were located in 310 genes involved in pathways such as GABA receptor signaling, protein kinase C signaling, dopamine receptor, and cAMP-mediated signaling [111].

There is scarce research investigating the cross-section of gene–epigenetic interactions in the development of chronification of pain in children. In 2021, a pilot study by Chidambaran et al. (2021) analyzed DNA methylation association with SNPs in 10–18-year-olds (average age of 14) undergoing spine fusion surgeries [112]. They found DNA methylation at 127 CpG sites mediated the association of 470 methylation quantitative trait (meQTL) loci with chronic pain [112]. Important CpG meQTL sites were located within 5 genes, namely, *SLC45A3, NUCKS1, RAB7, RAB7L1, SLC41A1,* and *PM20D1* [112]. Thus, these genes were deemed to be important in terms of epigenetic regulation risk for developing chronic pain after surgery in pediatric patients [112].

Transcriptomics and other -omics-related investigations of pain chronification in children are also lacking in the literature. The RNA sequencing of peripheral blood in adolescents undergoing pediatric spinal fusion surgeries revealed the increased expression of *HLA-DRB3* in adolescents who experienced chronic postoperative pain compared to those who did not, albeit the authors concluded they may have had a low sample size [113].

(d) Neuroendocrine evidence

Stress-associated biomarkers also play a role in the chronification of pediatric pain. Allostatic load [153] is a biological indicator of chronic stress. It is evaluated as a summed clinical index of neuroendocrine, cardiovascular, metabolic [154], immune, and inflammatory markers [155–157]. In a study of 61 children and adolescents with chronic pain, over 50% were classified as at high risk for allostatic load, indicating the role of chronic stress in chronic pain [156]. Although stress could be related to the pain condition itself, we also know that allostatic load correlates with adverse childhood events (ACE) and socioeconomic status, which indicates the possibility of stress preceding the development of chronic pain [158,159]. In fact, children with exposure to one or more ACEs had higher rates of chronic pain (8.7%) as compared to those with no reported ACEs (4.8%) [160]. Since ACEs are also associated with post-traumatic stress, which mediates the association of ACEs with mental health problems, it is important to assess ACEs [161,162] in children with chronic pain to inform mitigating strategies.

In patients with a history of early childhood trauma, increased methylation of CpG sites within the *TRPA1* promoter was later associated with increased mechanical pain thresholds in female adult patients with chronic pain [163]; the *FKBP5* variant rs3800373 was associated with right hippocampal volume in adults with musculoskeletal pain [164]; and altered *DRD2* expression in female children and altered *COMT* expression in male children was found [165]. It was speculated that epigenetic changes conferred by the parents' early adverse experiences were inherited in their children in a sex-dependent manner [165]. In another study conducted in the Netherlands involving 2980 adults, early life stress before the age of 16 was associated with higher musculoskeletal pain scores in adulthood [166]. This provides aa rationale for the investigation of stress-related genomic, and other, mechanisms in pain development (which has a lot in common with certain mental health conditions) along the childhood–adult continuum [167,168].

(e) Sex differences

Female sex has been shown to have a higher risk of acute to chronic pain transitions in adults [169–171]. Since female adolescents have a higher predilection for chronic pain conditions [172,173], one would hypothesize a higher risk for female sex for pain chronification in adolescents as well. Most studies in children undergoing surgery have not identified sex as a predictor of acute to chronic pain [6,174,175]. Suryakumar et al. did find a higher incidence of females developing chronic postsurgical pain after spine fusion; however, scoliosis has a female preponderance [176], and this might have influenced the results. Genetic interactions with sex were mentioned in previous sections (Section 2.5, (d)). Sex differences based on psychophysical tests are also mentioned in the next paragraph (Section 2.5, (f)). For a more comprehensive review on future priority areas to understand sex and gender differences in chronic pain, the reader is referred to these excellent reviews [177,178]. Further investigations are needed to understand the role of sex, hormonal mechanisms, and gender identity in acute to chronic pain transitions in pediatrics, especially given the pubertal transitions happening through adolescence.

(f) Psychophysical mechanisms

Quantitative sensory testing (QST) may reveal mechanisms of chronification from alterations in pain processing. QST provides non-invasive ways to interrogate large fiber function (Aβ), nociceptive small fiber (Aδ, C) function, and the spinothalamic pathways involved in pain chronification. A prospective longitudinal study in children aged 10–17 years conducted QSTs and followed participants for 4 months after acute musculoskeletal pain complaints. The incidence of chronification was 35%. They found that poor conditioned pain modulation using hot and cold thermal tasks was predictive of chronic pain [179], suggesting that impairment in inhibitory pain modulation may predict children's nonrecovery from acute musculoskeletal pain. Further studies are warranted evaluating mechanisms of central sensitization (using temporal summation) along with other pain paradigms (e.g., pressure pain). The evidence in adults suggest QST may be useful in a mechanism-based classification of pain [180], but there are gaps in our current understanding of QST in pediatric populations and age limitations in its applicability. Of note, QST protocol of the German research network on neuropathic pain (DFNS) encompassing all somatosensory modalities with modification of instructions and pain rating was evaluated for use in 176 children aged 6–12 years. This study by Blankenburg et al. found that QST was feasible for children over 5 years of age [181]. There were differences by body site (face more sensitive than the hand and/or foot), age (children aged 6–8 years were less sensitive to all thermal and mechanical detection stimuli but more sensitive to all pain stimuli than children aged 9–12 years who were similar to adolescents [13–17 years]), and sex (girls were more sensitive to thermal detection and pain stimuli, but not to mechanical detection and pain stimuli). Reference values were shown to differ from adults, but distribution properties (range, variance, and side differences) were similar and plausible for statistical factors. This seminal study demonstrated that developmental changes influenced reference values in children differently than from adults', while other properties were similar to adults.

Clinicians need further evidence-based QST protocols that are feasible and meaningful in clinical settings with high sensitivity and specificity for pain sub-types.

3. Future Directions for Research

The field of preclinical pediatric pain research has provided high-quality evidence for the development of maladaptive nociception and the effect of early injury on the development of inflammatory and neuropathic pain [54,84,182–185]. However, there are gaps in understanding prenatal and early postnatal insults across the continuum of a child's life [76]. While numerous animal studies suggest nociceptive priming related to stressful/painful experiences in early life and maladaptive pain responses in later life, human studies are not conclusive. Some find that long-term neuropsychological effects were only in those with highest opioid exposure, while others reinforce susceptibility to chronic pain by 10 years of age in 13% of children exposed to early life pain. On one hand, this also points to the need for better predictive preclinical models mimicking real life in NICU, the need for reliable objective measures of pain chronification, and a paucity of mechanism-based validated targets. On the other hand, they suggest the need for continued research to determine dose response of preemptive morphine and other medications targeting mechanistic pathways in attenuating long-term, behavioral impact of neonatal pain and preventing hyperalgesia [79]. While psychophysical tests to determine mechanisms can be used in children as young as 5 years, epigenetic tests and neuroimaging/EEG biomarkers could be relevant in younger children to understand the risk for chronic pain development in those with exposure to early life stressors.

There is also a dire need for multisite longitudinal pediatric studies with inclusion of diverse patient populations that are heterogeneous across multiple pain conditions, thus generating "big data" shared warehouses with well-defined phenotypes and well-characterized mechanisms accessible to all pain researchers. The multidimensional nature of pain emphasizes the need for investigations of multi-modal composite pain biomarker signatures for pain sub-phenotypes [186]. Recent advances in innovative analytical tools in artificial intelligence and machine learning, such as deep learning with neural networks, may allow pattern detection using several parameters from patient electronic databases. Patterns could be leveraged for the automated risk prediction of sub-phenotypes. Quantifying risk and understanding mechanisms could then guide healthcare providers to use tailored preventive strategies, despite the paucity of validated targets. Furthermore, artificial intelligence can be used to discover new drug molecules, and precision gene therapy practices may be utilized. The emphasis on pain biomarkers has been amplified by the National Institute of Health Helping to End Addiction Long-term (HEAL) initiative, the Biomarkers Consortium, and the National Institute of Health Blueprint for Neuroscience Research Grand Challenge of Pain. Currently, there are no clinical biomarkers for pain approved by the FDA. This further emphasizes the need for basic science, translational, and clinical researchers to collaborate on these efforts to develop qualitative and quantitative biomarkers to supplement patient self-reported outcomes for a more comprehensive assessment of treatment responders.

Thus, future research needs to target genetic, epigenetic, immune, electrophysiological and imagining biomarkers in appropriate pain models. For example, antagonists of voltage-gated sodium channel NaV1.7 are under investigation for treatment of certain pain conditions [187]. Given the implications for *KCNS1* channel genes and *PM20D1* in CPSP transition, future studies targeting these mechanisms may reveal new therapeutics [188,189]. In addition, tenazemub, an anti-NGF antibody (phase 3 trials), and inhibitors targeting TRPV1, TRPA1, and TRPM2 receptors (pre-clinical phase), are being investigated for pain conditions but mechanistically could be useful for pain chronification as well [190,191]. For example, treatment with TRP antagonists in mice with acute pancreatitis slowed progress to chronic pain [192]. Research is still needed to identify molecules that can enhance *KCNS1* function. In addition, it is possible that several nutritional, environmental, and psychological factors have shared epigenetic underpinnings with pain sensitization (for example, vitamin D deficiency, socioeconomic status, anxiety sensitivity) [193]. Epigenetic biomarkers can thus serve as prognostic indicators of therapy response [194–197]. Some examples of epigenetic drugs with successful clinical use for the treatment of hematologic malignancies are DNA methylation transferase (DNMT) inhibitors (5-azacytidine and decitabine). Similarly, inhibitors of DNMT, histone acetyl transferase (HAT), and histone deacetylase (HDAC), enzymes involved in methylation and histone acetylation, as well as CRISPR-mediated methylation or demethylation of specific genes [198], are promising targets to be pursued [199]. Continued exploration of epigenetic drugs is warranted with the means to avoid off-target negative effects. Integration of DNA methylation studies with transcriptomics, proteomics, and chromatin accessibility will allow better inferences regarding druggable targets such as transcription factors. Future research could leverage systems biology and bioinformatics to understand downstream signaling effects of drug targets to enable innovation in a cost-effective manner. Lastly, while evidence of sex–genome interactions in pain chronification have been reported in previous sections, it needs further study in pediatric populations.

4. Future Directions for Clinical Practice

To enable the implementation of research informed strategies, clinicians will need to elicit a detailed patient history regarding early life circumstances, previous pain experiences, socioeconomic environmental factors, etc., when children present with acute pain conditions or surgery. We need more validated, easy-to-use psychosocial measures for risk stratification in the clinic, for example, the Pediatric Pain Screening Tool for CPSP [176]. Psychophysical testing tools and standards need to be adapted for implementation at bedside for children. For example, in adults, use of von Frey filaments for temporal summation, pressure pain sensitivity using an algometer or a modified approach using a blood pressure cuff, and Neuropen for mechanical pain detection have been shown to identify sub-phenotypes [200,201]. Knowing baseline QST phenotypes may be able to predict efficacy of pregabalin, lidocaine, oxycodone, and placebo analgesia [202,203]. In addition, point-of-care genetic/epigenetic testing using blood or saliva samples would enable modification of analgesia regimens targeting altered genomic pathways, rather than the current trial-and-error approach [194,196,204]. Finally, we need to consolidate consensus guidelines derived from clinical evidence to support the choice of treatment intervention, based on mechanisms [205–207]. Future trials to prevent CPSP should investigate efficacy of interventions based on patient risk and mechanisms. For example, presurgical interventions to address psychosocial risk factors using behavioral interventions [208], functional disability using physical therapy, peripheral sensitization using regional analgesia, and/or central sensitization using NMDA antagonists or calcium channel blockers such as gabapentinoids [209–211]. Of note, current literature is inconclusive about the efficacy of pharmacological modalities or regional analgesia in preventing CPSP, mostly due to the heterogeneity of pain conditions, populations, small study sizes, variations in dosage, timing and duration of treatment, and variations in outcome measures [210–215]. Future studies with risk stratification and longer-term follow-up for multimodal pain protocols are warranted. In the case of children, family-centered care approaches are needed as impaired parental responses may also reinforce the child's pain response when parents have been involved with the NICU experience, indicating the need for parental education as well [216]. Importantly, we need policies supporting biomarker development and implementation, improved reimbursement for evidence-backed pain management practices, improved leverage of electronic media for education, assessments and management, and most importantly the support within the electronic medical record infrastructure to enable automated clinical decision support tools based on risk stratification.

Furthermore, the plasticity of the developing nervous system and mechanistic approaches imply reversibility. Thus, there is potential for modulating the processes favorably by use of physiologic interventions such as neuromodulation, virtual reality (VR), and psychological therapies [217]. Neurostimulation is a neuromodulatory method in which electrical impulses are delivered invasively or non-invasively to stimulate peripheral nerves, the spinal cord, or specific brain regions [218,219]. Ilfeld et al. have published extensively on the use of peripheral nerve stimulation as an opioid-sparing technique for postoperative pain [220,221]. However, its benefits for children and prevention of chronification remain to be proven. Central stimulation techniques have been investigated for the management of acute postoperative pain and prevention of chronic migraine, and they hold promise for the prevention of pain chronification [222]. Further work is needed to prove safety/efficacy in children for the prevention of pain chronification [223,224]. In addition, VR, a technology that provides an immersive experience in a simulated and interactive environment using multimodal sensory stimuli inputs, is increasingly being used in pain management [225]. Its application for post-traumatic distress and anxiety, as well as improvement in conditioned pain modulation efficiency, suggest it can influence central sensitization mechanisms and brain modulation of pain with the potential for long-lasting effects [226]. Although the concern may be that need for patient participation may limit its utility to developmentally mature children, VR has been used successfully in children as young as five years of age and children with cerebral palsy [227]. As children's brains process VR differently and fantasies might be confused with reality, virtual environments may need to be contextualized specifically to enable this distinction [228]. Other non-pharmacological modalities with positive effects on maladaptive pain processing are cognitive behavioral therapy (CBT) and mindfulness-based approaches, which have been used in adolescents. CBT for 4–11 weeks has been shown to restore RS-FC between the insula and somatosensory regions, with long-standing effects on pain outcomes and pain catastrophizing [132,229]. A Cochrane review of the use of psychological therapies for children with recurrent/chronic pain concluded that face-to-face psychological therapies are effective for reducing pain for children with headaches, as well as reducing pain intensity and disability in children with mixed chronic pain conditions [230]. However, the evidence for effects on anxiety and depression, as well as the long-term effects, were inadequate. In addition, integrative care and music therapy are effective treatment paradigms for the treatment of pediatric pain in different contexts [231–233], but they are less explored in the context of chronic pain transitions. Thus, the evidence for the effectiveness of most treatment paradigms is mixed [234]. It is likely that mechanistic trials of treatment paradigms stratified by genetic, psychophysical, and psychological risk assessments may improve the ability to discern responders. Table 1 lists the several mechanism-based available and potential pharmacologic and non-pharmacologic therapies in pain chronification [216]. However, early identification, prevention, and management are of utmost importance.

Table 1. Examples for mechanism-based (available and potential) approaches to the management of children at risk for pediatric chronic pain transitions.

Targeted Mechanisms	Pharmacological Interventions * (Examples)	Non-Pharmacological Interventions (Examples) Neuromodulation and Behavioral Therapy
Peripheral sensitization	Non-steroidal anti-inflammatory drugs such as ibuprofen, celecoxib	Peripheral nerve stimulation (PNS) Vagal nerve stimulation
	Regional analgesia techniques including peripheral nerve blocks and neuraxial analgesia	
	Capsaicin cream	
	Topical application/infiltration of local anesthetics such as lidocaine	
	In phases of trials: anti-NGF antibody (phase 3); TrkA receptor antagonist (phase 2)	
	Potential: TNF blockers such as adalimumab	

Table 1. *Cont.*

Targeted Mechanisms	Pharmacological Interventions * (Examples)	Non-Pharmacological Interventions (Examples) Neuromodulation and Behavioral Therapy	
Central sensitization/pain facilitation	Agonists at $\alpha2\delta$ (alpha-2-delta) subunit of presynaptic voltage-sensitive Ca^{2+} channels: gabapentin and pregabalin	Spinal cord stimulation (SCS) Transcutaneous electrical nerve stimulation (TENS)	
	NMDA antagonists (ketamine, methadone, dextromethorphan)		
Descending pain inhibition	Tricyclic antidepressants (amitriptyline)		
	Serotonin norepinephrine reuptake inhibitors (duloxetine)		
	Clonidine/dexmedetomidine		
Cortical modulation of pain	Anxiety medications such as benzodiazepines	Invasive neurostimulation: deep brain stimulation (DBS)	Virtual reality immersive therapy; distraction cognitive behavioral approaches; mindfulness integrative care relaxation, music, etc.
		Noninvasive brain stimulation: transcranial magnetic stimulation (TMS) and transcranial direct current stimulation (tDCS)	

* Opioids can potentially influence all mechanisms.

5. Conclusions

This state-of-the-art review article describes the evidence for the complex interplay between genetic, epigenetic, chemical, neuronal, and immune factors that interact synergistically to influence the development and maintenance of chronic pain in children. While innate pain perception and responses may be determined by genetic underpinnings, environmental experiences are encoded through functional and structural reorganizational processes in the plastic, developing nervous system to shape memory and behaviors through central and peripheral sensitization mechanisms. These can be detected using several psychophysical, imaging, and genomic tests, and reversed using tailored precision medicine approaches. Critical gaps in research and its translation into clinical practice were identified. These are barriers that need to be surmounted for successful innovation in the promising field of pain chronification in children. The implication for clinicians is that developmental aspects and mechanism-based treatment should be considered while caring for pediatric age groups. In caring for neonates undergoing painful/stressful procedures, there is an imperative to consider soothing therapies (sucrose analgesia, skin-to-skin care), and for neonates undergoing surgeries, the use of regional analgesia, as well as the judicious use of opioids and other analgesics to prevent hyperalgesic priming. This is especially important given that the risk is higher during the critical time of early development. In addition, since pain behavior may not correlate with brain markers during stress in neonates, reliance solely on pain behaviors may lead to undertreatment. Knowing that there is a risk for pain sensitization by 7–10 years of age, it is important to consider the history of early life stress and ACE factors while planning care management for future painful procedures, for behavioral optimization, and to prevent amplified pain responses and sustenance. Although genomic biomarkers for pain chronification are not validated and there are no FDA-approved biomarkers, the use of psychosocial screeners, currently available genetic tests for opioid PK/PD, bedside QST, and portable EEG hold promise to inform clinicians of potential sensitization. This will allow targeted and tailored measures to prevent chronification of pain upon exposure to another acute pain/stress episode by optimizing cerebral responses using non-pharmacological, behavioral, and neuromodulation therapies. Thus, mechanism-guided multimodal pharmacological therapies and regional techniques to provide analgesia and prevent exaggerated responses is especially important as the brain areas involved in pain chronification may also overlap with risk-reward salience areas involved in addiction. Future studies should focus on biomarker-guided risk stratification and the development of personalized non-opioid strategies for pain management. Another emerging concern at the crossroads of pain chronification and mental health stems from the potential overlap of primed pain responses and long-term risk for neurobehavioral and neuropsychiatric outcomes after exposure to early life stress. Future efforts to further understand this risk and mitigate it are warranted.

Supplementary Materials: The supplementary file supporting Figure 2 can be downloaded at: https://www.mdpi.com/article/10.3390/jcm12165176/s1.

Author Contributions: Conceptualization, I.T.D. and V.C.; methodology, I.T.D. and K.N.K.; data curation, I.T.D., K.N.K. and V.C.; writing—original draft preparation, I.T.D. and K.N.K.; writing—review and editing, V.C., I.T.D., K.N.K. and H.M.M.; visualization, H.M.M., K.N.K. and I.T.D.; supervision, V.C.; project administration, I.T.D. and K.N.K.; funding acquisition, V.C. All authors have read and agreed to the published version of the manuscript.

Funding: Research reported in this manuscript was supported by National Institute of Arthritis and Musculoskeletal and Skin Diseases under award number 5R01AR075857.

Institutional Review Board Statement: Not applicable.

Informed Consent Statement: Informed consent is not applicable to this article.

Data Availability Statement: Not applicable.

Conflicts of Interest: The authors declare no conflict of interest.

References

1. Hassett, A.L.; Hilliard, P.E.; Goesling, J.; Clauw, D.J.; Harte, S.E.; Brummett, C.M. Reports of chronic pain in childhood and adolescence among patients at a tertiary care pain clinic. *J. Pain* **2013**, *14*, 1390–1397. [CrossRef]
2. El-Metwally, A.; Salminen, J.J.; Auvinen, A.; Kautiainen, H.; Mikkelsson, M. Lower limb pain in a preadolescent population: Prognosis and risk factors for chronicity—A prospective 1- and 4-year follow-up study. *Pediatrics* **2005**, *116*, 673–681. [CrossRef]
3. Gobina, I.; Villberg, J.; Välimaa, R.; Tynjälä, J.; Whitehead, R.; Cosma, A.; Brooks, F.; Cavallo, F.; Ng, K.; de Matos, M.G.; et al. Prevalence of self-reported chronic pain among adolescents: Evidence from 42 countries and regions. *Eur. J. Pain* **2019**, *23*, 316–326. [CrossRef]
4. Chidambaran, V.; Zhang, X.; Martin, L.; Ding, L.; Weirauch, M.; Geisler, K.; Stubbeman, B.; Sadhasivam, S.; Ji, H. DNA methylation at the mu-1 opioid receptor gene (*OPRM1*) promoter predicts preoperative, acute, and chronic postsurgical pain after spine fusion. *Pharmacogenom. Pers. Med.* **2017**, *10*, 157–168. [CrossRef]
5. Chidambaran, V.; Pilipenko, V.; Jegga, A.G.; Geisler, K.; Martin, L.J. Systems Biology Guided Gene Enrichment Approaches Improve Prediction of Chronic Post-surgical Pain After Spine Fusion. *Front. Genet.* **2021**, *12*, 594250. [CrossRef]
6. Rabbitts, J.A.; Fisher, E.; Rosenbloom, B.N.; Palermo, T.M. Prevalence and Predictors of Chronic Postsurgical Pain in Children: A Systematic Review and Meta-Analysis. *J. Pain* **2017**, *18*, 605–614. [CrossRef]
7. Brattberg, G. Do pain problems in young school children persist into early adulthood? A 13-year follow-up. *Eur. J. Pain* **2004**, *8*, 187–199. [CrossRef]
8. Groenewald, C.B.; Essner, B.S.; Wright, D.; Fesinmeyer, M.D.; Palermo, T.M. The Economic Costs of Chronic Pain Among a Cohort of Treatment-Seeking Adolescents in the United States. *Pain* **2014**, *15*, 925–933. [CrossRef]
9. Brown, D.; Schenk, S.; Genent, D.; Zernikow, B.; Wager, J. A scoping review of chronic pain in emerging adults. *Pain Rep.* **2021**, *6*, e920. [CrossRef]
10. Kashikar-Zuck, S.; Goldschneider, K.R.; Powers, S.W.; Vaught, M.H.; Hershey, A.D. Depression and functional disability in chronic pediatric pain. *Clin. J. Pain* **2001**, *17*, 341–349. [CrossRef]
11. Kucyi, A.; Davis, K.D. The dynamic pain connectome. *Trends Neurosci.* **2015**, *38*, 86–95. [CrossRef]
12. Baliki, M.N.; Mansour, A.R.; Baria, A.T.; Apkarian, A.V. Functional reorganization of the default mode network across chronic pain conditions. *PLoS ONE* **2014**, *9*, e106133. [CrossRef]
13. Treede, R.D.; Rief, W.; Barke, A.; Aziz, Q.; Bennett, M.I.; Benoliel, R.; Cohen, M.; Evers, S.; Finnerup, N.B.; First, M.B.; et al. Chronic pain as a symptom or a disease: The IASP Classification of Chronic Pain for the International Classification of Diseases (ICD-11). *Pain* **2019**, *160*, 19–27. [CrossRef] [PubMed]
14. Wager, J.; Fabrizi, L.; Tham, S.W. Need for pediatric specifications for chronic pain diagnoses in the International Classification of Diseases (ICD-11). *Pain* **2023**, *164*, 1705–1708. [CrossRef] [PubMed]

5. Rabbitts, J.A.; Palermo, T.M.; Lang, E.A. A Conceptual Model of Biopsychosocial Mechanisms of Transition from Acute to Chronic Postsurgical Pain in Children and Adolescents. *J. Pain Res.* **2020**, *13*, 3071–3080. [CrossRef] [PubMed]

6. Sieberg, C.B.; Karunakaran, K.D.; Kussman, B.; Borsook, D. Preventing pediatric chronic postsurgical pain: Time for increased rigor. *Can. J. Pain* **2022**, *6*, 73–84. [CrossRef] [PubMed]

7. Farmer, M.A.; Baliki, M.N.; Apkarian, A.V. A dynamic network perspective of chronic pain. *Neurosci. Lett.* **2012**, *520*, 197–203. [CrossRef]

8. McGrath, P.J.; Walco, G.A.; Turk, D.C.; Dworkin, R.H.; Brown, M.T.; Davidson, K.; Eccleston, C.; Finley, G.A.; Goldschneider, K.; Haverkos, L.; et al. Core outcome domains and measures for pediatric acute and chronic/recurrent pain clinical trials: PedIMMPACT recommendations. *J. Pain* **2008**, *9*, 771–783. [CrossRef]

9. Palermo, T.M.; Walco, G.A.; Paladhi, U.R.; Birnie, K.A.; Crombez, G.; de la Vega, R.; Eccleston, C.; Kashikar-Zuck, S.; Stone, A.L. Core outcome set for pediatric chronic pain clinical trials: Results from a Delphi poll and consensus meeting. *Pain* **2021**, *162*, 2539–2547. [CrossRef]

10. FDA-NIH Biomarker Working Group. *BEST (Biomarkers, EndpointS, and other Tools) Resource*; Food and Drug Administration (US): National Institutes of Health (US): Silver Spring, MD, USA; Bethesda, MD, USA, 2016.

11. Douglas, S.R.; Shenoda, B.B.; Qureshi, R.A.; Sacan, A.; Alexander, G.M.; Perreault, M.; Barrett, J.E.; Aradillas-Lopez, E.; Schwartzman, R.J.; Ajit, S.K. Analgesic Response to Intravenous Ketamine Is Linked to a Circulating microRNA Signature in Female Patients with Complex Regional Pain Syndrome. *J. Pain* **2015**, *16*, 814–824. [CrossRef]

12. Lewis, C.M.; Vassos, E. Polygenic risk scores: From research tools to clinical instruments. *Genome Med.* **2020**, *12*, 44. [CrossRef] [PubMed]

23. Kuchenbaecker, K.; Telkar, N.; Reiker, T.; Walters, R.G.; Lin, K.; Eriksson, A.; Gurdasani, D.; Gilly, A.; Southam, L.; Tsafantakis, E.; et al. The transferability of lipid loci across African, Asian and European cohorts. *Nat. Commun.* **2019**, *10*, 4330. [CrossRef] [PubMed]

24. Ming, X.; Zhang, Z.; Zou, Z.; Lv, C.; Dong, Q.; He, Q.; Yi, Y.; Li, Y.; Wang, H.; Zhu, B. Kinetics and mechanisms of mitotic inheritance of DNA methylation and their roles in aging-associated methylome deterioration. *Cell Res.* **2020**, *30*, 980–996. [CrossRef] [PubMed]

25. Felix, J.F.; Cecil, C.A.M. Population DNA methylation studies in the Developmental Origins of Health and Disease (DOHaD) framework. *J. Dev. Orig. Health Dis.* **2019**, *10*, 306–313. [CrossRef]

26. Branham, E.M.; McLean, S.A.; Deliwala, I.; Mauck, M.C.; Zhao, Y.; McKibben, L.A.; Lee, A.; Spencer, A.B.; Zannas, A.S.; Lechner, M.; et al. CpG Methylation Levels in HPA Axis Genes Predict Chronic Pain Outcomes Following Trauma Exposure. *J. Pain* **2023**, *24*, 1127–1141. [CrossRef]

27. Chidambaran, V.; Ashton, M.; Martin, L.J.; Jegga, A.G. Systems biology-based approaches to summarize and identify novel genes and pathways associated with acute and chronic postsurgical pain. *J. Clin. Anesth.* **2020**, *62*, 109738. [CrossRef]

28. Bosak, N.; Branco, P.; Kuperman, P.; Buxbaum, C.; Cohen, R.M.; Fadel, S.; Zubeidat, R.; Hadad, R.; Lawen, A.; Saadon-Grosman, N.; et al. Brain Connectivity Predicts Chronic Pain in Acute Mild Traumatic Brain Injury. *Ann. Neurol.* **2022**, *92*, 819–833. [CrossRef]

29. Fragiadakis, G.K.; Gaudillière, B.; Ganio, E.A.; Aghaeepour, N.; Tingle, M.; Nolan, G.P.; Angst, M.S. Patient-specific Immune States before Surgery Are Strong Correlates of Surgical Recovery. *Anesthesiology* **2015**, *123*, 1241–1255. [CrossRef]

30. Chapman, C.R.; Vierck, C.J. The Transition of Acute Postoperative Pain to Chronic Pain: An Integrative Overview of Research on Mechanisms. *J. Pain* **2017**, *18*, 359.e1–359.e38. [CrossRef]

31. Arendt-Nielsen, L.; Morlion, B.; Perrot, S.; Dahan, A.; Dickenson, A.; Kress, H.G.; Wells, C.; Bouhassira, D.; Drewes, A.M. Assessment and manifestation of central sensitisation across different chronic pain conditions. *Eur. J. Pain* **2018**, *22*, 216–241. [CrossRef]

32. Bhatt, R.R.; Gupta, A.; Mayer, E.A.; Zeltzer, L.K. Chronic pain in children: Structural and resting-state functional brain imaging within a developmental perspective. *Pediatr. Res.* **2020**, *88*, 840–849. [CrossRef] [PubMed]

33. Constantinou, J.; Reynolds, M.L.; Woolf, C.J.; Safieh-Garabedian, B.; Fitzgerald, M. Nerve growth factor levels in developing rat skin: Upregulation following skin wounding. *Neuroreport* **1994**, *5*, 2281–2284. [CrossRef] [PubMed]

34. Howard, R.F.; Walker, S.M.; Mota, M.P.; Fitzgerald, M. The ontogeny of neuropathic pain: Postnatal onset of mechanical allodynia in rat spared nerve injury (SNI) and chronic constriction injury (CCI) models. *Pain* **2005**, *115*, 382–389. [CrossRef]

35. Lee, D.H.; Chung, J.M. Neuropathic pain in neonatal rats. *Neurosci. Lett.* **1996**, *209*, 140–142. [CrossRef]

36. McKelvey, R.; Berta, T.; Old, E.; Ji, R.R.; Fitzgerald, M. Neuropathic pain is constitutively suppressed in early life by anti-inflammatory neuroimmune regulation. *J. Neurosci.* **2015**, *35*, 457–466. [CrossRef]

37. Dourson, A.J.; Willits, A.; Raut, N.G.R.; Kader, L.; Young, E.; Jankowski, M.P.; Chidambaran, V. Genetic and epigenetic mechanisms influencing acute to chronic postsurgical pain transitions in pediatrics: Preclinical to clinical evidence. *Can. J. Pain* **2022**, *6*, 85–107. [CrossRef] [PubMed]

38. Anseloni, V.C.; He, F.; Novikova, S.I.; Turnbach Robbins, M.; Lidow, I.A.; Ennis, M.; Lidow, M.S. Alterations in stress-associated behaviors and neurochemical markers in adult rats after neonatal short-lasting local inflammatory insult. *Neuroscience* **2005**, *131*, 635–645. [CrossRef]

39. Victoria, N.C.; Inoue, K.; Young, L.J.; Murphy, A.Z. A single neonatal injury induces life-long deficits in response to stress. *Dev. Neurosci.* **2013**, *35*, 326–337. [CrossRef]

40. Yan, S.; Kentner, A.C. Mechanical allodynia corresponds to *OPRM1* downregulation within the descending pain network of male and female rats exposed to neonatal immune challenge. *Brain Behav. Immun.* **2017**, *63*, 148–159. [CrossRef]
41. Barr, G.A.; Wang, S.; Weisshaar, C.L.; Winkelstein, B.A. Developmental Changes in Pain and Spinal Immune Gene Expression after Radicular Trauma in the Rat. *Front. Neurol.* **2016**, *7*, 223. [CrossRef]
42. Moss, A.; Beggs, S.; Vega-Avelaira, D.; Costigan, M.; Hathway, G.J.; Salter, M.W.; Fitzgerald, M. Spinal microglia and neuropathic pain in young rats. *Pain* **2007**, *128*, 215–224. [CrossRef]
43. Cichon, J.; Sun, L.; Yang, G. Spared Nerve Injury Model of Neuropathic Pain in Mice. *Bio-Protocol* **2018**, *8*, e2777. [CrossRef]
44. Knaepen, L.; Patijn, J.; van Kleef, M.; Mulder, M.; Tibboel, D.; Joosten, E.A. Neonatal repetitive needle pricking: Plasticity of the spinal nociceptive circuit and extended postoperative pain in later life. *Dev. Neurobiol.* **2013**, *73*, 85–97. [CrossRef]
45. Burenkova, O.V.; Aleksandrova, E.A.; Zarayskaya, I.Y. Effects of early-life stress and HDAC inhibition on maternal behavior in mice. *Behav. Neurosci.* **2019**, *133*, 39–49. [CrossRef]
46. Loizzo, S.; Campana, G.; Vella, S.; Fortuna, A.; Galietta, G.; Guarino, I.; Costa, L.; Capasso, A.; Renzi, P.; Frajese, G.V.; et al. Post-natal stress-induced endocrine and metabolic alterations in mice at adulthood involve different pro-opiomelanocortin-derived peptides. *Peptides* **2010**, *31*, 2123–2129. [CrossRef]
47. Zuke, J.T.; Rice, M.; Rudlong, J.; Paquin, T.; Russo, E.; Burman, M.A. The Effects of Acute Neonatal Pain on Expression of Corticotropin-Releasing Hormone and Juvenile Anxiety in a Rodent Model. *eNeuro* **2019**, *6*. [CrossRef]
48. Moriarty, O.; Tu, Y.; Sengar, A.S.; Salter, M.W.; Beggs, S.; Walker, S.M. Priming of Adult Incision Response by Early-Life Injury: Neonatal Microglial Inhibition Has Persistent But Sexually Dimorphic Effects in Adult Rats. *J. Neurosci.* **2019**, *39*, 3081–3093. [CrossRef]
49. Ding, X.; Liang, Y.J.; Su, L.; Liao, F.F.; Fang, D.; Tai, J.; Xing, G.G. BDNF contributes to the neonatal incision-induced facilitation of spinal long-term potentiation and the exacerbation of incisional pain in adult rats. *Neuropharmacology* **2018**, *137*, 114–132. [CrossRef]
50. Segelcke, D.; Reichl, S.; Neuffer, S.; Zapp, S.; Rüther, T.; Evers, D.; Zahn, P.K.; Pogatzki-Zahn, E.M. The role of the spinal cyclooxygenase (COX) for incisional pain in rats at different developmental stages. *Eur. J. Pain* **2020**, *24*, 312–324. [CrossRef]
51. Anand, K.J.; Coskun, V.; Thrivikraman, K.V.; Nemeroff, C.B.; Plotsky, P.M. Long-term behavioral effects of repetitive pain in neonatal rat pups. *Physiol. Behav.* **1999**, *66*, 627–637. [CrossRef]
52. Ren, K.; Anseloni, V.; Zou, S.P.; Wade, B.E.; Novikova, I.S.; Ennis, M.; Traub, J.R.; Gold, S.M.; Dubner, R.; Lidow, S.M. Characterization of basal and re-inflammation-associated long-term alteration in pain responsivity following short-lasting neonatal local inflammatory insult. *Pain* **2004**, *110*, 588–596. [CrossRef]
53. Alvares, D.; Torsney, C.; Beland, B.; Reynolds, M.; Fitzgerald, M. Modelling the prolonged effects of neonatal pain. *Prog. Brain Res.* **2000**, *129*, 365–373. [CrossRef]
54. Bhutta, A.T.; Rovnaghi, C.; Simpson, P.M.; Gossett, J.M.; Scalzo, F.M.; Anand, K.J. Interactions of inflammatory pain and morphine in infant rats: Long-term behavioral effects. *Physiol. Behav.* **2001**, *73*, 51–58. [CrossRef] [PubMed]
55. Sternberg, W.F.; Ridgway, C.G. Effects of gestational stress and neonatal handling on pain, analgesia, and stress behavior of adult mice. *Physiol. Behav.* **2003**, *78*, 375–383. [CrossRef] [PubMed]
56. Al-Chaer, E.D.; Kawasaki, M.; Pasricha, P.J. A new model of chronic visceral hypersensitivity in adult rats induced by colon irritation during postnatal development. *Gastroenterology* **2000**, *119*, 1276–1285. [CrossRef] [PubMed]
57. Li, J.; Baccei, M.L. Neonatal tissue damage facilitates nociceptive synaptic input to the developing superficial dorsal horn via NGF-dependent mechanisms. *Pain* **2011**, *152*, 1846–1855. [CrossRef] [PubMed]
58. Li, J.; Baccei, M.L. Excitatory synapses in the rat superficial dorsal horn are strengthened following peripheral inflammation during early postnatal development. *Pain* **2009**, *143*, 56–64. [CrossRef]
59. Li, J.; Walker, S.M.; Fitzgerald, M.; Baccei, M.L. Activity-dependent modulation of glutamatergic signaling in the developing rat dorsal horn by early tissue injury. *J. Neurophysiol.* **2009**, *102*, 2208–2219. [CrossRef]
60. Li, J.; Baccei, M.L. Neonatal Tissue Damage Promotes Spike Timing-Dependent Synaptic Long-Term Potentiation in Adult Spinal Projection Neurons. *J. Neurosci.* **2016**, *36*, 5405–5416. [CrossRef]
61. Baccei, M.L.; Fitzgerald, M. Development of GABAergic and glycinergic transmission in the neonatal rat dorsal horn. *J. Neurosci.* **2004**, *24*, 4749–4757. [CrossRef]
62. Waldenström, A.; Thelin, J.; Thimansson, E.; Levinsson, A.; Schouenborg, J. Developmental learning in a pain-related system: Evidence for a cross-modality mechanism. *J. Neurosci.* **2003**, *23*, 7719–7725. [CrossRef] [PubMed]
63. Zouikr, I.; Karshikoff, B. Lifetime Modulation of the Pain System via Neuroimmune and Neuroendocrine Interactions. *Front. Immunol.* **2017**, *8*, 276. [CrossRef]
64. Brewer, C.L.; Baccei, M.L. The development of pain circuits and unique effects of neonatal injury. *J. Neural Transm.* **2020**, *127*, 467–479. [CrossRef]
65. Hathway, G.J.; Koch, S.; Low, L.; Fitzgerald, M. The changing balance of brainstem-spinal cord modulation of pain processing over the first weeks of rat postnatal life. *J. Physiol.* **2009**, *587*, 2927–2935. [CrossRef] [PubMed]
66. Walker, S.M.; Tochiki, K.K.; Fitzgerald, M. Hindpaw incision in early life increases the hyperalgesic response to repeat surgical injury: Critical period and dependence on initial afferent activity. *Pain* **2009**, *147*, 99–106. [PubMed]

7. Duff, E.P.; Moultrie, F.; van der Vaart, M.; Goksan, S.; Abos, A.; Fitzgibbon, S.P.; Baxter, L.; Wager, T.D.; Slater, R. Inferring pain experience in infants using quantitative whole-brain functional MRI signatures: A cross-sectional, observational study. *Lancet Digit. Health* **2020**, *2*, e458–e467. [CrossRef]

8. Baliki, M.N.; Petre, B.; Torbey, S.; Herrmann, K.M.; Huang, L.; Schnitzer, T.J.; Fields, H.L.; Apkarian, A.V. Corticostriatal functional connectivity predicts transition to chronic back pain. *Nat. Neurosci.* **2012**, *15*, 1117–1119. [CrossRef]

9. Menon, V. Developmental pathways to functional brain networks: Emerging principles. *Trends Cogn. Sci.* **2013**, *17*, 627–640. [CrossRef]

10. Fair, D.A.; Cohen, A.L.; Power, J.D.; Dosenbach, N.U.; Church, J.A.; Miezin, F.M.; Schlaggar, B.L.; Petersen, S.E. Functional brain networks develop from a "local to distributed" organization. *PLoS Comput. Biol.* **2009**, *5*, e1000381. [CrossRef]

11. Jolles, D.D.; van Buchem, M.A.; Crone, E.A.; Rombouts, S.A. A comprehensive study of whole-brain functional connectivity in children and young adults. *Cereb. Cortex* **2011**, *21*, 385–391. [CrossRef]

12. Dourson, A.; Hofmann, M.; Jankowski, M. Early life neuroimmune interactions modulate neonatal nociceptive priming. *Pain* **2021**, *22*, 578. [CrossRef]

13. Dourson, A.J.; Fadaka, A.O.; Warshak, A.M.; Paranjpe, A.; Weinhaus, B.; Queme, L.F.; Hofmann, M.C.; Evans, H.M.; Donmez, O.A.; Forney, C.; et al. Macrophage epigenetic memories of early life injury drive neonatal nociceptive priming. *bioRxiv* **2023**. [CrossRef]

14. Alvarado, S.; Tajerian, M.; Suderman, M.; Machnes, Z.; Pierfelice, S.; Millecamps, M.; Stone, L.S.; Szyf, M. An epigenetic hypothesis for the genomic memory of pain. *Front. Cell. Neurosci.* **2015**, *9*, 88. [CrossRef] [PubMed]

15. Carbajal, R.; Rousset, A.; Danan, C.; Coquery, S.; Nolent, P.; Ducrocq, S.; Saizou, C.; Lapillonne, A.; Granier, M.; Durand, P.; et al. Epidemiology and treatment of painful procedures in neonates in intensive care units. *JAMA* **2008**, *300*, 60–70. [CrossRef]

16. Peters, J.W.B.; Schouw, R.; Anand, K.J.S.; van Dijk, M.; Duivenvoorden, H.J.; Tibboel, D. Does neonatal surgery lead to increased pain sensitivity in later childhood? *Pain* **2005**, *114*, 444–454. [CrossRef] [PubMed]

17. Van den Bosch, G.E.; White, T.; El Marroun, H.; Simons, S.H.; van der Lugt, A.; van der Geest, J.N.; Tibboel, D.; van Dijk, M. Prematurity, Opioid Exposure and Neonatal Pain: Do They Affect the Developing Brain? *Neonatology* **2015**, *108*, 8–15. [CrossRef]

18. Tauzin, M.; Gouyon, B.; Hirt, D.; Carbajal, R.; Gouyon, J.B.; Brunet, A.C.; Ortala, M.; Goro, S.; Jung, C.; Durrmeyer, X. Frequencies, Modalities, Doses and Duration of Computerized Prescriptions for Sedative, Analgesic, Anesthetic and Paralytic Drugs in Neonates Requiring Intensive Care: A Prospective Pharmacoepidemiologic Cohort Study in 30 French NICUs From 2014 to 2020. *Front. Pharmacol.* **2022**, *13*, 939869. [CrossRef]

19. Laprairie, J.L.; Johns, M.E.; Murphy, A.Z. Preemptive Morphine Analgesia Attenuates the Long-Term Consequences of Neonatal Inflammation in Male and Female Rats. *Pediatr. Res.* **2008**, *64*, 625–630. [CrossRef]

20. Dührsen, L.; Simons, S.H.P.; Dzietko, M.; Genz, K.; Bendix, I.; Boos, V.; Sifringer, M.; Tibboel, D.; Felderhoff-Mueser, U. Effects of Repetitive Exposure to Pain and Morphine Treatment on the Neonatal Rat Brain. *Neonatology* **2012**, *103*, 35–43. [CrossRef]

21. Steinbauer, P.; Monje, F.J.; Kothgassner, O.; Goreis, A.; Eva, C.; Wildner, B.; Schned, H.; Deindl, P.; Seki, D.; Berger, A.; et al. The consequences of neonatal pain, stress and opiate administration in animal models: An extensive meta-analysis concerning neuronal cell death, motor and behavioral outcomes. *Neurosci. Biobehav. Rev.* **2022**, *137*, 104661. [CrossRef]

22. Van den Bosch, G.E.; Dijk, M.V.; Tibboel, D.; de Graaff, J.C. Long-term Effects of Early Exposure to Stress, Pain, Opioids and Anaesthetics on Pain Sensitivity and Neurocognition. *Curr. Pharm. Des.* **2017**, *23*, 5879–5886. [CrossRef] [PubMed]

23. Van den Bosch, G.; Tibboel, D.; Graaff, J.; El Marroun, H.; Lugt, A.; White, T.; van Dijk, M. Neonatal Pain, Opioid, and Anesthetic Exposure; What Remains in the Human Brain After the Wheels of Time? *Front. Pediatr.* **2022**, *10*, 825725. [CrossRef] [PubMed]

24. Verriotis, M.; Chang, P.; Fitzgerald, M.; Fabrizi, L. The development of the nociceptive brain. *Neuroscience* **2016**, *338*, 207–219. [CrossRef] [PubMed]

25. Giedd, J.N.; Rapoport, J.L. Structural MRI of pediatric brain development: What have we learned and where are we going? *Neuron* **2010**, *67*, 728–734. [CrossRef]

26. Sowell, E.R.; Peterson, B.S.; Thompson, P.M.; Welcome, S.E.; Henkenius, A.L.; Toga, A.W. Mapping cortical change across the human life span. *Nat. Neurosci.* **2003**, *6*, 309–315. [CrossRef] [PubMed]

27. Vinall, J.; Miller, S.P.; Bjornson, B.H.; Fitzpatrick, K.P.; Poskitt, K.J.; Brant, R.; Synnes, A.R.; Cepeda, I.L.; Grunau, R.E. Invasive procedures in preterm children: Brain and cognitive development at school age. *Pediatrics* **2014**, *133*, 412–421. [CrossRef]

28. Hohmeister, J.; Kroll, A.; Wollgarten-Hadamek, I.; Zohsel, K.; Demirakça, S.; Flor, H.; Hermann, C. Cerebral processing of pain in school-aged children with neonatal nociceptive input: An exploratory fMRI study. *Pain* **2010**, *150*, 257–267. [CrossRef]

29. Ranger, M.; Chau, C.M.; Garg, A.; Woodward, T.S.; Beg, M.F.; Bjornson, B.; Poskitt, K.; Fitzpatrick, K.; Synnes, A.R.; Miller, S.P.; et al. Neonatal pain-related stress predicts cortical thickness at age 7 years in children born very preterm. *PLoS ONE* **2013**, *8*, e76702. [CrossRef]

30. Slater, R.; Fabrizi, L.; Worley, A.; Meek, J.; Boyd, S.; Fitzgerald, M. Premature infants display increased noxious-evoked neuronal activity in the brain compared to healthy age-matched term-born infants. *Neuroimage* **2010**, *52*, 583–589. [CrossRef]

31. Jones, L.; Fabrizi, L.; Laudiano-Dray, M.; Whitehead, K.; Meek, J.; Verriotis, M.; Fitzgerald, M. Nociceptive Cortical Activity Is Dissociated from Nociceptive Behavior in Newborn Human Infants under Stress. *Curr. Biol.* **2017**, *27*, 3846–3851.e3843. [CrossRef]

32. Crettaz, B.; Marziniak, M.; Willeke, P.; Young, P.; Hellhammer, D.; Stumpf, A.; Burgmer, M. Stress-induced allodynia—Evidence of increased pain sensitivity in healthy humans and patients with chronic pain after experimentally induced psychosocial stress. *PLoS ONE* **2013**, *8*, e69460. [CrossRef] [PubMed]

93. Ozawa, M.; Kanda, K.; Hirata, M.; Kusakawa, I.; Suzuki, C. Influence of repeated painful procedures on prefrontal cortical pain responses in newborns. *Acta Paediatr.* **2011**, *100*, 198–203. [CrossRef]
94. Johnston, C.C.; Stevens, B.J. Experience in a neonatal intensive care unit affects pain response. *Pediatrics* **1996**, *98*, 925–930. [CrossRef]
95. Taddio, A.; Shah, V.; Gilbert-MacLeod, C.; Katz, J. Conditioning and hyperalgesia in newborns exposed to repeated heel lances. *JAMA* **2002**, *288*, 857–861. [CrossRef] [PubMed]
96. Taddio, A.; Shah, V.; Hancock, R.; Smith, R.W.; Stephens, D.; Atenafu, E.; Beyene, J.; Koren, G.; Stevens, B.; Katz, J. Effectiveness of sucrose analgesia in newborns undergoing painful medical procedures. *CMAJ* **2008**, *179*, 37–43. [CrossRef] [PubMed]
97. Johnston, C.; Campbell-Yeo, M.; Fernandes, A.; Inglis, D.; Streiner, D.; Zee, R. Skin-to-skin care for procedural pain in neonates. *Cochrane Database Syst. Rev.* **2014**, Cd008435. [CrossRef]
98. Hohmeister, J.; Demirakca, S.; Zohsel, K.; Flor, H.; Hermann, C. Responses to pain in school-aged children with experience in a neonatal intensive care unit: Cognitive aspects and maternal influences. *Eur. J. Pain* **2009**, *13*, 94–101. [CrossRef]
99. Doesburg, S.M.; Chau, C.M.; Cheung, T.P.L.; Moiseev, A.; Ribary, U.; Herdman, A.T.; Miller, S.P.; Cepeda, I.L.; Synnes, A.; Grunau, R.E. Neonatal pain-related stress, functional cortical activity and visual-perceptual abilities in school-age children born at extremely low gestational age. *Pain* **2013**, *154*, 1946–1952. [CrossRef]
100. Moiseev, A.; Doesburg, S.M.; Herdman, A.T.; Ribary, U.; Grunau, R.E. Altered Network Oscillations and Functional Connectivity Dynamics in Children Born Very Preterm. *Brain Topogr.* **2015**, *28*, 726–745. [CrossRef]
101. Sarnthein, J.; Stern, J.; Aufenberg, C.; Rousson, V.; Jeanmonod, D. Increased EEG power and slowed dominant frequency in patients with neurogenic pain. *Brain* **2006**, *129*, 55–64. [CrossRef]
102. Llinas, R.R.; Ribary, U.; Jeanmonod, D.; Kronberg, E.; Mitra, P.P. Thalamocortical dysrhythmia: A neurological and neuropsychiatric syndrome characterized by magnetoencephalography. *Proc. Natl. Acad. Sci. USA* **1999**, *96*, 15222–15227. [CrossRef] [PubMed]
103. Di Martino, A.; Shehzad, Z.; Kelly, C.; Roy, A.K.; Gee, D.G.; Uddin, L.Q.; Gotimer, K.; Klein, D.F.; Castellanos, F.X.; Milham, M.P. Relationship Between Cingulo-Insular Functional Connectivity and Autistic Traits in Neurotypical Adults. *Am. J. Psychiatry* **2009**, *166*, 891–899. [CrossRef] [PubMed]
104. Victoria, N.C.; Murphy, A.Z. Exposure to Early Life Pain: Long Term Consequences and Contributing Mechanisms. *Curr. Opin. Behav. Sci.* **2016**, *7*, 61–68. [CrossRef]
105. Steinbauer, P.; Deindl, P.; Fuiko, R.; Unterasinger, L.; Cardona, F.; Wagner, M.; Edobor, J.; Werther, T.; Berger, A.; Olischar, M.; et al. Long-term impact of systematic pain and sedation management on cognitive, motor, and behavioral outcomes of extremely preterm infants at preschool age. *Pediatr. Res.* **2021**, *89*, 540–548. [CrossRef]
106. Provenzi, L.; Guida, E.; Montirosso, R. Preterm behavioral epigenetics: A systematic review. *Neurosci. Biobehav. Rev.* **2018**, *84*, 262–271. [CrossRef]
107. Boggini, T.; Pozzoli, S.; Schiavolin, P.; Erario, R.; Mosca, F.; Brambilla, P.; Fumagalli, M. Cumulative procedural pain and brain development in very preterm infants: A systematic review of clinical and preclinical studies. *Neurosci. Biobehav. Rev.* **2021**, *123*, 320–336. [CrossRef]
108. Provenzi, L.; Fumagalli, M.; Scotto di Minico, G.; Giorda, R.; Morandi, F.; Sirgiovanni, I.; Schiavolin, P.; Mosca, F.; Borgatti, R.; Montirosso, R. Pain-related increase in serotonin transporter gene methylation associates with emotional regulation in 4.5-year-old preterm-born children. *Acta Paediatr.* **2020**, *109*, 1166–1174. [CrossRef]
109. Chau, C.M.; Ranger, M.; Sulistyoningrum, D.; Devlin, A.M.; Oberlander, T.F.; Grunau, R.E. Neonatal pain and *COMT* Val158Met genotype in relation to serotonin transporter (*SLC6A4*) promoter methylation in very preterm children at school age. *Front. Behav. Neurosci.* **2014**, *8*, 409. [CrossRef]
110. Chau, C.M.Y.; Ranger, M.; Bichin, M.; Park, M.T.M.; Amaral, R.S.C.; Chakravarty, M.; Poskitt, K.; Synnes, A.R.; Miller, S.P.; Grunau, R.E. Hippocampus, Amygdala, and Thalamus Volumes in Very Preterm Children at 8 Years: Neonatal Pain and Genetic Variation. *Front. Behav. Neurosci.* **2019**, *13*, 51. [CrossRef]
111. Chidambaran, V.; Zhang, X.; Geisler, K.; Stubbeman, B.L.; Chen, X.; Weirauch, M.T.; Meller, J.; Ji, H. Enrichment of Genomic Pathways Based on Differential DNA Methylation Associated with Chronic Postsurgical Pain and Anxiety in Children: A Prospective, Pilot Study. *Pain* **2019**, *20*, 771–785. [CrossRef]
112. Chidambaran, V.; Zhang, X.; Pilipenko, V.; Chen, X.; Wronowski, B.; Geisler, K.; Martin, L.J.; Barski, A.; Weirauch, M.T.; Ji, H. Methylation quantitative trait locus analysis of chronic postsurgical pain uncovers epigenetic mediators of genetic risk. *Epigenomics* **2021**, *13*, 613–630. [CrossRef]
113. Perry, M.; Sieberg, C.B.; Young, E.E.; Baumbauer, K.; Singh, V.; Wong, C.; Starkweather, A. The Potential Role of Preoperative Pain, Catastrophizing, and Differential Gene Expression on Pain Outcomes after Pediatric Spinal Fusion. *Pain Manag. Nurs.* **2021**, *22*, 44–49. [CrossRef] [PubMed]
114. Provenzi, L.; Fumagalli, M.; Sirgiovanni, I.; Giorda, R.; Pozzoli, U.; Morandi, F.; Beri, S.; Menozzi, G.; Mosca, F.; Borgatti, R.; et al. Pain-related stress during the Neonatal Intensive Care Unit stay and *SLC6A4* methylation in very preterm infants. *Front. Behav. Neurosci.* **2015**, *9*, 99. [CrossRef]
115. Provenzi, L.; Fumagalli, M.; Giorda, R.; Morandi, F.; Sirgiovanni, I.; Pozzoli, U.; Mosca, F.; Borgatti, R.; Montirosso, R. Maternal Sensitivity Buffers the Association between *SLC6A4* Methylation and Socio-Emotional Stress Response in 3-Month-Old Full Term, but not very Preterm Infants. *Front. Psychiatry* **2017**, *8*, 171. [CrossRef]

16. Provenzi, L.; Giorda, R.; Fumagalli, M.; Brambilla, M.; Mosca, F.; Borgatti, R.; Montirosso, R. Telomere length and salivary cortisol stress reactivity in very preterm infants. *Early Hum. Dev.* **2019**, *129*, 1–4. [CrossRef]
17. Provenzi, L.; Giorda, R.; Fumagalli, M.; Pozzoli, U.; Morandi, F.; Scotto di Minico, G.; Mosca, F.; Borgatti, R.; Montirosso, R. Pain exposure associates with telomere length erosion in very preterm infants. *Psychoneuroendocrinology* **2018**, *89*, 113–119. [CrossRef]
18. Mariani Wigley, I.L.C.; Mascheroni, E.; Fontana, C.; Giorda, R.; Morandi, F.; Bonichini, S.; McGlone, F.; Fumagalli, M.; Montirosso, R. The role of maternal touch in the association between *SLC6A4* methylation and stress response in very preterm infants. *Dev. Psychobiol.* **2021**, *63*, e22218. [CrossRef] [PubMed]
19. Grunau, R.E.; Cepeda, I.L.; Chau, C.M.; Brummelte, S.; Weinberg, J.; Lavoie, P.M.; Ladd, M.; Hirschfeld, A.F.; Russell, E.; Koren, G.; et al. Neonatal pain-related stress and *NFKBIA* genotype are associated with altered cortisol levels in preterm boys at school age. *PLoS ONE* **2013**, *8*, e73926. [CrossRef] [PubMed]
20. Dalal, P.G.; Doheny, K.K.; Klick, L.; Britcher, S.; Rebstock, S.; Bezinover, D.; Palmer, C.; Berlin, C.; Postula, M.; Kong, L.; et al. Analysis of acute pain scores and skin conductance measurements in infants. *Early Hum. Dev.* **2013**, *89*, 153–158. [CrossRef]
21. Hatfield, L.A.; Hoffman, R.K.; Polomano, R.C.; Conley, Y. Epigenetic Modifications Following Noxious Stimuli in Infants. *Biol. Res. Nurs.* **2018**, *20*, 137–144. [CrossRef]
22. Erbi, I.; Ciantelli, M.; Farinella, R.; Tuoni, C.; Gentiluomo, M.; Moscuzza, F.; Rizzato, C.; Bedini, A.; Faraoni, M.; Giusfredi, S.; et al. Role of *OPRM1*, clinical and anthropometric variants in neonatal pain reduction. *Sci. Rep.* **2020**, *10*, 7091. [CrossRef] [PubMed]
23. Harris, A.; Seckl, J. Glucocorticoids, prenatal stress and the programming of disease. *Horm. Behav.* **2011**, *59*, 279–289. [CrossRef] [PubMed]
24. Weaver, S.A.; Diorio, J.; Meaney, M.J. Maternal separation leads to persistent reductions in pain sensitivity in female rats. *J. Pain* **2007**, *8*, 962–969. [CrossRef]
25. Coutinho, S.V.; Plotsky, P.M.; Sablad, M.; Miller, J.C.; Zhou, H.; Bayati, A.I.; McRoberts, J.A.; Mayer, E.A. Neonatal maternal separation alters stress-induced responses to viscerosomatic nociceptive stimuli in rat. *Am. J. Physiol. Gastrointest. Liver Physiol.* **2002**, *282*, G307–G316. [CrossRef] [PubMed]
26. Green, P.G.; Chen, X.; Alvarez, P.; Ferrari, L.F.; Levine, J.D. Early-life stress produces muscle hyperalgesia and nociceptor sensitization in the adult rat. *Pain* **2011**, *152*, 2549–2556. [CrossRef] [PubMed]
27. Alvarez, P.; Green, P.G.; Levine, J.D. Stress in the Adult Rat Exacerbates Muscle Pain Induced by Early-Life Stress. *Biol. Psychiatry* **2013**, *74*, 688–695. [CrossRef]
28. Butler, R.K.; Finn, D.P. Stress-induced analgesia. *Prog. Neurobiol.* **2009**, *88*, 184–202. [CrossRef]
29. Grunau, R.E.; Holsti, L.; Haley, D.W.; Oberlander, T.; Weinberg, J.; Solimano, A.; Whitfield, M.F.; Fitzgerald, C.; Yu, W. Neonatal procedural pain exposure predicts lower cortisol and behavioral reactivity in preterm infants in the NICU. *Pain* **2005**, *113*, 293–300. [CrossRef] [PubMed]
30. Khasar, S.G.; Dina, O.A.; Green, P.G.; Levine, J.D. Sound stress-induced long-term enhancement of mechanical hyperalgesia in rats is maintained by sympathoadrenal catecholamines. *J. Pain* **2009**, *10*, 1073–1077. [CrossRef]
31. Ferrari, L.F.; Araldi, D.; Green, P.; Levine, J.D. Age-Dependent Sexual Dimorphism in Susceptibility to Develop Chronic Pain in the Rat. *Neuroscience* **2018**, *387*, 170–177. [CrossRef]
32. Lazaridou, A.; Kim, J.; Cahalan, C.M.; Loggia, M.L.; Franceschelli, O.; Berna, C.; Schur, P.; Napadow, V.; Edwards, R.R. Effects of Cognitive-Behavioral Therapy (CBT) on Brain Connectivity Supporting Catastrophizing in Fibromyalgia. *Clin. J. Pain* **2017**, *33*, 215–221. [CrossRef]
33. Brann, D.W.; Dhandapani, K.; Wakade, C.; Mahesh, V.B.; Khan, M.M. Neurotrophic and neuroprotective actions of estrogen: Basic mechanisms and clinical implications. *Steroids* **2007**, *72*, 381–405. [CrossRef]
34. Ferrari, L.F.; Araldi, D.; Levine, J.D. Regulation of Expression of Hyperalgesic Priming by Estrogen Receptor α in the Rat. *J. Pain* **2017**, *18*, 574–582. [CrossRef]
35. Heck, A.L.; Handa, R.J. Sex differences in the hypothalamic–pituitary–adrenal axis' response to stress: An important role for gonadal hormones. *Neuropsychopharmacology* **2019**, *44*, 45–58. [CrossRef] [PubMed]
36. Rabbitts, J.A.; Groenewald, C.B. Epidemiology of Pediatric Surgery in the United States. *Paediatr. Anaesth.* **2020**, *30*, 1083–1090. [CrossRef] [PubMed]
37. Sieberg, C.B.; Simons, L.E.; Edelstein, M.R.; DeAngelis, M.R.; Pielech, M.; Sethna, N.; Hresko, M.T. Pain prevalence and trajectories following pediatric spinal fusion surgery. *J. Pain* **2013**, *14*, 1694–1702. [CrossRef] [PubMed]
38. Jones, S.A.; Morales, A.M.; Holley, A.L.; Wilson, A.C.; Nagel, B.J. Default mode network connectivity is related to pain frequency and intensity in adolescents. *Neuroimage Clin.* **2020**, *27*, 102326. [CrossRef]
39. Baliki, M.N.; Geha, P.Y.; Fields, H.L.; Apkarian, A.V. Predicting value of pain and analgesia: Nucleus accumbens response to noxious stimuli changes in the presence of chronic pain. *Neuron* **2010**, *66*, 149–160. [CrossRef]
40. Koob, G.F. Neural mechanisms of drug reinforcement. *Ann. N. Y. Acad. Sci.* **1992**, *654*, 171–191. [CrossRef]
41. Apkarian, A.V.; Baliki, M.N.; Farmer, M.A. Predicting transition to chronic pain. *Curr. Opin. Neurol.* **2013**, *26*, 360–367. [CrossRef]
42. Mansour, A.R.; Baliki, M.N.; Huang, L.; Torbey, S.; Herrmann, K.M.; Schnitzer, T.J.; Apkarian, V.A. Brain white matter structural properties predict transition to chronic pain. *Pain* **2013**, *154*, 2160–2168. [CrossRef]
43. Zhao, X.; Xu, M.; Jorgenson, K.; Kong, J. Neurochemical changes in patients with chronic low back pain detected by proton magnetic resonance spectroscopy: A systematic review. *Neuroimage Clin.* **2017**, *13*, 33–38. [CrossRef]

144. Jung, Y.H.; Kim, H.; Lee, D.; Lee, J.Y.; Lee, W.J.; Moon, J.Y.; Choi, S.H.; Kang, D.H. Abnormal neurometabolites in fibromyalgia patients: Magnetic resonance spectroscopy study. *Mol. Pain* **2021**, *17*, 1744806921990946. [CrossRef]
145. Kim, S.H.; Lee, Y.; Lee, S.; Mun, C.W. Evaluation of the effectiveness of pregabalin in alleviating pain associated with fibromyalgia: Using functional magnetic resonance imaging study. *PLoS ONE* **2013**, *8*, e74099. [CrossRef]
146. Quaresima, V.; Bisconti, S.; Ferrari, M. A brief review on the use of functional near-infrared spectroscopy (fNIRS) for language imaging studies in human newborns and adults. *Brain Lang.* **2012**, *121*, 79–89. [CrossRef]
147. Karunakaran, K.D.; Peng, K.; Berry, D.; Green, S.; Labadie, R.; Kussman, B.; Borsook, D. NIRS measures in pain and analgesia: Fundamentals, features, and function. *Neurosci. Biobehav. Rev.* **2021**, *120*, 335–353. [CrossRef] [PubMed]
148. Ta Dinh, S.; Nickel, M.M.; Tiemann, L.; May, E.S.; Heitmann, H.; Hohn, V.D.; Edenharter, G.; Utpadel-Fischler, D.; Tölle, T.R.; Sauseng, P.; et al. Brain dysfunction in chronic pain patients assessed by resting-state electroencephalography. *Pain* **2019**, *160*, 2751–2765. [CrossRef] [PubMed]
149. Ocay, D.D.; Teel, E.F.; Luo, O.D.; Savignac, C.; Mahdid, Y.; Blain-Moraes, S.; Ferland, C.E. Electroencephalographic characteristics of children and adolescents with chronic musculoskeletal pain. *Pain Rep.* **2022**, *7*, e1054. [CrossRef]
150. Teel, E.F.; Ocay, D.D.; Blain-Moraes, S.; Ferland, C.E. Accurate classification of pain experiences using wearable electroencephalography in adolescents with and without chronic musculoskeletal pain. *Front. Pain Res.* **2022**, *3*, 991793. [CrossRef] [PubMed]
151. Ploner, M.; May, E.S. Electroencephalography and magnetoencephalography in pain research-current state and future perspectives. *Pain* **2018**, *159*, 206–211. [CrossRef]
152. Albertz, M.; Whitlock, P.; Yang, F.; Ding, L.; Uchtman, M.; Mecoli, M.; Olbrecht, V.; Moore, D.; McCarthy, J.; Chidambaran, V. Pragmatic comparative effectiveness study of multimodal fascia iliaca nerve block and continuous lumbar epidural-based protocols for periacetabular osteotomy. *J. Hip Preserv. Surg.* **2020**, *7*, 728–739. [CrossRef] [PubMed]
153. Geronimus, A.T.; Hicken, M.; Keene, D.; Bound, J. "Weathering" and age patterns of allostatic load scores among blacks and whites in the United States. *Am. J. Public Health* **2006**, *96*, 826–833. [CrossRef] [PubMed]
154. Seeman, T.E.; McEwen, B.S.; Rowe, J.W.; Singer, B.H. Allostatic load as a marker of cumulative biological risk: MacArthur studies of successful aging. *Proc. Natl. Acad. Sci. USA* **2001**, *98*, 4770–4775. [CrossRef] [PubMed]
155. Seeman, T.; Epel, E.; Gruenewald, T.; Karlamangla, A.; McEwen, B.S. Socio-economic differentials in peripheral biology: Cumulative allostatic load. *Ann. N. Y. Acad. Sci.* **2010**, *1186*, 223–239. [CrossRef]
156. Nelson, S.; Bento, S.; Enlow, M.B. Biomarkers of Allostatic Load as Correlates of Impairment in Youth with Chronic Pain: An Initial Investigation. *Children* **2021**, *8*, 709. [CrossRef]
157. Wallden, M.; Nijs, J. Before & beyond the pain—Allostatic load, central sensitivity and their role in health and function. *J. Bodyw. Mov. Ther.* **2021**, *27*, 388–392. [CrossRef]
158. Danese, A.; McEwen, B.S. Adverse childhood experiences, allostasis, allostatic load, and age-related disease. *Physiol. Behav.* **2012**, *106*, 29–39. [CrossRef] [PubMed]
159. Guidi, J.; Lucente, M.; Sonino, N.; Fava, G.A. Allostatic Load and Its Impact on Health: A Systematic Review. *Psychother. Psychosom.* **2021**, *90*, 11–27. [CrossRef]
160. Groenewald, C.B.; Murray, C.B.; Palermo, T.M. Adverse childhood experiences and chronic pain among children and adolescents in the United States. *Pain Rep.* **2020**, *5*, e839. [CrossRef]
161. Nelson, S.; Beveridge, J.K.; Mychasiuk, R.; Noel, M. Adverse Childhood Experiences (ACEs) and Internalizing Mental Health, Pain, and Quality of Life in Youth With Chronic Pain: A Longitudinal Examination. *J. Pain* **2021**, *22*, 1210–1220. [CrossRef]
162. Tidmarsh, L.V.; Harrison, R.; Ravindran, D.; Matthews, S.L.; Finlay, K.A. The Influence of Adverse Childhood Experiences in Pain Management: Mechanisms, Processes, and Trauma-Informed Care. *Front. Pain Res.* **2022**, *3*, 923866. [CrossRef] [PubMed]
163. Achenbach, J.; Rhein, M.; Gombert, S.; Meyer-Bockenkamp, F.; Buhck, M.; Eberhardt, M.; Leffler, A.; Frieling, H.; Karst, M. Childhood traumatization is associated with differences in TRPA1 promoter methylation in female patients with multisomatoform disorder with pain as the leading bodily symptom. *Clin. Epigenetics* **2019**, *11*, 126. [CrossRef] [PubMed]
164. Lobo, J.J.; Ayoub, L.J.; Moayedi, M.; Linnstaedt, S.D. Hippocampal volume, *FKBP5* genetic risk alleles, and childhood trauma interact to increase vulnerability to chronic multisite musculoskeletal pain. *Sci. Rep.* **2022**, *12*, 6511. [CrossRef] [PubMed]
165. Christensen, J.; Beveridge, J.K.; Wang, M.; Orr, S.L.; Noel, M.; Mychasiuk, R. A Pilot Study Investigating the Role of Gender in the Intergenerational Relationships between Gene Expression, Chronic Pain, and Adverse Childhood Experiences in a Clinical Sample of Youth with Chronic Pain. *Epigenomes* **2021**, *5*, 9. [CrossRef]
166. Generaal, E.; Milaneschi, Y.; Jansen, R.; Elzinga, B.M.; Dekker, J.; Penninx, B.W. The brain-derived neurotrophic factor pathway, life stress, and chronic multi-site musculoskeletal pain. *Mol. Pain* **2016**, *12*, 1744806916646783. [CrossRef]
167. Burke, N.N.; Finn, D.P.; McGuire, B.E.; Roche, M. Psychological stress in early life as a predisposing factor for the development of chronic pain: Clinical and preclinical evidence and neurobiological mechanisms. *J. Neurosci. Res.* **2017**, *95*, 1257–1270. [CrossRef]
168. Vinall, J.; Pavlova, M.; Asmundson, G.J.; Rasic, N.; Noel, M. Mental Health Comorbidities in Pediatric Chronic Pain: A Narrative Review of Epidemiology, Models, Neurobiological Mechanisms and Treatment. *Children* **2016**, *3*, 40. [CrossRef]
169. Liu, J.; Wang, C.; Gao, Y.; Tian, Y.; Wang, Y.; Wang, S. Sex-Specific Associations Between Preoperative Chronic Pain and Moderate to Severe Chronic Postoperative Pain in Patients 2 Years After Cardiac Surgery. *J. Pain Res.* **2022**, *15*, 4007–4015. [CrossRef]
170. Tighe, P.J.; Le-Wendling, L.T.; Patel, A.; Zou, B.; Fillingim, R.B. Clinically derived early postoperative pain trajectories differ by age, sex, and type of surgery. *Pain* **2015**, *156*, 609–617. [CrossRef]

71. Vasilopoulos, T.; Wardhan, R.; Rashidi, P.; Fillingim, R.B.; Wallace, M.R.; Crispen, P.L.; Parvataneni, H.K.; Prieto, H.A.; Machuca, T.N.; Hughes, S.J.; et al. Patient and Procedural Determinants of Postoperative Pain Trajectories. *Anesthesiology* **2021**, *134*, 421–434. [CrossRef]

72. Martin, A.L.; McGrath, P.A.; Brown, S.C.; Katz, J. Children with chronic pain: Impact of sex and age on long-term outcomes. *Pain* **2007**, *128*, 13–19. [CrossRef]

73. King, S.; Chambers, C.T.; Huguet, A.; MacNevin, R.C.; McGrath, P.J.; Parker, L.; MacDonald, A.J. The epidemiology of chronic pain in children and adolescents revisited: A systematic review. *Pain* **2011**, *152*, 2729–2738. [CrossRef]

74. Page, M.G.; Stinson, J.; Campbell, F.; Isaac, L.; Katz, J. Identification of pain-related psychological risk factors for the development and maintenance of pediatric chronic postsurgical pain. *J. Pain Res.* **2013**, *6*, 167–180. [CrossRef] [PubMed]

75. Connelly, M.; Fulmer, R.D.; Prohaska, J.; Anson, L.; Dryer, L.; Thomas, V.; Ariagno, J.E.; Price, N.; Schwend, R. Predictors of postoperative pain trajectories in adolescent idiopathic scoliosis. *Spine* **2014**, *39*, E174–E181. [CrossRef] [PubMed]

76. Narayanasamy, S.; Yang, F.; Ding, L.; Geisler, K.; Glynn, S.; Ganesh, A.; Sathyamoorthy, M.; Garcia, V.; Sturm, P.; Chidambaran, V. Pediatric Pain Screening Tool: A Simple 9-Item Questionnaire Predicts Functional and Chronic Postsurgical Pain Outcomes After Major Musculoskeletal Surgeries. *J. Pain* **2021**, *23*, 98–111. [CrossRef] [PubMed]

77. Ghazisaeidi, S.; Muley, M.M.; Salter, M.W. Neuropathic Pain: Mechanisms, Sex Differences, and Potential Therapies for a Global Problem. *Annu. Rev. Pharmacol. Toxicol.* **2023**, *63*, 565–583. [CrossRef]

78. Musey, P.I., Jr.; Linnstaedt, S.D.; Platts-Mills, T.F.; Miner, J.R.; Bortsov, A.V.; Safdar, B.; Bijur, P.; Rosenau, A.; Tsze, D.S.; Chang, A.K.; et al. Gender differences in acute and chronic pain in the emergency department: Results of the 2014 Academic Emergency Medicine consensus conference pain section. *Acad. Emerg. Med.* **2014**, *21*, 1421–1430. [CrossRef]

79. Holley, A.L.; Wilson, A.C.; Palermo, T.M. Predictors of the transition from acute to persistent musculoskeletal pain in children and adolescents: A prospective study. *Pain* **2017**, *158*, 794–801. [CrossRef]

80. Cruz-Almeida, Y.; Fillingim, R.B. Can Quantitative Sensory Testing Move Us Closer to Mechanism-Based Pain Management? *Pain Med.* **2014**, *15*, 61–72. [CrossRef]

81. Blankenburg, M.; Boekens, H.; Hechler, T.; Maier, C.; Krumova, E.; Scherens, A.; Magerl, W.; Aksu, F.; Zernikow, B. Reference values for quantitative sensory testing in children and adolescents: Developmental and gender differences of somatosensory perception. *Pain* **2010**, *149*, 76–88. [CrossRef]

82. Beland, B.; Fitzgerald, M. Influence of peripheral inflammation on the postnatal maturation of primary sensory neuron phenotype in rats. *J. Pain* **2001**, *2*, 36–45. [CrossRef]

83. Beggs, S.; Currie, G.; Salter, M.W.; Fitzgerald, M.; Walker, S.M. Priming of adult pain responses by neonatal pain experience: Maintenance by central neuroimmune activity. *Brain* **2012**, *135*, 404–417. [CrossRef]

84. Hathway, G.J.; Vega-Avelaira, D.; Fitzgerald, M. A critical period in the supraspinal control of pain: Opioid-dependent changes in brainstem rostroventral medulla function in preadolescence. *Pain* **2012**, *153*, 775–783. [CrossRef]

85. Fitzgerald, M.; McKelvey, R. Nerve injury and neuropathic pain—A question of age. *Exp. Neurol.* **2016**, *275 Pt 2*, 296–302. [CrossRef]

86. Borsook, D.; Becerra, L.; Hargreaves, R. Biomarkers for chronic pain and analgesia. Part 1: The need, reality, challenges, and solutions. *Discov. Med.* **2011**, *11*, 197–207.

87. Goldberg, Y.P.; Price, N.; Namdari, R.; Cohen, C.J.; Lamers, M.H.; Winters, C.; Price, J.; Young, C.E.; Verschoof, H.; Sherrington, R.; et al. Treatment of Na(v)1.7-mediated pain in inherited erythromelalgia using a novel sodium channel blocker. *Pain* **2012**, *153*, 80–85. [CrossRef] [PubMed]

88. Tsantoulas, C.; McMahon, S.B. Opening paths to novel analgesics: The role of potassium channels in chronic pain. *Trends Neurosci.* **2014**, *37*, 146–158. [CrossRef] [PubMed]

89. Long, J.Z.; Roche, A.M.; Berdan, C.A.; Louie, S.M.; Roberts, A.J.; Svensson, K.J.; Dou, F.Y.; Bateman, L.A.; Mina, A.I.; Deng, Z.; et al. Ablation of PM20D1 reveals N-acyl amino acid control of metabolism and nociception. *Proc. Natl. Acad. Sci. USA* **2018**, *115*, E6937–E6945. [CrossRef] [PubMed]

90. Markman, J.D.; Schnitzer, T.J.; Perrot, S.; Beydoun, S.R.; Ohtori, S.; Viktrup, L.; Yang, R.; Bramson, C.; West, C.R.; Verburg, K.M. Clinical Meaningfulness of Response to Tanezumab in Patients with Chronic Low Back Pain: Analysis From a 56-Week, Randomized, Placebo- and Tramadol-Controlled, Phase 3 Trial. *Pain Ther.* **2022**, *11*, 1267–1285. [CrossRef] [PubMed]

91. Koivisto, A.-P.; Belvisi, M.G.; Gaudet, R.; Szallasi, A. Advances in TRP channel drug discovery: From target validation to clinical studies. *Nat. Rev. Drug Discov.* **2022**, *21*, 41–59. [CrossRef] [PubMed]

92. Schwartz, E.S.; La, J.H.; Scheff, N.N.; Davis, B.M.; Albers, K.M.; Gebhart, G.F. TRPV1 and TRPA1 antagonists prevent the transition of acute to chronic inflammation and pain in chronic pancreatitis. *J. Neurosci.* **2013**, *33*, 5603–5611. [CrossRef]

93. Nirvanie-Persaud, L.; Millis, R.M. Epigenetics and Pain: New Insights to an Old Problem. *Cureus* **2022**, *14*, e29353. [CrossRef]

94. Denk, F.; McMahon, S.B. Chronic pain: Emerging evidence for the involvement of epigenetics. *Neuron* **2012**, *73*, 435–444. [CrossRef] [PubMed]

95. Doehring, A.; Geisslinger, G.; Lotsch, J. Epigenetics in pain and analgesia: An imminent research field. *Eur. J. Pain* **2011**, *15*, 11–16. [CrossRef] [PubMed]

96. Kanherkar, R.R.; Stair, S.E.; Bhatia-Dey, N.; Mills, P.J.; Chopra, D.; Csoka, A.B. Epigenetic Mechanisms of Integrative Medicine. *Evid. Based Complement. Alternat. Med.* **2017**, *2017*, 19. [CrossRef] [PubMed]

197. Niederberger, E.; Resch, E.; Parnham, M.J.; Geisslinger, G. Drugging the pain epigenome. *Nat. Rev. Neurol.* **2017**, *13*, 434–447. [CrossRef] [PubMed]
198. Sung, C.K.; Yim, H. CRISPR-mediated promoter de/methylation technologies for gene regulation. *Arch. Pharm. Res.* **2020**, *43*, 705–713. [CrossRef] [PubMed]
199. López-Muñoz, E.; Mejía-Terrazas, G.E. Epigenetics and Postsurgical Pain: A Scoping Review. *Pain Med.* **2021**, *23*, 246–262. [CrossRef] [PubMed]
200. Sachau, J.; Appel, C.; Reimer, M.; Sendel, M.; Vollert, J.; Hüllemann, P.; Baron, R. Test–retest reliability of a simple bedside quantitative sensory testing battery for chronic neuropathic pain. *Pain Rep.* **2023**, *8*, e1049. [CrossRef]
201. Reimer, M.; Sachau, J.; Forstenpointner, J.; Baron, R. Bedside testing for precision pain medicine. *Curr. Opin. Support. Palliat. Care* **2021**, *15*, 116–124. [CrossRef]
202. Edwards, R.R.; Dworkin, R.H.; Turk, D.C.; Angst, M.S.; Dionne, R.; Freeman, R.; Hansson, P.; Haroutounian, S.; Arendt-Nielsen, L.; Attal, N.; et al. Patient phenotyping in clinical trials of chronic pain treatments: IMMPACT recommendations. *Pain* **2016**, *157*, 1851–1871. [CrossRef] [PubMed]
203. Eisenberg, E.; Midbari, A.; Haddad, M.; Pud, D. Predicting the analgesic effect to oxycodone by 'static' and 'dynamic' quantitative sensory testing in healthy subjects. *Pain* **2010**, *151*, 104–109. [CrossRef] [PubMed]
204. Clarke, H.; Katz, J.; Flor, H.; Rietschel, M.; Diehl, S.R.; Seltzer, Z. Genetics of chronic post-surgical pain: A crucial step toward personal pain medicine. *Can. J. Anaesth.* **2015**, *62*, 294–303. [CrossRef]
205. Bernstein, B.E.; Stamatoyannopoulos, J.A.; Costello, J.F.; Ren, B.; Milosavljevic, A.; Meissner, A.; Kellis, M.; Marra, M.A.; Beaudet, A.L.; Ecker, J.R.; et al. The NIH Roadmap Epigenomics Mapping Consortium. *Nat. Biotechnol.* **2010**, *28*, 1045–1048. [CrossRef]
206. Caudle, K.E.; Sangkuhl, K.; Whirl-Carrillo, M.; Swen, J.J.; Haidar, C.E.; Klein, T.E.; Gammal, R.S.; Relling, M.V.; Scott, S.A.; Hertz, D.L.; et al. Standardizing *CYP2D6* Genotype to Phenotype Translation: Consensus Recommendations from the Clinical Pharmacogenetics Implementation Consortium and Dutch Pharmacogenetics Working Group. *Clin. Transl. Sci.* **2020**, *13*, 116–124. [CrossRef]
207. Crews, K.R.; Monte, A.A.; Huddart, R.; Caudle, K.E.; Kharasch, E.D.; Gaedigk, A.; Dunnenberger, H.M.; Leeder, J.S.; Callaghan, J.T.; Samer, C.F.; et al. Clinical Pharmacogenetics Implementation Consortium Guideline for *CYP2D6*, *OPRM1*, and *COMT* Genotypes and Select Opioid Therapy. *Clin. Pharmacol. Ther.* **2021**, *110*, 888–896. [CrossRef]
208. Chidambaran, V.; Simpson, B.; Brower, L.; Hanke, R.; Mecoli, M.; Lane, B.; Williams, S.; McKenna, E.; Bates, C.; Kraemer, A.; et al. Design and implementation of a novel patient-centered empowerment approach for pain optimisation in children undergoing major surgery. *BMJ Open Qual.* **2022**, *11*, e001874. [CrossRef] [PubMed]
209. Arendt-Nielsen, L.; Mansikka, H.; Staahl, C.; Rees, H.; Tan, K.; Smart, T.S.; Monhemius, R.; Suzuki, R.; Drewes, A.M. A translational study of the effects of ketamine and pregabalin on temporal summation of experimental pain. *Reg. Anesth. Pain Med.* **2011**, *36*, 585–591. [CrossRef]
210. Hayes, C.; Armstrong-Brown, A.; Burstal, R. Perioperative intravenous ketamine infusion for the prevention of persistent post-amputation pain: A randomized, controlled trial. *Anaesth. Intensive Care* **2004**, *32*, 330–338. [CrossRef]
211. Clarke, H.; Bonin, R.P.; Orser, B.A.; Englesakis, M.; Wijeysundera, D.N.; Katz, J. The prevention of chronic postsurgical pain using gabapentin and pregabalin: A combined systematic review and meta-analysis. *Anesth. Analg.* **2012**, *115*, 428–442. [CrossRef]
212. Steyaert, A.; Lavand'homme, P. Prevention and Treatment of Chronic Postsurgical Pain: A Narrative Review. *Drugs* **2018**, *78*, 339–354. [CrossRef] [PubMed]
213. Thapa, P.; Euasobhon, P. Chronic postsurgical pain: Current evidence for prevention and management. *Korean J. Pain* **2018**, *31*, 155–173. [CrossRef] [PubMed]
214. Chaparro, L.E.; Smith, S.A.; Moore, R.A.; Wiffen, P.J.; Gilron, I. Pharmacotherapy for the prevention of chronic pain after surgery in adults. *Cochrane Database Syst. Rev.* **2013**, *2013*, Cd008307. [CrossRef]
215. Clarke, H.; Poon, M.; Weinrib, A.; Katznelson, R.; Wentlandt, K.; Katz, J. Preventive analgesia and novel strategies for the prevention of chronic post-surgical pain. *Drugs* **2015**, *75*, 339–351. [CrossRef]
216. Bruneau, A.; Carrié, S.; Moscaritolo, L.; Ingelmo, P. Mechanism-Based Pharmacological Treatment for Chronic Non-cancer Pain in Adolescents: Current Approaches and Future Directions. *Pediatr. Drugs* **2022**, *24*, 573–583. [CrossRef]
217. Bazzari, A.H.; Bazzari, F.H. Advances in targeting central sensitization and brain plasticity in chronic pain. *Egypt. J. Neurol. Psychiatry Neurosurg.* **2022**, *58*, 38. [CrossRef]
218. Kaye, A.D.; Ridgell, S.; Alpaugh, E.S.; Mouhaffel, A.; Kaye, A.J.; Cornett, E.M.; Chami, A.A.; Shah, R.; Dixon, B.M.; Viswanath, O.; et al. Peripheral Nerve Stimulation: A Review of Techniques and Clinical Efficacy. *Pain Ther.* **2021**, *10*, 961–972. [CrossRef]
219. Moisset, X.; Lanteri-Minet, M.; Fontaine, D. Neurostimulation methods in the treatment of chronic pain. *J. Neural Transm.* **2020**, *127*, 673–686. [CrossRef]
220. Ilfeld, B.M.; Plunkett, A.; Vijjeswarapu, A.M.; Hackworth, R.; Dhanjal, S.; Turan, A.; Cohen, S.P.; Eisenach, J.C.; Griffith, S.; Hanling, S.; et al. Percutaneous Peripheral Nerve Stimulation (Neuromodulation) for Postoperative Pain: A Randomized, Sham-controlled Pilot Study. *Anesthesiology* **2021**, *135*, 95–110. [CrossRef]
221. García-Collado, A.; Valera-Calero, J.A.; Fernández-de-Las-Peñas, C.; Arias-Buría, J.L. Effects of Ultrasound-Guided Nerve Stimulation Targeting Peripheral Nerve Tissue on Pain and Function: A Scoping Review. *J. Clin. Med.* **2022**, *11*, 3753. [CrossRef]
222. Knotkova, H.; Hamani, C.; Sivanesan, E.; Le Beuffe, M.F.E.; Moon, J.Y.; Cohen, S.P.; Huntoon, M.A. Neuromodulation for chronic pain. *Lancet* **2021**, *397*, 2111–2124. [CrossRef]

23. Meeker, T.J.; Jupudi, R.; Lenz, F.A.; Greenspan, J.D. New Developments in Non-invasive Brain Stimulation in Chronic Pain. *Curr. Phys. Med. Rehabil. Rep.* **2020**, *8*, 280–292. [CrossRef] [PubMed]
24. Allen, C.H.; Kluger, B.M.; Buard, I. Safety of Transcranial Magnetic Stimulation in Children: A Systematic Review of the Literature. *Pediatr. Neurol.* **2017**, *68*, 3–17. [CrossRef] [PubMed]
25. Won, A.S.; Bailey, J.; Bailenson, J.; Tataru, C.; Yoon, I.A.; Golianu, B. Immersive Virtual Reality for Pediatric Pain. *Children* **2017**, *4*, 52. [CrossRef]
26. Orakpo, N.; Vieux, U.; Castro-Nuñez, C. Case Report: Virtual Reality Neurofeedback Therapy as a Novel Modality for Sustained Analgesia in Centralized Pain Syndromes. *Front. Psychiatry* **2021**, *12*, 660105. [CrossRef]
27. Bryanton, C.; Bossé, J.; Brien, M.; McLean, J.; McCormick, A.; Sveistrup, H. Feasibility, motivation, and selective motor control: Virtual reality compared to conventional home exercise in children with cerebral palsy. *Cyberpsychol. Behav.* **2006**, *9*, 123–128. [CrossRef] [PubMed]
28. Baumgartner, T.; Speck, D.; Wettstein, D.; Masnari, O.; Beeli, G.; Jäncke, L. Feeling present in arousing virtual reality worlds: Prefrontal brain regions differentially orchestrate presence experience in adults and children. *Front. Hum. Neurosci.* **2008**, *2*, 8. [CrossRef]
29. Shpaner, M.; Kelly, C.; Lieberman, G.; Perelman, H.; Davis, M.; Keefe, F.J.; Naylor, M.R. Unlearning chronic pain: A randomized controlled trial to investigate changes in intrinsic brain connectivity following Cognitive Behavioral Therapy. *Neuroimage Clin.* **2014**, *5*, 365–376. [CrossRef]
30. Fisher, E.; Law, E.; Dudeney, J.; Palermo, T.M.; Stewart, G.; Eccleston, C. Psychological therapies for the management of chronic and recurrent pain in children and adolescents. *Cochrane Database Syst. Rev.* **2018**, *9*, Cd003968. [CrossRef]
31. Cotton, S.; Luberto, C.M.; Bogenschutz, L.H.; Pelley, T.J.; Dusek, J. Integrative care therapies and pain in hospitalized children and adolescents: A retrospective database review. *J. Altern. Complement. Med.* **2014**, *20*, 98–102. [CrossRef]
32. Sommers, E.; D'Amico, S.; Goldstein, L.; Gardiner, P. Integrative Approaches to Pediatric Chronic Pain in an Urban Safety-Net Hospital: Cost Savings, Clinical Benefits, and Safety. *J. Integr. Complement. Med.* **2022**, *28*, 445–453. [CrossRef] [PubMed]
33. Ting, B.; Tsai, C.L.; Hsu, W.T.; Shen, M.L.; Tseng, P.T.; Chen, D.T.; Su, K.P.; Jingling, L. Music Intervention for Pain Control in the Pediatric Population: A Systematic Review and Meta-Analysis. *J. Clin. Med.* **2022**, *11*, 991. [CrossRef] [PubMed]
34. Jotwani, M.L.; Wu, Z.; Lunde, C.E.; Sieberg, C.B. The missing mechanistic link: Improving behavioral treatment efficacy for pediatric chronic pain. *Front. Pain Res.* **2022**, *3*, 1022699. [CrossRef] [PubMed]

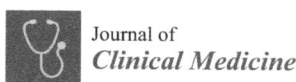

Journal of
Clinical Medicine

Article

The Role of Back Muscle Dysfunctions in Chronic Low Back Pain: State-of-the-Art and Clinical Implications

Thomas Matheve [1,2,*], Paul Hodges [3] and Lieven Danneels [1]

1   Spine, Head and Pain Research Unit Ghent, Department of Rehabilitation Sciences, Ghent University, 9000 Gent, Belgium; lieven.danneels@ugent.be
2   REVAL—Rehabilitation Research Center, Faculty of Rehabilitation Sciences, UHasselt, 3500 Diepenbeek, Belgium
3   NHMRC—Centre of Clinical Research Excellence in Spinal Pain, Injury & Health, School of Health & Rehabilitation Sciences, The University of Queensland, Brisbane 4072, Australia; p.hodges@uq.edu.au
*   Correspondence: thomas.matheve@ugent.be

Abstract: Changes in back muscle function and structure are highly prevalent in patients with chronic low back pain (CLBP). Since large heterogeneity in clinical presentation and back muscle dysfunctions exists within this population, the potential role of back muscle dysfunctions in the persistence of low back pain differs between individuals. Consequently, interventions should be tailored to the individual patient and be based on a thorough clinical examination taking into account the multidimensional nature of CLBP. Considering the complexity of this process, we will provide a state-of-the-art update on back muscle dysfunctions in patients with CLBP and their implications for treatment. To this end, we will first give an overview of (1) dysfunctions in back muscle structure and function, (2) the potential of exercise therapy to address these dysfunctions, and (3) the relationship between changes in back muscle dysfunctions and clinical parameters. In a second part, we will describe a framework for an individualised approach for back muscle training in patients with CLBP.

Keywords: back pain; muscle dysfunction; clinical implications

Citation: Matheve, T.; Hodges, P.; Danneels, L. The Role of Back Muscle Dysfunctions in Chronic Low Back Pain: State-of-the-Art and Clinical Implications. *J. Clin. Med.* **2023**, *12*, 5510. https://doi.org/10.3390/jcm12175510

Academic Editor: Icro Maremmani

Received: 13 July 2023
Revised: 21 August 2023
Accepted: 23 August 2023
Published: 24 August 2023

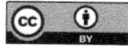

1. Introduction

Low back pain (LBP) is one of the leading causes of disability worldwide and has an enormous impact on a personal and societal level [1,2]. About 80% of the population will experience an episode of LBP during their lifetime [3]. Although an episode of acute LBP usually resolves within a few weeks, up to two thirds of patients report a flare-up within one year and about 15% will develop chronic low back pain (CLBP) [4–7], which is typically defined as LBP lasting for more than three months. The multidimensional nature of CLBP has been widely accepted [8,9]. Acknowledging the relative contribution of different factors to CLBP—including physical, emotional, cognitive, lifestyle, social, and behavioural aspects—is essential, as they will guide the assessment and treatment of the individual patient [10,11].

Two important physical factors are the structure and function of the back muscles, in particular of the lumbar multifidus and erector spinae (see Figure 1) [12,13]. The lumbar multifidus is the most medial back muscle in the lumbar region [13]. The multifidus muscle includes short deep fibres that span two intervertebral segments (referred to as the deep multifidus), and more superficially located muscle fibres that span three to five vertebral segments (referred to as superficial multifidus) [13]. The erector spinae is located laterally to the lumbar multifidus and consists of the lumbar and thoracic portions of the longissimus and iliocostalis muscles [13]. Due to its location and anatomy, the deep multifidus has little potential to extend the lumbar spine and mainly provides compressive forces that are important for segmental control [14]. Because of their more superficial location and longer lever arms, the superficial multifidus and erector spinae have a greater contribution to lumbar spine extension [13]. When they contract asymmetrically, they also contribute to sidebending and rotation [13,14].

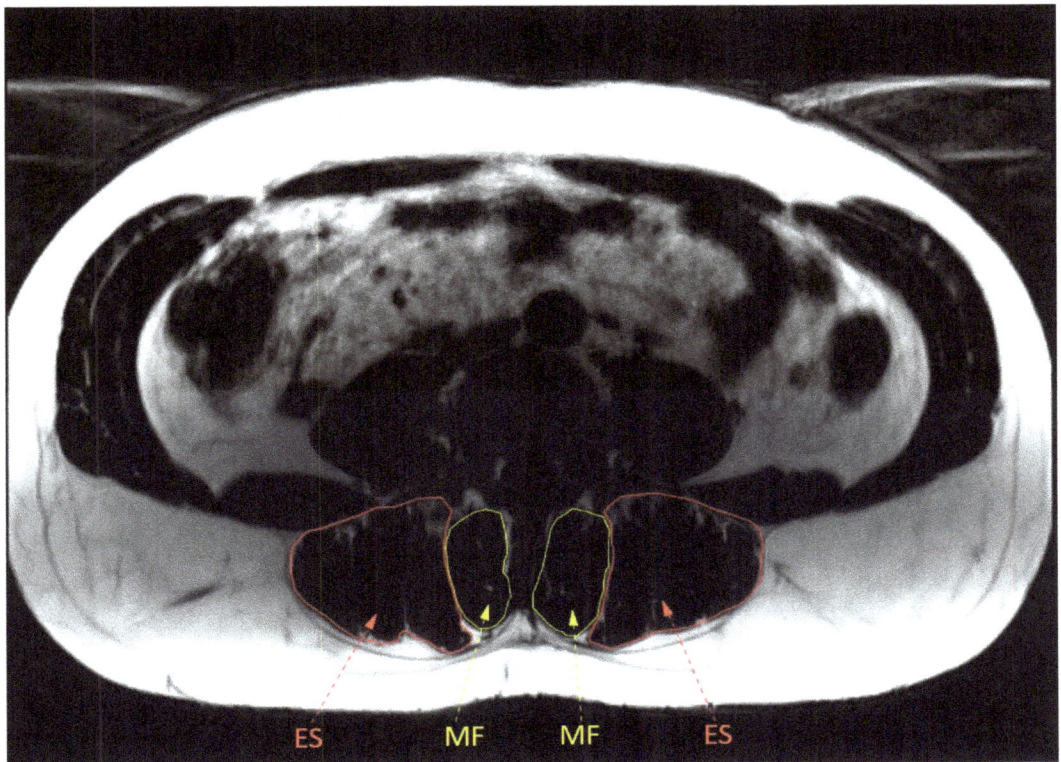

Figure 1. Anatomy of back muscles at L4 level. ES = erector spinae; MF = multifidus.

Evidence is emerging that changes in back muscle function and structure are time-dependent and exist on a continuum from acute to chronic LBP [12,15]. One potential implication of this is that different treatments are likely to be required to target these features depending on the timepoint on this trajectory towards chronicity. Of note, even within subgroups based on the time-course—and especially in patients with CLBP—there is large variability in the features of back muscle structure and function, and their role in the persistence of back problems is likely to differ between individuals [10]. This implies that interventions should always be based on a thorough examination taking into account the specific presentation of back muscle changes and the other multidimensional features of CLBP. This can be complex.

The objectives of this paper are to provide a state-of-the-art update of features of back muscle structure and function in patients with CLBP and their potential implications for treatment. To this end, the paper first gives an overview of (1) dysfunctions in back muscle structure and function, (2) the potential for exercise therapy to address these dysfunctions, and (3) the relationship between changes in back muscle dysfunctions and clinical parameters. In a second part, a framework is described for an individualised approach for back muscle training patients with CLBP.

2. Back Muscle Dysfunctions in Patients with Chronic Low Back Pain

2.1. Methods

To ensure the inclusion of the most recent and relevant information in this state-of-the-art overview of back muscle dysfunctions in CLBP, we conducted literature searches in the Pubmed and Web of Science databases up until April 2023. Search terms were partly derived from earlier conducted (systematic) reviews on the topics included in this overview (e.g., [16–19]). We selected papers including adults with CLBP that contained relevant information consistent with our three main objectives of this overview, i.e., to describe (1) dysfunctions in back muscle structure and function, (2) the potential for exercise therapy to address these dysfunctions, and (3) the relationship between changes in back muscle dysfunctions and clinical parameters. Both original research and literature reviews were considered.

2.2. Muscle Structure

Persistence of LBP is associated with extensive changes in the structure of the back muscles. Several studies have identified bilateral reduction in the multifidus cross-sectional area (CSA) and sometimes over several spinal levels in CLBP [20–24]. This differs from the more localized reduction of CSA (which can be specific to the painful side in unilateral conditions) in acute LBP. Findings for other muscles vary across studies [24]. Some studies report atrophy of the combined erector spinae and multifidus [25], whereas others report atrophy of the multifidus alone in CLBP [20,21]. Smaller CSAs of the multifidus, psoas, and quadratus lumborum muscle have been reported in some cases of LBP of longer duration [26]. Some studies comparing measures between individuals with continuous LBP and intermittent LBP in remission found no differences in the multifidus or erector spinae CSA [15,27].

Fatty infiltrations, either restricted to the multifidus or more widespread, have been shown using both qualitative [24,25,28] and quantitative [27] methods. Overall, patients with CLBP have a greater CSA of fat in the multifidus and to a lesser extent in erector spinae when compared to pain-free persons [24]. Moreover, the fat CSA and lean muscle fat index (indicating more fatty infiltration) are greater in the multifidus and erector spinae in cases of continuous CLBP (i.e., 7 pain days/week) than in individuals with recurrent LBP and noncontinuous CLBP (i.e., 3–4 pain days/week) [15]. Computed tomography measures have not found generalized fatty infiltration across the back muscles [21], but muscle density measures using computed tomography (which might be related to differences in fat content) show lower values in the multifidus and erector spinae at levels with facet joint osteoarthritis, spondylolisthesis, and intervertebral disc narrowing [29]. Experimental animal studies have shown a progression from localized to multisegmental changes in muscle structure over time after injury to a single intervertebral disc [30].

Findings regarding muscle-fibre-type proportions in CLBP are variable [14,16,17]. One study showed lower proportions of type I fibres and higher proportions of type II fibres in patients with CLBP scheduled for spinal surgery [31]. This study found no difference in the CSA of individual fibres, suggesting a smaller area occupied by type I fibres [31]. Another study in patients with CLBP scheduled for surgery also reported a higher proportion of type II fibres compared to pain-free persons, but found a smaller CSA of both Type I and Type II fibres in the CLBP group [32]. These results were independent of physical activity levels in the CLBP group [32]. A negative correlation between the proportion of type I fibres and the duration of pain, but a positive correlation with type IIx fibres, has also been observed [33]. T2 resting values also suggest a tendency towards a higher proportion of type II fibres in the multifidus and erector spinae in LBP [15]. Not all studies support these observations. Some studies found no differences in fibre size [34] or type I fibre proportion [34,35] in mild disabling LBP, despite poorer performance on a back muscle endurance test [34]. Variations in findings may be explained by symptom severity or the presence of spinal pathology. For instance, greater fibre II type proportions compared to pain-free persons have been reported for individuals undergoing surgery [31,32], whereas some studies in mild LBP found no differences [34,35]. Other aspects, such as variations in biopsy locations and the harvesting of control samples from cadavers with unclear LBP history may also contribute to variation in findings. Moreover, different methods have been used to classify muscle fibre types, such as myosin ATPase histochemical staining [31,33,34], expression of myosin heavy chain isoforms [35] or other methods [15,32]. This affects reported variations in type II classification [17], and some studies also do not specify the type II subclassification (e.g., IIa vs. IIx/d [36]) [15,32,34]. These issues complicate the interpretation of results and comparisons between studies. Finally, it is important to consider that all human studies are cross-sectional, and no longitudinal data are available. Longitudinal human studies are warranted to provide more insight into these aspects [12].

The mechanisms underlying structural muscle changes in CLBP are not completely understood, but are thought to differ over the time-course of the condition. In acute back pain, neurologically mediated reflex inhibition has been speculated in humans [37] and supported by animal data [38]. In the subacute period, there is emerging evidence from animal studies for changes mediated by the immune system [30] that have been supported by human data [39]. In the chronic phase, the features of muscle structure might be explained by deconditioning [12]. Reduced capacity due to earlier neural and inflammatory mechanisms may transition to reduced function [40,41]. Conditions that compromise the intervertebral foramen, such as spinal stenosis [42] and intervertebral disc disease [40], might lead to muscle atrophy and fat infiltration via mechanisms of denervation.

In sum, extensive changes in back muscle structure are present in patients with CLBP. In particular, the lumbar multifidus has a smaller bilateral CSA and increased fatty infiltration. These changes are less clear or less pronounced for other muscles. Findings regarding muscle-fibre-type proportions in CLBP are variable. When interpreting these results, it is important to consider the heterogeneity in the CLBP population as changes in muscle structure seem to be more pronounced in patients with more severe complaints (e.g., more continuous and/or more disabling LBP). See Table 1 for a summary of changes in back muscle structure in patients with CLBP.

Table 1. Summary of changes in back muscle structure in patients with chronic low back pain.

Parameter	Summary of Changes in Patients with Chronic Low Back Pain
Cross-sectional area (CSA)	- Smaller bilateral CSA of multifidus; unclear for erector spinae and other back muscles.
Fatty infiltration	- Increased fatty infiltration in multifidus and to a lesser extent in erector spinae. - More fatty infiltration in continuous CLBP compared to noncontinuous CLBP.
Muscle fibre type	- Inconsistent results, but potentially dependent on LBP severity. Increased type II fibre proportion in patients scheduled for spinal surgery; no differences with pain-free persons in mild disabling CLBP.

2.3. Back Muscle Function

There is a large body of literature that has evaluated and reviewed features of sensorimotor control of the back muscles that differ between individuals with and without back pain. This section considers some specific features, including recent observations, that have relevance for designing interventions. For comprehensive reviews see [12,43].

2.3.1. Sensorimotor Control

Back muscles make an important contribution to the control of spinal posture. They are activated in advance of perturbations that are predictable and react with short latency to perturbations that are not predictable. A recent systematic review concluded that differences in the reaction times of erector spinae to predictable and unpredictable perturbations were variable between individuals with and without low back pain—some studies show delayed reaction times and other studies found no differences [18]. There are many potential explanations for the variation including differences in recording electrodes, different task, back pain patients with different presentations, and different methods to quantify the timing of muscle activation. In the studies that do report differences in erector spinae reaction time, they are typically delayed [18,19]. Although these data appear to suggest some compromise in the activation of back muscles (which implies suboptimal control) [12], there are also data that suggest excessive recruitment of back muscles in response to experimental pain [44] and in individuals with chronic back pain during functional tasks [12,45], especially in those with unhelpful beliefs [46,47]. Increased activation appears to more consistently involve the more superficial erector spinae than deep (e.g., multifidus) muscles [12].

Other work has examined the sensorimotor mechanisms for control of back muscles by evaluation of the response of the muscles to transcranial magnetic stimulation over the motor cortex. Some studies have revealed reduced excitability of the descending pathways to the erector spinae [48] and alterations in the motor cortex representation of the back muscles [49]. Notably, this altered representation was characterized by the merging of distinct brain representations of the deep multifidus and superficial erector spinae muscles. This phenomenon has been found to correlate with the severity of LBP [50], particularly in individuals who have poorer capacity to differentiate between lumbar and thoracolumbar motion [51]. Changes in corticomotor function provide support for compromised multifidus muscle function in LBP. However, further research is necessary to fully comprehend the relationship between brain changes, motor function, and symptoms associated with LBP [12].

Studies that have investigated the somatosensory system in LBP have identified less disturbance to postural control from stimulation of proprioceptive signals from the back muscles in standing positions [52–54], which might indicate that information on back position/movement is weighted down. Patients with LBP also have impaired lumbar proprioception compared with controls when measured actively in sitting positions (especially when patients are categorised in direction-specific subgroups) or via a threshold to the detection of passive motion [55,56].

In conclusion, timing of erector spinae activation to predictable and unpredictable perturbations varies between patients with CLBP, but if impairments are present, they are characterized by delayed activation. Increased activity of erector spinae (as opposed to lumbar multifidus) during functional tasks is often observed in individuals with CLBP, which may represent a protective movement strategy. Motor cortex changes in areas representing the back muscles are related to compromised multifidus muscle function in LBP. Conversely, patients with LBP typically reduce the weighting of afferent proprioceptive information from the back muscles (mainly multifidus) for maintaining postural control. This indicates that changes in both 'top down' and 'bottom up' mechanisms are involved in sensorimotor control impairments in LBP. See Table 2 for a summary of changes in selected back muscle functions in patients with CLBP.

Table 2. Summary of changes in selected back muscle functions in patients with chronic low back pain.

Parameter	Summary of Changes in Patients with Chronic Low Back Pain
Sensorimotor control	
	- Reaction times of erector spinae to predictable and unpredictable perturbations are inconsistent. When changes in erector spinae reaction time are found, they are typically delayed. - Increased activity of erector spinae during functional tasks, especially in patients with unhelpful beliefs. - Alterations in the motor cortex representation of the back muscles are present. - Patients with LBP weight down afferent proprioceptive information from back muscles during postural control tasks.
Spatial distribution	
	- Patients with CLBP activate more cranially located regions of back extensors during fatiguing tasks. - Unclear whether differences in spatiotemporal changes are present in CLBP. Spatiotemporal changes seem to vary depending on the task and the individual.
Muscle strength and endurance	
	- Decreased in CLBP, but strong inter-individual variability.

2.3.2. Spatial Distribution of Lumbar Back Muscle Activity

Activity of superficial muscles is often assessed using bipolar surface electromyography, which limits the evaluation of muscle activity to a few separate lumbar areas. High-density surface electromyography can overcome this limitation, as this method uses a grid of multiple small electrodes (e.g., 5×13 electrodes) with small inter-electrode distance (e.g., 8 mm). Typically, the bottom end of this grid is placed 2 cm lateral to the L5 spinous process, covering the lumbar erector spinae up to approximately L2 [57–59]. This allows the measurement of the spatial distribution (i.e., which areas of the erector spinae are active) and spatiotemporal changes in superficial muscle activity during repeated or sustained tasks with more detail than traditional bipolar surface electromyography [58,60]. Some recent work with high-density surface electromyography has provided new insight into spatial distribution and spatiotemporal changes in erector spinae in patients with CLBP.

Alterations in spatial distribution of erector spinae muscle activity have been observed in CLBP, but differences appear to be task-dependent. During tasks that induce higher levels of muscle activity and muscle fatigue, such as repeated lifting or muscle endurance tests, individuals with CLBP typically use more cranially located regions of the erector spinae compared to pain-free persons [61–64]. Moreover, those with CLBP also have less dispersed erector spinae muscle activity during these type of tasks [63–65]. These differences relative to pain-free individuals have not been observed for low-load activities, such as walking or sit-to-stand [66]. The importance of muscle activity levels is shown by Arvanitidis et al. [62], who used a 15 s isometric back extension exercise at 20% and 50% of erector spinae MVC. During the low-load task, both patients with CLBP and pain-free persons used an equally dispersed activation pattern of erector spinae. During the high-load task, erector spinae activity was located more cranially in patients with CLBP, while the opposite pattern was observed in the pain-free persons.

In pain-free persons, spatiotemporal changes in erector spinae activity are typically present during repetitive or prolonged fatiguing tasks [59,63,65,67]. However, this redistribution of lumbar erector spinae activity does not seem to follow a stereotypical pattern, as both caudal and cranial shifts in erector spinae activity have been observed [59,63,67]. This suggests that motor control strategies to redistribute muscle activity might be specific to the individual and task. It is currently unclear whether there are differences in redistribution in erector spinae activity in patients with CLBP relative to that observed in pain-free persons because some studies have reported impairments [59,65] whereas others have not [61,68]. In studies that have reported impairments in spatial (re)distribution of erector spinae in CLBP, these impairments have been related to increased pain during [59,65] and poorer performance [63] on repetitive or endurance tasks. This failure to redistribute with fatigue appears consistent with the hypothesis that variation in muscle activation acts to reduce fatigue and prevent tissue overloading, thus protecting against the development of pain [69]. The absence of impairments of (re)distribution of erector spinae activity in 25–35% of patients with CLBP [59,63] might explain why some studies do not find between-group differences.

Both central and peripheral mechanisms have been put forward to explain impaired redistribution of back muscle activity [70]. Motor adaptations to acute pain that are driven by the nervous system are thought to protect body tissues from potential or actual injury [71]. Although it is not exactly clear why these adaptations may persist when protection is no longer necessary in the absence of nociceptive pain, pain-related psychological factors may play a role in this process [71,72]. Preliminary evidence supports a potential relationship with psychological features—spatial redistribution of erector spinae is less in patients with acute LBP [73] and was decreased during a repetitive lifting task in pain-free persons who perceived this task as more harmful [57]. Alternatively, redistribution of muscle activity may be hampered in patients with structural changes in the back muscles, such as increased fatty infiltration, fibrosis or fast-twitch muscle fibres [70]. These changes in muscle quality would be expected to increase metabolic demand and accelerate fatigue [15], and as these changes are more profound in caudal lumbar regions this might underlie the more cranial and less distributed activity.

In summary, individuals with CLBP appear to activate different and less diffuse areas of the back muscles during fatiguing tasks compared to pain-free controls. As impairments in spatial (re)distribution of erector spinae activity have been associated with pain and fatigue, these features could possibly be a potential treatment target [60].

2.3.3. Back Muscle Strength and Endurance

In their review, Steele et al. (2014) concluded that patients with (chronic) LBP have decreased lumbar extensor strength and endurance [74]. This has been confirmed by the recent literature [63,75–87]. However, this is not supported by all studies and the effect sizes of differences between individuals with and without CLBP are variable [86–88]. Although this may be partly due to variations in assessment protocols, such as differences in participant positioning (e.g., sit vs. stance) or type of exercise (e.g., isometric vs. isokinetic), this variability in between-group effect sizes is also observed when the same testing protocols are used. For example, small to very large effect sizes in differences in back muscle endurance have been reported between patients with CLBP and pain-free persons when measured with the Biering–Sorensen test [87,89]. Large variability is also present between results from studies using the same (or very similar) testing protocols in the same population. For example, time to failure during the Biering–Sorensen test in pain-free persons has been reported to range between 78 and 221 s [90,91], while in patients with CLBP, time to failure ranges between 39 and 144 s [84,90]. This variation is not unexpected as it would be naïve to assume that all patients with this highly heterogeneous condition would present in a similar manner. Many features can account for the variation.

Besides demographic (e.g., age or sex) and anthropometric (e.g., BMI) variables, it has frequently been suggested that pain-related psychological factors may substantially contribute to the variability in muscle strength and endurance in patients with CLBP [92]. For example, patients with higher levels of fear of movement may terminate the test prematurely; in a simple manner, this might relate to a belief that the task might cause pain or injury. Contrary to this hypothesis, a recent meta-analysis only found very small associations between pain-related psychological factors and muscle strength and endurance tests in patients with CLBP [93]. However, this might not tell the whole story—pain-related psychological factors are typically assessed using generic self-report measures, such as the Tampa Scale for Kinesiophobia [94,95] and these generic measures do not capture a patient's beliefs regarding specific activities or tasks [94]. It is plausible that muscle strength and endurance may be better predicted by task-specific psychological assessments instead of generic questionnaires, as has been shown for other types of movement behaviour (e.g., lumbar range of motion) [95,96].

In summary, interpretation of the performance on back muscle strength and endurance tests of an individual patient with CLBP is challenging. Interpretation is confounded by the many different methods to assess back muscle strength and endurance [74,97,98], variation in the patients' functional demands (e.g., physical job requirements), and the capacity of muscles outside the lumbar region (hip or thoracic extensor muscles) to contribute to test performance [74,99]. With respect to this latter point—some studies report that performance on the Biering–Sorensen test is determined by fatigue of the hip extensor muscles [100,101]. Since dysfunctions in back muscle strength and endurance are common in patients with CLBP, these aspects require assessment. Yet, test results need to be interpreted carefully, keeping in mind potential confounding.

2.4. Potential for Exercise Therapy to Address Back Muscle Dysfunctions

The literature summarized above supports the justification for consideration of the changes in structure and function of the back muscles as a component of a multifactorial program for the management of back pain. Addressing muscle changes in CLBP may involve strategies to reduce excessive protection, often involving overactivation of the more superficial erector spinae muscles, while also improving the function and structure of the deeper muscles, including the multifidus. Assessments of many aspects are likely to be necessary to identify the range of features that are critical to address in LBP treatment. These include, but are not limited to, assessments of movements [102], posture [103], psychological factors [94], and pain characteristics [10] to identify the specific aspects that need attention.

Specific exercises can improve the impaired back muscle functions that are targeted during treatment [104–106]. Although many studies have investigated muscle endurance and strength outcomes, there is also evidence that specific sensorimotor control training can change muscle recruitment of the back muscles [107].

Evidence of the impact of exercise for structural changes in back muscles is incomplete. Some evidence confirms the capacity of exercise to restore muscle size [108], and muscle fibrosis can be reduced by physical exercise in animals [109]. A recent systematic review concluded that the very limited evidence that is available suggests that fatty infiltration in back muscles might not be reversible with exercise therapy [110]. Interpretation of these data is not straightforward; the exercise programs used in some of the few available studies may have been too short and used insufficient loads to achieve structural changes [110], and whether the affected muscles were actually recruited during the training tasks was not addressed. Restoring fatty and fibrotic changes in muscle structure would likely require resistance training and be preceded by exercise to ensure adequate engagement of the affected muscles during the training tasks. Failure of a 16-week (3x/week; 6–10 RM) program of resistance training to reduce fatty infiltration at the lower lumbar spine (L5-S1) might relate to failure to engage these muscle areas in the training task [111]. In chronic LBP, it has also been shown that low-load motor control training alone is insufficient to restore muscle CSA [112], but combining it with controlled progressive overload training after low-load training can promote hypertrophy in the multifidus and reduce pain and disability [108]. This finding is supported by a more recent systematic review [113]. Considering the reduced proportion of type I muscle fibres in a subgroup of patients, endurance training may also be necessary. It is plausible to speculate that training for chronic LBP should initially focus on activation patterns tailored to individual adaptations, followed by resistance training for strength and endurance.

In conclusion, there is clear evidence that specific exercises can improve back muscle strength and endurance, and some studies also show that specific sensorimotor control training can change back muscle recruitment. The picture is less clear regarding the impact of exercise therapy on muscle structure, which may partly be explained by methodological limitations of the current literature. Exercise programmes of longer duration that initially focus on adequate muscle recruitment strategies followed by resistance training may be necessary to achieve changes in muscle structure.

2.5. Changes in Back Muscle Function and Clinical Parameters

Given the observed dysfunctions in patients with CLBP, lumbar back muscles are often targeted during exercise programmes. Because these exercise programmes typically lead to improvements in the targeted muscle-related (e.g., strength) and clinical (e.g., pain and disability) parameters [105,106,114], it is tempting to hypothesise that there is a causal relationship between these two. Although plausible, it remains unclear whether improvements in clinical parameters are contingent upon changes in lumbar back muscle function [115–119]. For example, Wong et al. (2014) concluded in their systematic review that the relationship between changes in multifidus (function) and clinical improvements are uncertain [115], although it must be acknowledged that many of the included studies used measures that lacked the capacity to evaluate the activation of the deep portion of the muscle. A systematic review by Steiger et al. (2012) showed that improvements in trunk extension strength were not associated with reductions in pain intensity and disability [116]. Again, the issue might be the lack of specificity of measures, as when the analysis is restricted to studies that evaluated lumbar extensor strength in isolation, positive correlations were found [120].

Various limitations of clinical studies require consideration when interpreting their results. First, clinical trials often do not consider the heterogeneity of the CLBP population. There is mounting evidence that patients with nociplastic pain (i.e., pain related to abnormal processing of nociceptive information [121]) or unhelpful beliefs (e.g., fear of movement) do not respond well to specific exercise therapy, such as muscle strengthening or motor control training [122–125]. Although these patients might achieve improvements in muscle function, this is unlikely to translate to clinical improvements [10].

Second, clinical trials typically assess movement behaviour (e.g., kinematics or muscle activity) in a generic manner, irrespective of patient presentation. If the movements and muscle-function parameters relevant for the individual patient are not considered, the relationships between changes in muscle function and clinical parameters are less likely to be observed [119,126]. In this respect, a systematic review by Wernli et al. (2020) showed that relationships between changes in movement behaviour and pain or disability in patients with LBP were only found in 31% of the comparisons in clinical trials [127]. In contrast, a different systematic review including only single-case designs—using more individualised measures—reported such relationships in 72% of the comparisons [126]. Although most studies have only assessed kinematic parameters (e.g., ROM), the few available case-studies assessing changes in back muscle activity in an individual manner also found relationships with clinical improvements [117,126]. An individualised approach may potentially lead to new insights regarding the relationships with clinical improvements.

In summary, there remains uncertainty whether changes in back muscle function after an exercise program are causally related to clinical improvements. Evaluating the impact of treatment by using assessments tailored to the individual patient is worthy of investigation and likely to provide a more promising investigation of the question.

3. Framework for an Individualised Approach to Back Muscle Training in Patients with CLBP

This section provides a framework for consideration of how back muscle training might be included in a comprehensive management plan for individuals with CLBP. An overview is provided in Figure 2.

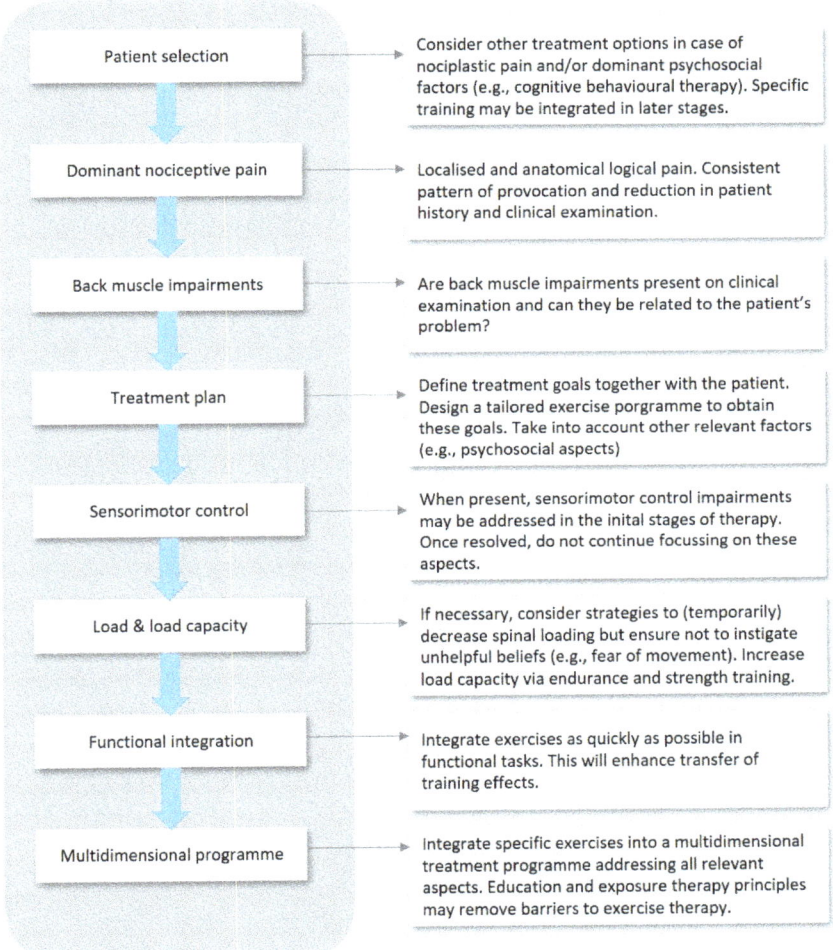

Figure 2. Overview of integrated framework for an individualised approach to back muscle training in patients with CLBP.

3.1. Take the Heterogeneity of the CLBP Population into Account

Although exercise therapy is effective in reducing pain and disability in patients with CLBP, effect sizes are modest at best and not all patients respond well to specific exercises [114,128]. Moreover, systematic reviews typically show that one type of exercise therapy is not superior to another [114,128]. An important limitation of many clinical trials is that they provide exercise therapy in a non-individualised manner, failing to take into account the heterogeneity of the CLBP population [123]. A major challenge is thus to target patients who are likely to benefit from a particular treatment.

There is increasing evidence that specific exercise therapy—i.e., sensorimotor control, muscle endurance and strength training—that focuses on changing how a patient uses their body and loads the spine is less effective for patients with strong unhelpful beliefs (e.g., fear of movement) or clear nociplastic pain characteristics [122–125,129,130] than for those with nociceptive pain (see below) [10]. For the former type of patients other treatments such as cognitive behavioural therapy (e.g., exposure therapy in vivo to tackle avoidance behaviour) or more general exercises (e.g., aerobic activities) may be recommended [94,124,125,131–133]. In that case, encouraging a patient to get back to function despite their pain and regardless of how they move might be most critical (although avoidance behaviour should be addressed). While it could eventually be useful to integrate more specific exercises into these programmes (e.g., to address deconditioning), it is unlikely that this would be an effective target in the initial stages of the therapy.

Specific exercises targeting the back muscles are probably more effective for patients with CLBP of predominantly nociceptive origin [122]. These patients have more localised pain with relatively clear patterns of provocation and reduction with specific postures and movements [134,135]. The premise is that suboptimal loading of spinal structures can be a cause of ongoing nociceptive input in many of these patients and a mechanism for the persistence of their CLBP. For individuals where this is related to postures and movements that involve activation of back extensors, addressing back muscle dysfunctions through specific exercise therapy has the potential to impact pain and disability secondary to optimised spinal loading [10]. This remains hypothetical and the exact mechanisms via which specific exercise therapy works are still largely unknown and are likely to be multifactorial [136].

Of note, within the subgroup of patients with nociceptive CLBP there is a large heterogeneity in clinical presentation and in back muscle dysfunctions. For instance, whether back muscles have high or low activity depends on clinical features of back pain, such as whether their pain is provoked by sitting in lumbar extension or flexion [103]. It would be expected that training to enhance back muscle structure and function would only be relevant for those who have clinical features that imply impaired structure and function and their relationship to pain provocation. Individualising exercise interventions based on a comprehensive patient history and clinical examination is paramount. A careful evaluation of the (painful) activities will guide treatment choices. For example, the modalities of back muscle endurance training can be different for patients who need to perform many repetitive flexion movements versus those who need to be able to maintain prolonged static semi-flex positions. In other words, effects of training are likely to be larger if treatments address features the patient lacks for participation in valued life activities.

In summary, a critical first step in designing an intervention that includes consideration of the back muscles is to critically judge the potential pain mechanisms that might explain a patient's pain. If nociceptive pain mechanisms are expected, then careful consideration of the patient's presenting movement, posture, and back muscle structure would be relevant.

3.2. Balancing Load and Load Capacity

In order to balance spinal loading and load capacity, patients with CLBP are often given advice and exercises that aim to protect the back and reduce spinal loading [137]. For example, they are taught to avoid sitting or lifting with a bent back. Although strategies to reduce spinal loading may be appropriate, it is critical that this does not lead to unhelpful beliefs such as 'my back is fragile and needs protection'. These types of messages from health care practitioners are an important way for patients with LBP to acquire such unhelpful beliefs [137,138].

As there is evidence that many patients with CLBP have reduced back muscle strength and endurance [74,97] and that changes in muscle structure might require loading to be changed [108], therapists should aim to train with loads sufficient to induce strength and endurance improvement. Although load is unlikely to be harmful, it might be painful. Teaching patients to modify their movement prior to loading might be required. Increasing the load capacity is essential for functional reintegration, as many daily life, leisure and job-related activities require repetitive or prolonged muscle contractions. A careful analysis of these requirements can guide decision making during therapy.

It is important to be aware that higher-load exercises might provoke transient back pain, and this is an important reason for patients to stop exercising [139,140]. Performance during strength exercises could also be impaired when patients expect them to be painful [93]. Pain education prior to participation in a (high-load) exercise programme may be helpful to remove barriers that may negatively affect adherence [141].

3.3. Sensorimotor Control Training

Earlier observations of structural and functional changes in the (deep) multifidus led to the development of specific sensorimotor control exercises targeting this muscle [37]. During these exercises, patients cognitively activate the (deep) lumbar multifidus independently from other back muscles [107]. It has been shown that changes in motor coordination could be reversed by these specific exercises, while this was not the case for simple back extensions activating all back muscles in a non-specific way [107]. Consequently, specific sensorimotor training of the multifidus has been advocated for patients with CLBP [12]. Although some have questioned whether such a specific approach is necessary because specific sensorimotor control exercises are not superior to general exercises to reduce pain and disability in patients with CLBP [142], other data suggest that this type of training might be more successful than general exercise when applied to patients with a consistent relationship between movements and pain (i.e., nociceptive type pain) [122]. This requires further investigation.

It is logical that an exercise programme should target multiple components (e.g., sensorimotor control and muscle strength) and multiple muscles when appropriate. When sensorimotor control impairments are present, it may be recommended to integrate selective activation exercises of the multifidus in the initial stages of therapy. This can restore muscle activation patterns at the lower lumbar spine [107], which in turn might help to engage more caudal regions of the back extensor muscles during fatiguing exercises. This is highly relevant, because patients with CLBP activate more cranial regions of the back extensor muscles during these tasks [61–64], resulting in earlier fatigue [63] and increased pain [59,65]. However, whether sensorimotor control exercises can affect spatial distribution of back muscle activity is unknown.

Once adequate sensorimotor control of the multifidus is achieved during selective activation exercises, it is unlikely to be necessary to continue to focus on this aspect and to transition to more functional training. Changes in muscle activation patterns obtained during selective training are likely to transfer to other activities [107]. Motor learning also needs to progress from an initial cognitive stage to more autonomous stages. A concern is that some individuals might become hypervigilant about the movements of their lower back as this may lead to unwanted protective movement behaviour [143].

3.4. Directed to Functional Integration

Analytical (non-functional) back muscle exercises can be useful when motor coordination is impaired or when the load capacity of the spine is low. In the last condition, analytical machine-based resistance exercises can be useful to create controlled overload in safe conditions in function of strength or endurance training [106]. However, training and rehabilitation should always be function-oriented. Therefore, we should, not hastily, but as soon as possible, start exercising in function of daily load and activities. In other words, training should integrate exercises into functional activities that are relevant for the individual patient and align exercise modalities with patient needs, as this allows for a better transfer of training effects.

Functional integration requires detailed assessment of the specific needs of a patient. This includes the functional evaluation of painful or frequently performed activities and adopted postures, with specific attention to habitual movement behaviour (for detailed description see [144]). The conclusions of this analysis should be translated to the choice of exercise modalities to individualise treatment. Examples include adaptation of movement speed, choice of functional positions, introduction of functional arm or leg movements, emphasis on static postures or dynamic movements, increased number of repetitions or introduction of dual cognitive tasks.

3.5. Integration of Back Muscle Training into a Multidimensional Treatment Plan

Although interventions that are limited to back muscle exercises have been shown to improve pain and disability [106], it is unlikely that this is ideal and that integration into a multidimensional treatment plan is likely to be more successful. There are multiple dimensions to consider.

Other physical aspects contributing to a patient's problem should be considered. This might include training of other muscle groups, proprioceptive and movement coordination exercises, improving general physical fitness, and changing 24 h movement behaviour. Obtaining long-term behavioural change is challenging [145], but small adaptations such as movement breaks to interrupt static postures might already be useful [146].

Patients with nociceptive CLBP typically do not have a generalised fear of movement, but they might be afraid of certain activities [94,95]. When introducing functional back muscle exercises, such as lifting loads with a bent back, some patients might be afraid to perform them because they perceive these tasks as harmful [95]. Although pain education may be useful, it is often not sufficient to tackle avoidance behaviour [147,148], so principles rooted in exposure therapy may be necessary to address potential avoidance behaviour [94,131]. By letting patients experience that the expected catastrophe ('My back will snap during lifting with a bent back') does not occur, their expectation will be violated and they can learn that these activities are safe to perform [149,150]. This will increase confidence in their ability to perform these activities and it will extinguish avoidance behaviour [149], which in turn will decrease disability. A recent randomised clinical trial showed that this approach is superior to general exercise therapy for reducing pain and disability in patients with chronic spinal pain [151].

It is also likely that many other elements require consideration that will differ between individuals. This might include consideration of sleep hygiene, stress management, diet, an many other aspects of an individual's lifestyle that can relate to pain [152,153]. Patients require a detailed assessment to guide individualised training.

3.6. Critical Appraisal

Although our framework for an individualised approach to back muscle training in patients with CLBP is based on the best available evidence, there remains uncertainty regarding various aspects that require clarification in future research. For example, the optimal exercise modalities to achieve changes in muscle function and structure are not always clear, and the relationships between these changes and clinical improvements require further investigation. Moreover, selecting patients that will benefit from a particular treatment is challenging given the heterogeneity of the CLBP population. Even within the subgroup of patients that is more likely to respond well to specific exercise therapy (i.e., those with dominant nociceptive pain characteristics), large variability in muscle function impairments is present. Careful analysis of muscle function is thus essential, yet not straightforward, especially in clinical settings where specialized equipment (e.g., electromyography) is often not available. Despite these limitations, the currently proposed framework provides clinicians with guidance on how to implement specific exercise tailored to the individual with CLBP.

3.7. Summary

Back muscle training is likely to be most effective if matched to the right patients and tailored to their needs and presentation. Exercise to target back muscle function and structure is likely to have its greatest impact on outcomes for patients with nociceptive CLBP.

Within this heterogeneous group, back muscle dysfunction is not uniform and treatment plans would depend on findings of thorough patient history and clinical examination. Specific sensorimotor control exercises at the initial stages of an exercise programme may be useful to optimise muscle activation patterns, but progression should be made towards back muscle endurance and strength training. Gradually increasing the load is safe for most patients and should be encouraged, rather than risking hypervigilance and excessive protection of the back. Exercises should be integrated into functional movements relevant for the patient. Because higher load (functional) exercises may cause transient back pain, education and the application of exposure therapy principles may be necessary to ensure adequate engagement of the patient. For an optimal outcome, back muscle exercises should be incorporated into an individualised multidimensional treatment plan.

4. Conclusions

This paper provides an overview of changes in muscle structure and muscle function in patients with CLBP. The integrated framework proposed for back muscle training in this population is based on current knowledge. It is essential to acknowledge the large variability in back muscle dysfunctions between patients with CLBP, and to carefully interpret their role in the persistence of back problems for the individual person. A multidimensional approach to low back pain management is likely to be optimal.

Author Contributions: Conceptualization, T.M. and L.D.; writing—original draft preparation, T.M. and L.D.; writing review and editing, T.M., L.D. and P.H. All authors have read and agreed to the published version of the manuscript.

Funding: P.H. is supported by a fellowship (APP1194937) from the National Health and Medical Research Council (NHMRC) of Australia.

Institutional Review Board Statement: Not applicable.

Informed Consent Statement: Not applicable.

Data Availability Statement: Not applicable.

Conflicts of Interest: The authors declare no conflict of interest.

References

1. Maher, C.; Underwood, M.; Buchbinder, R. Non-specific low back pain. *Lancet* **2017**, *389*, 736–747. [CrossRef] [PubMed]
2. Dagenais, S.; Caro, J.; Haldeman, S. A systematic review of low back pain cost of illness studies in the United States and internationally. *Spine J.* **2008**, *8*, 8–20. [CrossRef] [PubMed]
3. Airaksinen, O.; Brox, J.I.; Cedraschi, C.; Hildebrandt, J.; Klaber-Moffett, J.; Kovacs, F.; Mannion, A.F.; Reis, S.; Staal, J.B.; Ursin, H.; et al. Chapter 4. European guidelines for the management of chronic nonspecific low back pain. *Eur. Spine J.* **2006**, *15* (Suppl. S2), S192–S300. [CrossRef]
4. Mehling, W.E.; Gopisetty, V.; Bartmess, E.; Acree, M.; Pressman, A.; Goldberg, H.; Hecht, F.M.; Carey, T.; Avins, A.L. The prognosis of acute low back pain in primary care in the United States: A 2-year prospective cohort study. *Spine* **2012**, *37*, 678–684. [CrossRef] [PubMed]
5. Henschke, N.; Maher, C.G.; Refshauge, K.M.; Herbert, R.D.; Cumming, R.G.; Bleasel, J.; York, J.; Das, A.; McAuley, J.H. Prognosis in patients with recent onset low back pain in Australian primary care: Inception cohort study. *BMJ* **2008**, *337*, a171. [CrossRef] [PubMed]
6. da Silva, T.; Mills, K.; Brown, B.T.; Pocovi, N.; de Campos, T.; Maher, C.; Hancock, M.J. Recurrence of low back pain is common: A prospective inception cohort study. *J. Physiother.* **2019**, *65*, 159–165. [CrossRef] [PubMed]
7. Downie, A.S.; Hancock, M.J.; Rzewuska, M.; Williams, C.M.; Lin, C.C.; Maher, C.G. Trajectories of acute low back pain: A latent class growth analysis. *Pain* **2016**, *157*, 225–234. [CrossRef]
8. Vlaeyen, J.W.S.; Maher, C.G.; Wiech, K.; Van Zundert, J.; Meloto, C.B.; Diatchenko, L.; Battie, M.C.; Goossens, M.; Koes, B.; Linton, S.J. Low back pain. *Nat. Rev. Dis. Primers* **2018**, *4*, 52. [CrossRef]
9. Hartvigsen, J.; Hancock, M.J.; Kongsted, A.; Louw, Q.; Ferreira, M.L.; Genevay, S.; Hoy, D.; Karppinen, J.; Pransky, G.; Sieper, J.; et al. What low back pain is and why we need to pay attention. *Lancet* **2018**, *391*, 2356–2367. [CrossRef]
10. Hodges, P.W. Hybrid Approach to Treatment Tailoring for Low Back Pain: A Proposed Model of Care. *J. Orthop. Sports Phys. Ther.* **2019**, *49*, 453–463. [CrossRef]

11. Tagliaferri, S.D.; Miller, C.T.; Owen, P.J.; Mitchell, U.H.; Brisby, H.; Fitzgibbon, B.; Masse-Alarie, H.; Van Oosterwijck, J.; Belavy D.L. Domains of Chronic Low Back Pain and Assessing Treatment Effectiveness: A Clinical Perspective. *Pain Pract. Off. J. World Inst. Pain* **2020**, *20*, 211–225. [CrossRef]
12. Hodges, P.W.; Danneels, L. Changes in Structure and Function of the Back Muscles in Low Back Pain: Different Time Points Observations, and Mechanisms. *J. Orthop. Sports Phys. Ther.* **2019**, *49*, 464–476. [CrossRef] [PubMed]
13. Bogduk, N. The Lumbar Muscles and Their Fascia. In *Physical Therapy of the Low Back*, 3rd ed.; Twomey, L.T., Taylor, J.M., Eds. Churchill Livingstone: Philidelphia, PA, USA, 2000.
14. MacDonald, D.A.; Moseley, G.L.; Hodges, P.W. The lumbar multifidus: Does the evidence support clinical beliefs? *Man. Ther.* **2006**, *11*, 254–263. [CrossRef] [PubMed]
15. Goubert, D.; De Pauw, R.; Meeus, M.; Willems, T.; Cagnie, B.; Schouppe, S.; Van Oosterwijck, J.; Dhondt, E.; Danneels, L. Lumbar muscle structure and function in chronic versus recurrent low back pain: A cross-sectional study. *Spine J.* **2017**, *17*, 1285–1296 [CrossRef] [PubMed]
16. Cagnie, B.; Dhooge, F.; Schumacher, C.; De Meulemeester, K.; Petrovic, M.; van Oosterwijck, J.; Danneels, L. Fiber Typing of the Erector Spinae and Multifidus Muscles in Healthy Controls and Back Pain Patients: A Systematic Literature Review. *J. Manip. Physiol. Ther.* **2015**, *38*, 653–663. [CrossRef]
17. Purushotham, S.; Stephenson, R.S.; Sanderson, A.; Abichandani, D.; Greig, C.; Gardner, A.; Falla, D. Microscopic changes in the spinal extensor musculature in people with chronic spinal pain: A systematic review. *Spine J.* **2022**, *22*, 1205–1221. [CrossRef]
18. Knox, M.F.; Chipchase, L.S.; Schabrun, S.M.; Romero, R.J.; Marshall, P.W.M. Anticipatory and compensatory postural adjustments in people with low back pain: A systematic review and meta-analysis. *Spine J.* **2018**, *18*, 1934–1949. [CrossRef]
19. Prins, M.R.; Griffioen, M.; Veeger, T.T.J.; Kiers, H.; Meijer, O.G.; van der Wurff, P.; Bruijn, S.M.; van Dieën, J.H. Evidence of splinting in low back pain? A systematic review of perturbation studies. *Eur. Spine J.* **2018**, *27*, 40–59. [CrossRef]
20. Beneck, G.J.; Kulig, K. Multifidus atrophy is localized and bilateral in active persons with chronic unilateral low back pain. *Arch. Phys. Med. Rehabil.* **2012**, *93*, 300–306. [CrossRef]
21. Danneels, L.A.; Vanderstraeten, G.G.; Cambier, D.C.; Witvrouw, E.E.; De Cuyper, H.J. CT imaging of trunk muscles in chronic low back pain patients and healthy control subjects. *Eur. Spine J.* **2000**, *9*, 266–272. [CrossRef]
22. Fortin, M.; Macedo, L.G. Multifidus and paraspinal muscle group cross-sectional areas of patients with low back pain and control patients: A systematic review with a focus on blinding. *Phys. Ther.* **2013**, *93*, 873–888. [CrossRef] [PubMed]
23. Wallwork, T.L.; Stanton, W.R.; Freke, M.; Hides, J.A. The effect of chronic low back pain on size and contraction of the lumbar multifidus muscle. *Man. Ther.* **2009**, *14*, 496–500. [CrossRef] [PubMed]
24. Seyedhoseinpoor, T.; Taghipour, M.; Dadgoo, M.; Sanjari, M.A.; Takamjani, I.E.; Kazemnejad, A.; Khoshamooz, Y.; Hides, J. Alteration of lumbar muscle morphology and composition in relation to low back pain: A systematic review and meta-analysis. *Spine J.* **2022**, *22*, 660–676. [CrossRef] [PubMed]
25. Parkkola, R.; Rytökoski, U.; Kormano, M. Magnetic resonance imaging of the discs and trunk muscles in patients with chronic low back pain and healthy control subjects. *Spine* **1993**, *18*, 830–836. [CrossRef]
26. Kamaz, M.; Kireşi, D.; Oğuz, H.; Emlik, D.; Levendoğlu, F. CT measurement of trunk muscle areas in patients with chronic low back pain. *Diagn. Interv. Radiol.* **2007**, *13*, 144–148. [CrossRef]
27. Hultman, G.; Nordin, M.; Saraste, H.; Ohlsèn, H. Body composition, endurance, strength, cross-sectional area, and density of MM erector spinae in men with and without low back pain. *J. Spinal Disord.* **1993**, *6*, 114–123. [CrossRef]
28. Kader, D.F.; Wardlaw, D.; Smith, F.W. Correlation between the MRI changes in the lumbar multifidus muscles and leg pain. *Clin. Radiol.* **2000**, *55*, 145–149. [CrossRef]
29. Kalichman, L.; Hodges, P.; Li, L.; Guermazi, A.; Hunter, D.J. Changes in paraspinal muscles and their association with low back pain and spinal degeneration: CT study. *Eur. Spine J.* **2010**, *19*, 1136–1144. [CrossRef]
30. Hodges, P.W.; James, G.; Blomster, L.; Hall, L.; Schmid, A.; Shu, C.; Little, C.; Melrose, J. Multifidus Muscle Changes After Back Injury Are Characterized by Structural Remodeling of Muscle, Adipose and Connective Tissue, but Not Muscle Atrophy: Molecular and Morphological Evidence. *Spine* **2015**, *40*, 1057–1071. [CrossRef]
31. Mannion, A.F.; Weber, B.R.; Dvorak, J.; Grob, D.; Müntener, M. Fibre type characteristics of the lumbar paraspinal muscles in normal healthy subjects and in patients with low back pain. *J. Orthop. Res. Off. Publ. Orthop. Res. Soc.* **1997**, *15*, 881–887. [CrossRef]
32. Mazis, N.; Papachristou, D.J.; Zouboulis, P.; Tyllianakis, M.; Scopa, C.D.; Megas, P. The effect of different physical activity levels on muscle fiber size and type distribution of lumbar multifidus. A biopsy study on low back pain patient groups and healthy control subjects. *Eur. J. Phys. Rehabil. Med.* **2009**, *45*, 459–467. [CrossRef]
33. Mannion, A.F.; Käser, L.; Weber, E.; Rhyner, A.; Dvorak, J.; Müntener, M. Influence of age and duration of symptoms on fibre type distribution and size of the back muscles in chronic low back pain patients. *Eur. Spine J.* **2000**, *9*, 273–281. [CrossRef] [PubMed]
34. Crossman, K.; Mahon, M.; Watson, P.J.; Oldham, J.A.; Cooper, R.G. Chronic low back pain-associated paraspinal muscle dysfunction is not the result of a constitutionally determined "adverse" fiber-type composition. *Spine* **2004**, *29*, 628–634. [CrossRef] [PubMed]
35. Agten, A.; Stevens, S.; Verbrugghe, J.; Timmermans, A.; Vandenabeele, F. Biopsy samples from the erector spinae of persons with nonspecific chronic low back pain display a decrease in glycolytic muscle fibers. *Spine J.* **2020**, *20*, 199–206. [CrossRef] [PubMed]

36. Blaauw, B.; Schiaffino, S.; Reggiani, C. Mechanisms modulating skeletal muscle phenotype. *Compr. Physiol.* **2013**, *3*, 1645–1687. [CrossRef]
37. Hides, J.A.; Richardson, C.A.; Jull, G.A. Multifidus muscle recovery is not automatic after resolution of acute, first-episode low back pain. *Spine* **1996**, *21*, 2763–2769. [CrossRef]
38. Hodges, P.W.; Galea, M.P.; Holm, S.; Holm, A.K. Corticomotor excitability of back muscles is affected by intervertebral disc lesion in pigs. *Eur. J. Neurosci.* **2009**, *29*, 1490–1500. [CrossRef]
39. James, G.; Chen, X.; Diwan, A.; Hodges, P.W. Fat infiltration in the multifidus muscle is related to inflammatory cytokine expression in the muscle and epidural adipose tissue in individuals undergoing surgery for intervertebral disc herniation. *Eur. Spine J.* **2021**, *30*, 837–845. [CrossRef]
40. Yoshihara, K.; Nakayama, Y.; Fujii, N.; Aoki, T.; Ito, H. Atrophy of the multifidus muscle in patients with lumbar disk herniation: Histochemical and electromyographic study. *Orthopedics* **2003**, *26*, 493–495. [CrossRef]
41. Sihvonen, T.; Lindgren, K.A.; Airaksinen, O.; Manninen, H. Movement disturbances of the lumbar spine and abnormal back muscle electromyographic findings in recurrent low back pain. *Spine* **1997**, *22*, 289–295. [CrossRef]
42. Haig, A.J. Paraspinal denervation and the spinal degenerative cascade. *Spine J.* **2002**, *2*, 372–380. [CrossRef] [PubMed]
43. van Dieën, J.H.; Reeves, N.P.; Kawchuk, G.; van Dillen, L.R.; Hodges, P.W. Motor Control Changes in Low Back Pain: Divergence in Presentations and Mechanisms. *J. Orthop. Sports Phys. Ther.* **2019**, *49*, 370–379. [CrossRef] [PubMed]
44. Devecchi, V.; Falla, D.; Cabral, H.V.; Gallina, A. Neuromuscular adaptations to experimentally induced pain in the lumbar region: Systematic review and meta-analysis. *Pain* **2023**, *164*, 1159–1180. [CrossRef] [PubMed]
45. Arendt-Nielsen, L.; Graven-Nielsen, T.; Svarrer, H.; Svensson, P. The influence of low back pain on muscle activity and coordination during gait: A clinical and experimental study. *Pain* **1996**, *64*, 231–240. [CrossRef] [PubMed]
46. Christe, G.; Crombez, G.; Edd, S.; Opsommer, E.; Jolles, B.M.; Favre, J. Relationship between psychological factors and spinal motor behaviour in low back pain: A systematic review and meta-analysis. *Pain* **2021**, *162*, 672–686. [CrossRef]
47. Ippersiel, P.; Teoli, A.; Wideman, T.H.; Preuss, R.A.; Robbins, S.M. The Relationship Between Pain-Related Threat and Motor Behavior in Nonspecific Low Back Pain: A Systematic Review and Meta-Analysis. *Phys. Ther.* **2022**, *102*, pzab274. [CrossRef]
48. Strutton, P.H.; Theodorou, S.; Catley, M.; McGregor, A.H.; Davey, N.J. Corticospinal excitability in patients with chronic low back pain. *J. Spinal Disord. Tech.* **2005**, *18*, 420–424. [CrossRef]
49. Tsao, H.; Danneels, L.A.; Hodges, P.W. ISSLS prize winner: Smudging the motor brain in young adults with recurrent low back pain. *Spine* **2011**, *36*, 1721–1727. [CrossRef]
50. Schabrun, S.M.; Elgueta-Cancino, E.L.; Hodges, P.W. Smudging of the Motor Cortex Is Related to the Severity of Low Back Pain. *Spine* **2017**, *42*, 1172–1178. [CrossRef]
51. Elgueta-Cancino, E.; Schabrun, S.; Hodges, P. Is the Organization of the Primary Motor Cortex in Low Back Pain Related to Pain, Movement, and/or Sensation? *Clin. J. Pain* **2018**, *34*, 207–216. [CrossRef]
52. Pijnenburg, M.; Caeyenberghs, K.; Janssens, L.; Goossens, N.; Swinnen, S.P.; Sunaert, S.; Brumagne, S. Microstructural integrity of the superior cerebellar peduncle is associated with an impaired proprioceptive weighting capacity in individuals with non-specific low back pain. *PLoS ONE* **2014**, *9*, e100666. [CrossRef]
53. Brumagne, S.; Janssens, L.; Knapen, S.; Claeys, K.; Suuden-Johanson, E. Persons with recurrent low back pain exhibit a rigid postural control strategy. *Eur. Spine J.* **2008**, *17*, 1177–1184. [CrossRef]
54. Claeys, K.; Brumagne, S.; Dankaerts, W.; Kiers, H.; Janssens, L. Decreased variability in postural control strategies in young people with non-specific low back pain is associated with altered proprioceptive reweighting. *Eur. J. Appl. Physiol.* **2011**, *111*, 115–123. [CrossRef] [PubMed]
55. Tong, M.H.; Mousavi, S.J.; Kiers, H.; Ferreira, P.; Refshauge, K.; van Dieen, J. Is there a relationship between lumbar proprioception and low back pain? A systematic review with meta-analysis. *Arch. Phys. Med. Rehabil.* **2016**, *98*, 120–136.e2. [CrossRef]
56. Korakakis, V.; O'Sullivan, K.; Kotsifaki, A.; Sotiralis, Y.; Giakas, G. Lumbo-pelvic proprioception in sitting is impaired in subgroups of low back pain-But the clinical utility of the differences is unclear. A systematic review and meta-analysis. *PLoS ONE* **2021**, *16*, e0250673. [CrossRef] [PubMed]
57. Liechti, M.; von Arx, M.; Eichelberger, P.; Bangerter, C.; Meier, M.L.; Schmid, S. Spatial distribution of erector spinae activity is related to task-specific pain-related fear during a repetitive object lifting task. *J. Electromyogr. Kinesiol. Off. J. Int. Soc. Electrophysiol. Kinesiol.* **2022**, *65*, 102678. [CrossRef] [PubMed]
58. Besomi, M.; Hodges, P.W.; Van Dieën, J.; Carson, R.G.; Clancy, E.A.; Disselhorst-Klug, C.; Holobar, A.; Hug, F.; Kiernan, M.C.; Lowery, M.; et al. Consensus for experimental design in electromyography (CEDE) project: Electrode selection matrix. *J. Electromyogr. Kinesiol. Off. J. Int. Soc. Electrophysiol. Kinesiol.* **2019**, *48*, 128–144. [CrossRef] [PubMed]
59. Falla, D.; Gizzi, L.; Tschapek, M.; Erlenwein, J.; Petzke, F. Reduced task-induced variations in the distribution of activity across back muscle regions in individuals with low back pain. *Pain* **2014**, *155*, 944–953. [CrossRef]
60. Falla, D.; Gallina, A. New insights into pain-related changes in muscle activation revealed by high-density surface electromyography. *J. Electromyogr. Kinesiol. Off. J. Int. Soc. Electrophysiol. Kinesiol.* **2020**, *52*, 102422. [CrossRef]
61. Arvanitidis, M.; Bikinis, N.; Petrakis, S.; Gkioka, A.; Tsimpolis, D.; Falla, D.; Martinez-Valdes, E. Spatial distribution of lumbar erector spinae muscle activity in individuals with and without chronic low back pain during a dynamic isokinetic fatiguing task. *Clin. Biomech.* **2021**, *81*, 105214. [CrossRef]

62. Arvanitidis, M.; Jiménez-Grande, D.; Haouidji-Javaux, N.; Falla, D.; Martinez-Valdes, E. People with chronic low back pain display spatial alterations in high-density surface EMG-torque oscillations. *Sci. Rep.* **2022**, *12*, 15178. [CrossRef] [PubMed]

63. Sanderson, A.; Martinez-Valdes, E.; Heneghan, N.R.; Murillo, C.; Rushton, A.; Falla, D. Variation in the spatial distribution of erector spinae activity during a lumbar endurance task in people with low back pain. *J. Anat.* **2019**, *234*, 532–542. [CrossRef] [PubMed]

64. Sanderson, A.; Cescon, C.; Heneghan, N.R.; Kuithan, P.; Martinez-Valdes, E.; Rushton, A.; Barbero, M.; Falla, D. People With Low Back Pain Display a Different Distribution of Erector Spinae Activity During a Singular Mono-Planar Lifting Task. *Front. Sports Act. Living* **2019**, *1*, 65. [CrossRef] [PubMed]

65. Abboud, J.; Nougarou, F.; Pagé, I.; Cantin, V.; Massicotte, D.; Descarreaux, M. Trunk motor variability in patients with non-specific chronic low back pain. *Eur. J. Appl. Physiol.* **2014**, *114*, 2645–2654. [CrossRef] [PubMed]

66. Serafino, F.; Trucco, M.; Occhionero, A.; Cerone, G.L.; Chiarotto, A.; Vieira, T.; Gallina, A. Understanding regional activation of thoraco-lumbar muscles in chronic low back pain and its relationship to clinically relevant domains. *BMC Musculoskelet. Disord.* **2021**, *22*, 432. [CrossRef]

67. Tucker, K.; Falla, D.; Graven-Nielsen, T.; Farina, D. Electromyographic mapping of the erector spinae muscle with varying load and during sustained contraction. *J. Electromyogr. Kinesiol. Off. J. Int. Soc. Electrophysiol. Kinesiol.* **2009**, *19*, 373–379. [CrossRef]

68. Ringheim, I.; Indahl, A.; Roeleveld, K. Reduced muscle activity variability in lumbar extensor muscles during sustained sitting in individuals with chronic low back pain. *PLoS ONE* **2019**, *14*, e0213778. [CrossRef]

69. Hamill, J.; Palmer, C.; Van Emmerik, R.E. Coordinative variability and overuse injury. *Sports Med. Arthrosc. Rehabil. Ther. Technol. SMARTT* **2012**, *4*, 45. [CrossRef]

70. Hodges, P.W. To redistribute muscle activity in pain, or not: That is the question. *Pain* **2014**, *155*, 849–850. [CrossRef]

71. Hodges, P.W.; Smeets, R.J. Interaction between pain, movement, and physical activity: Short-term benefits, long-term consequences, and targets for treatment. *Clin. J. Pain* **2015**, *31*, 97–107. [CrossRef]

72. Thomas, J.S.; France, C.R. The relationship between pain-related fear and lumbar flexion during natural recovery from low back pain. *Eur. Spine J.* **2008**, *17*, 97–103. [CrossRef] [PubMed]

73. Martinez-Valdes, E.; Wilson, F.; Fleming, N.; McDonnell, S.J.; Horgan, A.; Falla, D. Rowers with a recent history of low back pain engage different regions of the lumbar erector spinae during rowing. *J. Sci. Med. Sport/Sports Med. Aust.* **2019**, *22*, 1206–1212. [CrossRef] [PubMed]

74. Steele, J.; Bruce-Low, S.; Smith, D. A reappraisal of the deconditioning hypothesis in low back pain: Review of evidence from a triumvirate of research methods on specific lumbar extensor deconditioning. *Curr. Med. Res. Opin.* **2014**, *30*, 865–911. [CrossRef] [PubMed]

75. Conway, R.; Behennah, J.; Fisher, J.; Osborne, N.; Steele, J. A Comparison of Isolated Lumbar Extension Strength Between Healthy Asymptomatic Participants and Chronic Low Back Pain Participants Without Previous Lumbar Spine Surgery. *Spine* **2018**, *43*, E1232–E1237. [CrossRef]

76. Mingorance, J.A.; Montoya, P.; Miranda, J.G.V.; Riquelme, I. An Observational Study Comparing Fibromyalgia and Chronic Low Back Pain in Somatosensory Sensitivity, Motor Function and Balance. *Healthcare* **2021**, *9*, 1533. [CrossRef]

77. Moreno Catalá, M.; Schroll, A.; Laube, G.; Arampatzis, A. Muscle Strength and Neuromuscular Control in Low-Back Pain: Elite Athletes Versus General Population. *Front. Neurosci.* **2018**, *12*, 436. [CrossRef]

78. Rossi, D.M.; Morcelli, M.H.; Cardozo, A.C.; Denadai, B.S.; Gonçalves, M.; Navega, M.T. Discriminant analysis of neuromuscular variables in chronic low back pain. *J. Back. Musculoskelet. Rehabil.* **2015**, *28*, 239–246. [CrossRef]

79. da Silva, R.A.; Vieira, E.R.; Cabrera, M.; Altimari, L.R.; Aguiar, A.F.; Nowotny, A.H.; Carvalho, A.F.; Oliveira, M.R. Back muscle fatigue of younger and older adults with and without chronic low back pain using two protocols: A case-control study. *J. Electromyogr. Kinesiol. Off. J. Int. Soc. Electrophysiol. Kinesiol.* **2015**, *25*, 928–936. [CrossRef]

80. Han, G.; Zhou, S.; Wang, W.; Li, W.; Qiu, W.; Li, X.; Fan, X.; Li, W. Correlations between paraspinal extensor muscle endurance and clinical outcomes in preoperative LSS patients and clinical value of an endurance classification. *J. Orthop. Transl.* **2022**, *35*, 81–86. [CrossRef]

81. Jubany, J.; Marina, M.; Angulo-Barroso, R. Electromyographic and Kinematic Analysis of Trunk and Limb Muscles During a Holding Task in Individuals With Chronic Low Back Pain and Healthy Controls. *PM&R* **2017**, *9*, 1106–1116. [CrossRef]

82. Langenfeld, A.; Wirth, B.; Scherer-Vrana, A.; Riner, F.; Gaehwiler, K.; Valdivieso, P.; Humphreys, B.K.; Scholkmann, F.; Flueck, M.; Schweinhardt, P. No alteration of back muscle oxygenation during isometric exercise in individuals with non-specific low back pain. *Sci. Rep.* **2022**, *12*, 8306. [CrossRef] [PubMed]

83. Miñambres-Martín, D.; Martín-Casas, P.; López-de-Uralde-Villanueva, I.; Fernández-de-Las-Peñas, C.; Valera-Calero, J.A.; Plaza-Manzano, G. Physical Function in Amateur Athletes with Lumbar Disc Herniation and Chronic Low Back Pain: A Case-Control Study. *Int. J. Environ. Res. Public. Health* **2022**, *19*, 3743. [CrossRef] [PubMed]

84. Pilz, B.; Vasconcelos, R.A.; Teixeira, P.P.; Mello, W.; Oliveira, I.O.; Ananias, J.; Timko, M.; Grossi, D.B. Comparison of Hip and Lumbopelvic Performance Between Chronic Low Back Pain Patients Suited for the Functional Optimization Approach and Healthy Controls. *Spine* **2020**, *45*, E37–E44. [CrossRef] [PubMed]

85. Rose-Dulcina, K.; Armand, S.; Dominguez, D.E.; Genevay, S.; Vuillerme, N. Asymmetry of lumbar muscles fatigability with non-specific chronic low back pain patients. *Eur. Spine J.* **2019**, *28*, 2526–2534. [CrossRef]

96. Rostami, M.; Ansari, M.; Noormohammadpour, P.; Mansournia, M.A.; Kordi, R. Ultrasound assessment of trunk muscles and back flexibility, strength and endurance in off-road cyclists with and without low back pain. *J. Back. Musculoskelet. Rehabil.* **2015**, *28*, 635–644. [CrossRef]

97. Tavares, J.M.A.; Rodacki, A.L.F.; Hoflinger, F.; Dos Santos Cabral, A.; Paulo, A.C.; Rodacki, C.L.N. Physical Performance, Anthropometrics and Functional Characteristics Influence the Intensity of Nonspecific Chronic Low Back Pain in Military Police Officers. *Int. J. Environ. Res. Public. Health* **2020**, *17*, 6434. [CrossRef]

98. Pranata, A.; Perraton, L.; El-Ansary, D.; Clark, R.; Fortin, K.; Dettmann, T.; Brandham, R.; Bryant, A. Lumbar extensor muscle force control is associated with disability in people with chronic low back pain. *Clin. Biomech.* **2017**, *46*, 46–51. [CrossRef]

99. Behennah, J.; Conway, R.; Fisher, J.; Osborne, N.; Steele, J. The relationship between balance performance, lumbar extension strength, trunk extension endurance, and pain in participants with chronic low back pain, and those without. *Clin. Biomech.* **2018**, *53*, 22–30. [CrossRef]

100. Simmonds, M.J.; Olson, S.L.; Jones, S.; Hussein, T.; Lee, C.E.; Novy, D.; Radwan, H. Psychometric characteristics and clinical usefulness of physical performance tests in patients with low back pain. *Spine* **1998**, *23*, 2412–2421. [CrossRef]

101. Gruther, W.; Wick, F.; Paul, B.; Leitner, C.; Posch, M.; Matzner, M.; Crevenna, R.; Ebenbichler, G. Diagnostic accuracy and reliability of muscle strength and endurance measurements in patients with chronic low back pain. *J. Rehabil. Med.* **2009**, *41*, 613–619. [CrossRef]

102. Huijnen, I.P.J.; Verbunt, J.A.; Wittink, H.M.; Smeets, R.J.E.M. Physical performance measurement in chronic low back pain: Measuring physical capacity or pain-related behaviour? *Eur. J. Physiother.* **2013**, *15*, 103–110. [CrossRef]

103. Matheve, T.; Janssens, L.; Goossens, N.; Danneels, L.; Willems, T.; Van Oosterwijck, J.; De Baets, L. The Relationship Between Pain-Related Psychological Factors and Maximal Physical Performance in Low Back Pain: A Systematic Review and Meta-Analysis. *J. Pain. Off. J. Am. Pain. Soc.* **2022**, *23*, 2036–2051. [CrossRef]

104. De Baets, L.; Meulders, A.; Van Damme, S.; Caneiro, J.P.; Matheve, T. Understanding discrepancies in a person's fear of movement and avoidance behaviour: A guide for musculoskeletal rehabilitation clinicians who support people with chronic musculoskeletal pain. *J. Orthop. Sports Phys. Ther.* **2023**, *53*, 307–316. [CrossRef]

105. Matheve, T.; De Baets, L.; Bogaerts, K.; Timmermans, A. Lumbar range of motion in chronic low back pain is predicted by task-specific, but not by general measures of pain-related fear. *Eur. J. Pain* **2019**, *23*, 1171–1184. [CrossRef]

106. Wildenbeest, M.H.; Kiers, H.; Tuijt, M.; van Dieën, J.H. Associations of low-back pain and pain-related cognitions with lumbar movement patterns during repetitive seated reaching. *Gait Posture* **2021**, *91*, 216–222. [CrossRef]

107. Demoulin, C.; Vanderthommen, M.; Duysens, C.; Crielaard, J.M. Spinal muscle evaluation using the Sorensen test: A critical appraisal of the literature. *Jt. Bone Spine Rev. Rhum.* **2006**, *73*, 43–50. [CrossRef] [PubMed]

108. Althobaiti, S.; Rushton, A.; Aldahas, A.; Falla, D.; Heneghan, N.R. Practicable performance-based outcome measures of trunk muscle strength and their measurement properties: A systematic review and narrative synthesis. *PLoS ONE* **2022**, *17*, e0270101. [CrossRef] [PubMed]

99. Pitcher, M.J.; Behm, D.G.; Mackinnon, S.N. Neuromuscular fatigue during a modified biering-sørensen test in subjects with and without low back pain. *J. Sports Sci. Med.* **2007**, *6*, 549–559. [PubMed]

100. Kankaanpää, M.; Laaksonen, D.; Taimela, S.; Kokko, S.M.; Airaksinen, O.; Hänninen, O. Age, sex, and body mass index as determinants of back and hip extensor fatigue in the isometric Sørensen back endurance test. *Arch. Phys. Med. Rehabil.* **1998**, *79*, 1069–1075. [CrossRef]

101. Moffroid, M.; Reid, S.; Henry, S.M.; Haugh, L.D.; Ricamato, A. Some endurance measures in persons with chronic low back pain. *J. Orthop. Sports Phys. Ther.* **1994**, *20*, 81–87. [CrossRef]

102. Elgueta-Cancino, E.; Schabrun, S.; Danneels, L.; van den Hoorn, W.; Hodges, P. Validation of a Clinical Test of Thoracolumbar Dissociation in Chronic Low Back Pain. *J. Orthop. Sports Phys. Ther.* **2015**, *45*, 703–712. [CrossRef]

103. Dankaerts, W.; O'Sullivan, P.; Burnett, A.; Straker, L. Altered patterns of superficial trunk muscle activation during sitting in nonspecific chronic low back pain patients: Importance of subclassification. *Spine* **2006**, *31*, 2017–2023. [CrossRef] [PubMed]

104. Claes, S.; Campos, L.F.; Correia, K.L.; de Lucena, J.M.S.; Gentil, P.; Durigan, J.L.; Ribeiro, A.L.A.; Martins, W.R. Exercise interventions can improve muscle strength, endurance, and electrical activity of lumbar extensors in individuals with non-specific low back pain: A systematic review with meta-analysis. *Sci. Rep.* **2021**, *11*, 16842. [CrossRef] [PubMed]

105. Wood, L.; Foster, N.E.; Lewis, M.; Bronfort, G.; Groessl, E.J.; Hewitt, C.; Miyamoto, G.C.; Reme, S.E.; Bishop, A. Matching the Outcomes to Treatment Targets of Exercise for Low Back Pain: Does it Make a Difference? Results of Secondary Analyses From Individual Patient Data of Randomised Controlled Trials and Pooling of Results Across Trials in Comparative Meta-analysis. *Arch. Phys. Med. Rehabil.* **2023**, *104*, 218–228. [CrossRef] [PubMed]

106. Steele, J.; Bruce-Low, S.; Smith, D. A review of the specificity of exercises designed for conditioning the lumbar extensors. *Br. J. Sports Med.* **2015**, *49*, 291–297. [CrossRef] [PubMed]

107. Tsao, H.; Druitt, T.R.; Schollum, T.M.; Hodges, P.W. Motor training of the lumbar paraspinal muscles induces immediate changes in motor coordination in patients with recurrent low back pain. *J. Pain Off. J. Am. Pain Soc.* **2010**, *11*, 1120–1128. [CrossRef] [PubMed]

108. Danneels, L.A.; Vanderstraeten, G.G.; Cambier, D.C.; Witvrouw, E.E.; Bourgois, J.; Dankaerts, W.; De Cuyper, H.J. Effects of three different training modalities on the cross sectional area of the lumbar multifidus muscle in patients with chronic low back pain. *Br. J. Sports Med.* **2001**, *35*, 186–191. [CrossRef]

109. Kwak, H.B.; Kim, J.H.; Joshi, K.; Yeh, A.; Martinez, D.A.; Lawler, J.M. Exercise training reduces fibrosis and matrix metalloproteinase dysregulation in the aging rat heart. *FASEB J.* **2011**, *25*, 1106–1117. [CrossRef]
110. Wesselink, E.O.; Pool, J.J.M.; Mollema, J.; Weber, K.A., 2nd; Elliott, J.M.; Coppieters, M.W.; Pool-Goudzwaard, A.L. Is fatty infiltration in paraspinal muscles reversible with exercise in people with low back pain? A systematic review. *Eur. Spine J.* **2023**, *32*, 787–796. [CrossRef]
111. Welch, N.; Moran, K.; Antony, J.; Richter, C.; Marshall, B.; Coyle, J.; Falvey, E.; Franklyn-Miller, A. The effects of a free-weight-based resistance training intervention on pain, squat biomechanics and MRI-defined lumbar fat infiltration and functional cross-sectional area in those with chronic low back. *BMJ Open Sport. Exerc. Med.* **2015**, *1*, e000050. [CrossRef]
112. Danneels, L.A.; Cools, A.M.; Vanderstraeten, G.G.; Cambier, D.C.; Witvrouw, E.E.; Bourgois, J.; de Cuyper, H.J. The effects of three different training modalities on the cross-sectional area of the paravertebral muscles. *Scand. J. Med. Sci. Sports* **2001**, *11*, 335–341. [CrossRef] [PubMed]
113. Shahtahmassebi, B.; Hebert, J.J.; Stomski, N.J.; Hecimovich, M.; Fairchild, T.J. The effect of exercise training on lower trunk muscle morphology. *Sports Med.* **2014**, *44*, 1439–1458. [CrossRef] [PubMed]
114. Hayden, J.A.; Ellis, J.; Ogilvie, R.; Malmivaara, A.; van Tulder, M.W. Exercise therapy for chronic low back pain. *Cochrane Database Syst. Rev.* **2021**, *9*, Cd009790. [CrossRef] [PubMed]
115. Wong, A.Y.; Parent, E.C.; Funabashi, M.; Kawchuk, G.N. Do changes in transversus abdominis and lumbar multifidus during conservative treatment explain changes in clinical outcomes related to nonspecific low back pain? A systematic review. *J. Pain Off. J. Am. Pain Soc.* **2014**, *15*, 377.e1–377.e35. [CrossRef] [PubMed]
116. Steiger, F.; Wirth, B.; de Bruin, E.D.; Mannion, A.F. Is a positive clinical outcome after exercise therapy for chronic non-specific low back pain contingent upon a corresponding improvement in the targeted aspect(s) of performance? A systematic review. *Eur. Spine J.* **2012**, *21*, 575–598. [CrossRef] [PubMed]
117. Wernli, K.; O'Sullivan, P.; Smith, A.; Campbell, A.; Kent, P. Movement, posture and low back pain. How do they relate? A replicated single-case design in 12 people with persistent, disabling low back pain. *Eur. J. Pain* **2020**, *24*, 1831–1849. [CrossRef]
118. McGorry, R.W.; Lin, J.H. Flexion relaxation and its relation to pain and function over the duration of a back pain episode. *PLoS ONE* **2012**, *7*, e39207. [CrossRef]
119. Laird, R.A.; Kent, P.; Keating, J.L. Modifying patterns of movement in people with low back pain -does it help? A systematic review. *BMC Musculoskelet. Disord.* **2012**, *13*, 169. [CrossRef]
120. Steele, J.; Fisher, J.; Perrin, C.; Conway, R.; Bruce-Low, S.; Smith, D. Does change in isolated lumbar extensor muscle function correlate with good clinical outcome? A secondary analysis of data on change in isolated lumbar extension strength, pain, and disability in chronic low back pain. *Disabil. Rehabil.* **2019**, *41*, 1287–1295. [CrossRef]
121. Fitzcharles, M.A.; Cohen, S.P.; Clauw, D.J.; Littlejohn, G.; Usui, C.; Häuser, W. Nociplastic pain: Towards an understanding of prevalent pain conditions. *Lancet* **2021**, *397*, 2098–2110. [CrossRef]
122. Macedo, L.G.; Maher, C.G.; Hancock, M.J.; Kamper, S.J.; McAuley, J.H.; Stanton, T.R.; Stafford, R.; Hodges, P.W. Predicting response to motor control exercises and graded activity for patients with low back pain: Preplanned secondary analysis of a randomized controlled trial. *Phys. Ther.* **2014**, *94*, 1543–1554. [CrossRef] [PubMed]
123. Falla, D.; Hodges, P.W. Individualized Exercise Interventions for Spinal Pain. *Exerc. Sport Sci. Rev.* **2017**, *45*, 105–115. [CrossRef] [PubMed]
124. Ferro Moura Franco, K.; Lenoir, D.; Dos Santos Franco, Y.R.; Jandre Reis, F.J.; Nunes Cabral, C.M.; Meeus, M. Prescription of exercises for the treatment of chronic pain along the continuum of nociplastic pain: A systematic review with meta-analysis. *Eur. J. Pain* **2021**, *25*, 51–70. [CrossRef] [PubMed]
125. de Zoete, R.M.J.; Nikles, J.; Coombes, J.S.; Onghena, P.; Sterling, M. The effectiveness of aerobic versus strengthening exercise therapy in individuals with chronic whiplash-associated disorder: A randomised single case experimental design study. *Disabil. Rehabil.* **2022**, 1–10. [CrossRef] [PubMed]
126. Wernli, K.; Tan, J.; O'Sullivan, P.; Smith, A.; Campbell, A.; Kent, P. The Relationship Between Changes in Movement and Changes in Low Back Pain: A Systematic Review of Single-Case Designs. *JOSPT Cases* **2021**, *1*, 199–219. [CrossRef]
127. Wernli, K.; Tan, J.S.; O'Sullivan, P.; Smith, A.; Campbell, A.; Kent, P. Does Movement Change When Low Back Pain Changes? A Systematic Review. *J. Orthop. Sports Phys. Ther.* **2020**, *50*, 664–670. [CrossRef]
128. Saragiotto, B.T.; Maher, C.G.; Yamato, T.P.; Costa, L.O.; Costa, L.C.; Ostelo, R.W.; Macedo, L.G. Motor Control Exercise for Nonspecific Low Back Pain: A Cochrane Review. *Spine* **2016**, *41*, 1284–1295. [CrossRef]
129. Wertli, M.M.; Burgstaller, J.M.; Weiser, S.; Steurer, J.; Kofmehl, R.; Held, U. Influence of catastrophizing on treatment outcome in patients with nonspecific low back pain: A systematic review. *Spine* **2014**, *39*, 263–273. [CrossRef]
130. Wertli, M.M.; Rasmussen-Barr, E.; Weiser, S.; Bachmann, L.M.; Brunner, F. The role of fear avoidance beliefs as a prognostic factor for outcome in patients with nonspecific low back pain: A systematic review. *Spine J.* **2014**, *14*, 816–836.e814. [CrossRef]
131. den Hollander, M.; Smeets, R.; van Meulenbroek, T.; van Laake-Geelen, C.C.M.; Baadjou, V.A.; Timmers, I. Exposure in Vivo as a Treatment Approach to Target Pain-Related Fear: Theory and New Insights From Research and Clinical Practice. *Phys. Ther.* **2022**, *102*, pzab270. [CrossRef]
132. Woods, M.P.; Asmundson, G.J. Evaluating the efficacy of graded in vivo exposure for the treatment of fear in patients with chronic back pain: A randomized controlled clinical trial. *Pain* **2008**, *136*, 271–280. [CrossRef] [PubMed]

33. López-de-Uralde-Villanueva, I.; Muñoz-García, D.; Gil-Martínez, A.; Pardo-Montero, J.; Muñoz-Plata, R.; Angulo-Díaz-Parreño, S.; Gómez-Martínez, M.; La Touche, R. A Systematic Review and Meta-Analysis on the Effectiveness of Graded Activity and Graded Exposure for Chronic Nonspecific Low Back Pain. *Pain Med.* **2016**, *17*, 172–188. [CrossRef] [PubMed]

34. Smart, K.M.; Blake, C.; Staines, A.; Thacker, M.; Doody, C. Mechanisms-based classifications of musculoskeletal pain: Part 3 of 3: Symptoms and signs of nociceptive pain in patients with low back (+/− leg) pain. *Man. Ther.* **2012**, *17*, 352–357. [CrossRef] [PubMed]

35. Freynhagen, R.; Rey, R.; Argoff, C. When to consider "mixed pain"? The right questions can make a difference! *Curr. Med. Res. Opin.* **2020**, *36*, 2037–2046. [CrossRef]

36. McDevitt, A.W.; O'Halloran, B.; Cook, C.E. Cracking the code: Unveiling the specific and shared mechanisms behind musculoskeletal interventions. *Arch. Physiother.* **2023**, *13*, 14. [CrossRef]

37. Christe, G.; Nzamba, J.; Desarzens, L.; Leuba, A.; Darlow, B.; Pichonnaz, C. Physiotherapists' attitudes and beliefs about low back pain influence their clinical decisions and advice. *Musculoskelet. Sci. Pract.* **2021**, *53*, 102382. [CrossRef]

38. Darlow, B.; Dowell, A.; Baxter, G.D.; Mathieson, F.; Perry, M.; Dean, S. The enduring impact of what clinicians say to people with low back pain. *Ann. Fam. Med.* **2013**, *11*, 527–534. [CrossRef]

39. Palazzo, C.; Klinger, E.; Dorner, V.; Kadri, A.; Thierry, O.; Boumenir, Y.; Martin, W.; Poiraudeau, S.; Ville, I. Barriers to home-based exercise program adherence with chronic low back pain: Patient expectations regarding new technologies. *Ann. Phys. Rehabil. Med.* **2016**, *59*, 107–113. [CrossRef]

40. Jack, K.; McLean, S.M.; Moffett, J.K.; Gardiner, E. Barriers to treatment adherence in physiotherapy outpatient clinics: A systematic review. *Man. Ther.* **2010**, *15*, 220–228. [CrossRef]

141. Louw, A.; Sluka, K.A.; Nijs, J.; Courtney, C.A.; Zimney, K. Revisiting the Provision of Pain Neuroscience Education: An Adjunct Intervention for Patients but a Primary Focus of Clinician Education. *J. Orthop. Sports Phys. Ther.* **2021**, *51*, 57–59. [CrossRef]

142. Saragiotto, B.T.; Maher, C.G.; Yamato, T.P.; Costa, L.O.; Menezes Costa, L.C.; Ostelo, R.W.; Macedo, L.G. Motor control exercise for chronic non-specific low-back pain. *Cochrane Database Syst. Rev.* **2016**, Cd012004. [CrossRef] [PubMed]

143. O'Sullivan, P.B.; Caneiro, J.P.; O'Keeffe, M.; Smith, A.; Dankaerts, W.; Fersum, K.; O'Sullivan, K. Cognitive Functional Therapy: An Integrated Behavioral Approach for the Targeted Management of Disabling Low Back Pain. *Phys. Ther.* **2018**, *98*, 408–423. [CrossRef] [PubMed]

144. Hodges, P.W.; Van Dillen, L.R.; McGill, S.M.; Brumagne, S.; Hides, J.A.; Moseley, G.L. Integrated Clinical Approach to Motor Control Interventions in Low Back and Pelvic Pain. In *Spinal Control: The Rehabilitation of Back Pain. State of the Art and Science*, 1st ed.; Hodges, P.W., Cholewicki, J., Van dieen, J.H., Eds.; Churchill Livingstone: London, UK, 2013; pp. 243–309.

145. Schwarzer, R.; Luszczynska, A. How to overcome health-compromising behaviors: The health action process approach. *Eur. Psychol.* **2008**, *13*, 141–151. [CrossRef]

146. Gallagher, K.M.; Payne, M.; Daniels, B.; Caldwell, A.R.; Ganio, M.S. Walking breaks can reduce prolonged standing induced low back pain. *Hum. Mov. Sci.* **2019**, *66*, 31–37. [CrossRef] [PubMed]

147. Gatzounis, R.; den Hollander, M.; Meulders, A. Optimizing Long-term Outcomes of Exposure for Chronic Primary Pain from the Lens of Learning Theory. *J. Pain Off. J. Am. Pain Soc.* **2021**, *22*, 1315–1327. [CrossRef]

148. Schemer, L.; Vlaeyen, J.W.S.; Doerr, J.M.; Skoluda, N.; Nater, U.M.; Rief, W.; Glombiewski, J.A. Treatment processes during exposure and cognitive-behavioral therapy for chronic back pain: A single-case experimental design with multiple baselines. *Behav. Res. Ther.* **2018**, *108*, 58–67. [CrossRef]

149. Craske, M.G.; Treanor, M.; Conway, C.C.; Zbozinek, T.; Vervliet, B. Maximizing exposure therapy: An inhibitory learning approach. *Behav. Res. Ther.* **2014**, *58*, 10–23. [CrossRef]

150. Craske, M.G.; Treanor, M.; Zbozinek, T.D.; Vervliet, B. Optimizing exposure therapy with an inhibitory retrieval approach and the OptEx Nexus. *Behav. Res. Ther.* **2022**, *152*, 104069. [CrossRef]

151. Malfliet, A.; Kregel, J.; Coppieters, I.; De Pauw, R.; Meeus, M.; Roussel, N.; Cagnie, B.; Danneels, L.; Nijs, J. Effect of Pain Neuroscience Education Combined With Cognition-Targeted Motor Control Training on Chronic Spinal Pain: A Randomized Clinical Trial. *JAMA Neurol.* **2018**, *75*, 808–817. [CrossRef]

152. Nijs, J.; D'Hondt, E.; Clarys, P.; Deliens, T.; Polli, A.; Malfliet, A.; Coppieters, I.; Willaert, W.; Tumkaya Yilmaz, S.; Elma, Ö.; et al. Lifestyle and Chronic Pain across the Lifespan: An Inconvenient Truth? *PM&R J. Inj. Funct. Rehabil.* **2020**, *12*, 410–419. [CrossRef]

153. Craige, E.A.; Memon, A.R.; Belavy, D.L.; Vincent, G.E.; Owen, P.J. Effects of non-pharmacological interventions on sleep in chronic low back pain: A systematic review and meta-analysis of randomised controlled trials. *Sleep. Med. Rev.* **2023**, *68*, 101761. [CrossRef] [PubMed]

MDPI

St. Alban-Anlage 66

4052 Basel

Switzerland

www.mdpi.com

Journal of Clinical Medicine Editorial Office

E-mail: jcm@mdpi.com

www.mdpi.com/journal/jcm

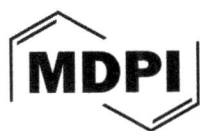